Neurobiology of Violence

Second Edition

Neurobiology of Violence

Second Edition

Jan Volavka, M.D., Ph.D.
Chief, Clinical Research Division
The Nathan S. Kline Institute for Psychiatric Research
Professor, Department of Psychiatry
New York University Medical Center
New York, New York

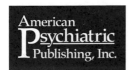
Washington, DC
London, England

Manufactured in the United States of America on acid-free paper
06 05 04 03 02   5 4 3 2 1
Second Edition

Typeset in Adobe's New Baskerville and Optima

American Psychiatric Publishing, Inc.
1400 K Street, N.W.
Washington, DC 20005
www.appi.org

Library of Congress Cataloging-in-Publication Data
Volavka, Jan, 1934–
    Neurobiology and violence / Jan Volavka.—2nd ed.
        p. ; cm.
    Includes bibliographical references and index.
    ISBN 1-58562-081-5 (alk. paper)
        1. Violence—Physiological aspects. 2. Violence—Psychological aspects. I. Title.
    [DNLM: 1. Violence. 2. Neurobiology. BF 575.A3 V899n 2002]
    RC569.5.V55 V65 2002
    616.85'82—dc21

                                                                2002067895

British Library Cataloguing in Publication Data
A CIP record is available from the British Library.

Contents

Preface to the Second Edition

The second edition is coming out at a time when neurobiological bases of aggression have become more accepted and less controversial. These developments are primarily due to the profusion of excellent research in this area published during the past decade. Many of these studies in the neurobiology of violence were made possible by breakthroughs in genomics and technological improvements in imaging methods, as well as by new developments in psychopharmacology. Large-scale longitudinal prospective studies that had taken years to set up have yielded valuable information. Accordingly, chapters dealing with these rapidly developing areas have been thoroughly revised. Some of these new developments were covered in various reviews that my colleague, Dr. Citrome, and I published over the past 5 years. The second edition of this book expands, updates, and integrates this published material.

A word of explanation regarding references to older research is in order. I have elected to keep in the book information on work that was done a long time ago, as long as the research is still relevant and the results have not been disproved. Some of these references date back to the first half of the twentieth century. Had I excluded them, these references could become lost to the current and future generations of researchers and practitioners who rely largely on searches of electronic databases for their reviews of the field. This is so because most of the existing databases go back only to the 1960s, with abstracts and full texts available only for more recent publications. It is essential that researchers be familiar with the most important older work to prevent unwittingly repetitive research and to understand the roots of current thinking.

Preface to the First Edition

My preparation for this book started in 1944 when I was 10 years old. I was doing time in a Nazi prison not too far from Prague. The place was brutal and frightening. I would not recommend such experience to future researchers into violence, but it certainly did focus my mind on the problem. After the war, my fear dissipated and was replaced by curiosity: How was this possible? What made them do this?

When yet another foreign army invaded Prague in 1968, I had enough of state-supported violence and left for New York. It took me less than a week to realize that I exchanged one type of violence for another. My first mugging was swift and predictable, as were the assaults by patients in my hospital. I was amazed by the pervasiveness of random violence in American life. What amazed me even more was that nobody I met seemed interested in this issue beyond the development of individual survival strategies: understanding violence appeared to be somebody else's business. I was attracted to the problem.

My interest in violence increased during the early 1970s when I ran a small ward that specialized in rapid detoxification of opioid-dependent individuals; acute withdrawal was accompanied by irritability and sometimes overt aggression. Later on, I accepted Dr. Mednick's invitation to collaborate on genetic studies in Denmark (including an XYY study).

In 1983, I was given the opportunity to use a special ward at the Manhattan Psychiatric Center as a research site. The ward, called Intensive Psychiatric Service, housed the most violent patients from the borough of Manhattan. Within several years, that ward became the focus of a group of psychiatric researchers specializing in studies of violence.

The book expands and updates our recent reviews (Volavka 1990; Volavka et al. 1992b). Portions of the reviews are used (with permission) with relatively little change. Some concepts used in this book were developed and published in our earlier reviews (Mednick and Volavka 1980; Mednick et al. 1982).

Violent behavior and, specifically, violent crime in the community have caused major concern in this country for decades; their recent upswing in the cities of Eastern and Western Europe has been widely publicized. Violence has persistently resisted policies intended to control it. It is possible that these policies have been failing because they address the consequences rather than the origins of violence.

Violent behavior in psychiatric facilities has also increased. It makes the hospitals unsafe, makes a mockery of the therapeutic environment, consumes time and effort that should be used for clinical care, and causes fear, demoralization, and ultimately burnout among the staff.

Obviously, violence has multiple causes. There is no doubt that societal causes such as poverty and discrimination play a major role in the development of violent behavior. Most of the literature on violence deals with such societal factors. However, it is clear (and fortunate) that not everybody afflicted by poverty or discrimination will become a violent individual. Conversely, violent people who are rich do exist. Thus, additional factors must be involved in the generation of violent behavior.

The evidence for psychobiological origins of violence has been mounting steadily, and a large number of journal articles on this topic were published in the past decade. Edited volumes with chapters by individual contributors have appeared, but there has not been a large-scale critical presentation since that by Moyer (1976), whose book was largely concerned with aggression in nonhuman mammals. The present book was written to update, summarize, and critically evaluate the field of neurobiology of violence (defined as a form of human aggression).

The literature dealing with this topic is scattered across many specialized fields. Neurotransmitters, electroencephalograms, hallucinations, arrests, epidemiological surveys, psychopharmacology, and stereotactic surgery—all these disparate subjects related to violence are discussed by authors using different tools, vocabularies, and points of view. Many experts in these fields who apply their specialized knowledge to the problem of violence do not seem to know or care very much about what the experts in the other fields have to say about the topic. This is regrettable because violence is a complex problem, unlikely to be explained by any unidimensional approach. The advantage of a single-authored book is the opportunity to provide an integrated view of the multifaceted literature.

Acknowledgments

Drs. Anderson, Brizer, Citrome, Convit, Crowner, Douyon, Gaztanaga, Greenberg, Hoptman, Jaeger, Krakowski, Kunz, Nemes, Nolan, Roy, and others who worked at the Intensive Psychiatric Service and the Nathan Kline Institute have made significant contributions. Parts of the book are based on the work done by various members of this group in collaboration with me or independently. Our work at the Manhattan Psychiatric Center and Rockland Psychiatric Center would have been impossible without the consistent support of the respective hospital directors, Michael Ford, M.D., and James H. Bopp, M.A. Current research is being conducted largely at the Clinical Research and Evaluation Facility (CREF), an inpatient unit operated by the Nathan Kline Institute and the Rockland Psychiatric Center. Much of the credit for this work goes to Leslie Citrome, M.D., M.P.H., Director of the CREF.

Max Fink, M.D., suggested that I write the book, edited most of the chapters, and provided advice and encouragement from start to finish. Pal Czobor, Ph.D., provided statistical consultation for most chapters and wrote the appended statistical part of the section on actuarial prediction. Mr. T.B. Cooper and Drs. Anderson, Cancro, Chou, Citrome, Czobor, Ford, Hoptman, Krakowski, Kunz, Libiger, Malhotra, Martell, Mednick, and Nolan critiqued drafts of various chapters. Klaus Miczek, Ph.D., generously shared his reference database.

Ms. Czoborne and Drs. Libigerova and Vitrai provided technical assistance. There is a library behind each scientific book. I could not have written this book without the support of librarians at the Nathan Kline Institute: Mr. Stuart Moss, Ms. Lois Cohan, Ms. Sharon Sternbach, Ms. Juliet Peterson, and Ms. Judith Allen.

Finally, I am indebted to the reviewers of the first edition of this book. They pointed out various areas that needed improvement; if the second edition is better than the first one, it is at least partly due to their insightful comments.

Introduction

Attempts to explain violent behavior, violent crime, or crime in general by biological factors have a stormy history. Science, ideology, and politics blend in a volatile solution that always seems ready to explode and frequently does. The intensity of disagreements increases when the argument is framed in terms of genetic (or constitutional) versus environmental effects. To understand how this polarization of views came about, we have to go back to Charles Darwin's *The Origin of Species* (1859) and *The Descent of Man* (1871). In the following paragraphs, I discuss crime (which includes violent crime) because specific data on violent crime or violent behavior were not available until recently and because the debate was not focused on violence.

SCIENCE GONE AWRY: 1859–1953

Darwin's theory of evolution influenced Cesare Lombroso (1836–1909), an Italian forensic physician, who developed the first modern biological theory of criminality. Lombroso observed various physical anomalies in some of the criminals he examined. Some of the signs were related to the cranial shape and facial features (e.g., sloping forehead). He interpreted these anomalies as *atavisms* (recurrences of phylogenetically earlier forms). In its initial form, the theory said that criminals (or at least some of them) were inferior throwbacks to a more primitive stage in the development of the human race. Having said that, he made an assumption that moral inferiority of criminals (thought to be the basis of their propensity to break the law) was just another consequence of the primitive stage of their development: an atavistic cranium sheltered an atavistic brain that reached only a primitive, inferior level of moral development.

Lombroso's initial theory (which remains historically more important than its later modifications) was soon discredited. This was not difficult because the theory was wrong essentially in all its aspects: few criminals had the Lombrosian anomalies, but some noncriminals did; the anomalies could not be interpreted as atavisms; moral development was a tautology because it was defined by criminality. Inadequacies of Lombroso's measurement and sampling methods contributed to his errors.

Nevertheless, Lombroso's theory had a great impact. Anthropometric measurements and somatotyping of criminals have continued into the second half of the twentieth century, and this type of work was given a surprising amount of respectful attention in a leading book on the causes of crime (J. Q. Wilson and Herrnstein 1986, pp. 70–90). It is unfortunate that the first modern attempt to trace the cause of crime to physical attributes of individuals was so inadequate. Lombroso's errors undermined the credibility of the biology of crime for generations to come.

Another deleterious effect of this type was caused by Lombroso's description of criminals as atavistic, primitive, and inferior. The notion that there are national, racial, or religious subgroups that can be "scientifically" labeled as inferior is extremely dangerous.

Social Darwinism, a vulgar misapplication of the idea of natural selection, has developed these notions in detail. Herbert Spencer (1820–1903), an English philosopher, substituted his slogan "survival of the fittest" for Darwin's natural selection. Thus, a process invoked by Darwin to explain evolution of the species was misapplied to sociology. Spencer's slogan was used to justify the cutthroat struggle "for survival" among individuals and groups. Linked to the naive "genetics" of the times, social Darwinism was used to rationalize European imperialism as well as American racist social policies at home. Such policies included barring or restricting immigration of racially undesirable people (such as the Chinese or Eastern Europeans) and the segregation of blacks. Blacks already were considered to be inferior to whites; now there seemed to be "scientific" support for that notion and, consequently, for racial discrimination.

The malignant consequences of dividing humans into "superior" and "inferior" racial groups were demonstrated by the Holocaust. Nazi theoreticians considered the physical characteristics of Jews as important landmarks confirming their subhuman (*untermensch*) nature. Conversely, people endowed with "Nordic" physical characteristics (tall stature, blond hair, blue eyes, etc.) were "scientifically" considered fit to rule over others. The racial superiority of the Nordic types could be further enhanced, the Nazis thought, by controlled human mating. Thus, a theory linking biology and human behavior was used to justify classification of people according to their biological characteristics, systematic extermination of those groups that were considered inferior, and—incidentally—eugenic attempts to improve the genetic stock. Pseudoscientific misinterpretations of biology (and, specifically, genetics) were used to support ideological systems justifying oppression and genocide.

Soviet theoreticians also misinterpreted biology and genetics in support of an ideological system justifying oppression and genocide. Trofim Denisovich Lysenko (1898–1976) declared that conventional genetics (which he called "morganism-mendelism") was a bourgeois pseudoscience. To replace genetics, he developed a variation of Lamarck's theory: he posited that heritability of acquired characteristics was the major force of evolution. Very few people in the Soviet Union dared to criticize this theory because, from the late 1930s until well after Stalin's death (1953), those who did lost their jobs and sometimes their lives (Graham 1993, p. 130).

Although Lysenko did not apply his genetic theories to humans, they formed a part of a more general ideological system generated by the Communist Party of the Soviet Union. Genetics was seen as a bourgeois way to justify the existence of capitalism because the oppressors blamed an inadequate genetic endowment of the oppressed for their plight. A dominance of environmental (in this case, social) over constitutional (genetic) factors was an important assumption behind the Party's effort to create a "New Soviet Man." That effort was partly based on Lenin's postulate that crime would essentially disappear in the Communist society. There would be some isolated individual "excesses," but these would be so minor that no law enforcement apparatus would be needed to suppress them (Lenin 1932, p. 75).

The application of this extreme environmentalist theory to criminology precluded any role of constitutional factors in crime. Crime was due to oppression and exploitation of the workers by the bourgeoisie. Biological or biopsychological theories of crime only served to "discount the possibility of a liquidation of crime, and, protecting the pillars of capitalism, transfer the fight against crime from the social to the biological level" (Gercenzon 1965, p. 37).

In summary, theories linking genetic characteristics of individuals and racial groups to behaviors seen as undesirable have a long and disturbing history. They were used to justify Nazi policies of racial discrimination and genocide. On the other hand, ideological denials of genetic influences set Soviet Russian science back, and an exclusive emphasis on environmental factors failed to fulfill its promise of a crime-free society. Both types of pseudoscience—Nazi and Soviet—were invoked to justify the ideology of mass murder. These lessons of history should not be forgotten, but they should not paralyze our thinking about the relations between genes and environment in the development of violent behavior.

GENETIC AND ENVIRONMENTAL FACTORS

Much of the past discussions and ideological controversies regarding the respective roles of genes and environment had been framed in the terms of child development. Thus, the genetic (or "constitutional") factors were subsumed under the term "nature," whereas the environmental factors were called "nurture." Many ideological battles of the past were "nature versus nurture" controversies. In their original primitive shape, the argument was presented in an "either-or" form: either "nature" (genes) is destiny and the environment does not matter, or "nurture" (environment) completely determines the outcome and "nature" is irrelevant.

Although some of the public discussion is still caught in this obsolete "either-or" framework, it has become clear that genes and environment continuously interact. The transcriptional function of the gene is regulated, in part, by environmental factors. Thus, changes in gene expression can be elicited as the child learns good or bad habits in his or her rearing environment. Learned behavior then has an impact on the environment and causes it to change; that change, in turn, affects gene expression. Serial transactions between genes and environment thus shape both, and "all of "nurture" is ultimately expressed as "nature" (Kandel 1998, p. 460).

TOPICS AND STRUCTURE OF THIS BOOK

Much of the confusion in the literature on violence stems from inadequate definitions of aggression, violence, and violent crime. Many authors without adequate understanding use crime statistics. It was obvious that these issues needed to be clarified in Chapter 1.

Reading the animal literature on aggression, I was surprised to see that many phenomena observed in humans relatively recently had animal analogs that have been known for decades. The relationship between serotonin and aggression is a case in point. Many other aspects of animal aggression, particularly among nonhuman primates, are shared with humans. For these and other reasons, Chapter 2 is devoted to animal aggression.

Subsequent chapters deal with the human brain and violent behavior. Searching for a model that would help me organize the material, I considered a proposal for the classification of aggression: The Carolina Nosology of Destructive Behavior (Eichelman and Hartwig 1990). This multiaxial system is interesting, but it is not particularly suitable for the presentation of nonclinical material. I found no other model to follow. It was obvious that it would be good to have a theory that would govern the organization of the book and the selection of its topics.

If we had a Grand Unified Theory of Aggression, the facts would have been logically presented as they fit the theory. Unfortunately, this theory is not yet available. The next most logical organization, called "From Molecules to Behavior and Back," would be centered on neurotransmitters. I would first describe the neurotransmitters and their receptors; then I would track these transmitter systems in various brain structures and describe how the disturbance in these systems causes aggression as a symptom or neuropsychiatric diseases that then manifest themselves in aggression; and finally, I would add a pharmacology section describing how these disturbances of specific systems can be corrected (back from behavior to molecules). I started this approach in Chapter 3, but when I tried to continue to brain structures and diseases, it became obvious that this method was beyond the current state of knowledge.

Chapter 4 therefore starts with the brain structures and proceeds to neurological diagnostic categories. A separate presentation of the large amount of electrophysiologic literature on aggression was chosen because the methods needed to be explained, and the literature could not easily fit the section on brain structures (because many electroencephalographic findings cannot be definitively tied to any structure) or the section on diseases (beyond epilepsy, most of the electroencephalographic abnormalities in aggressive patients are nonspecific).

The subsequent three chapters (Chapter 5, "Congenital and Demographic Factors," Chapter 6, "Developmental Antecedents of Violent Behavior," and Chapter 7, "Personality Disorders and Impulse Control") track in time, from conception to adulthood, the interplay between constitutional and environmental factors in the evolution of violent behavior. Chapter 8, on substance abuse, forms a transition between the previous chapter on personality disorders and the subsequent chapters on major mental disorders. This position of the chapter is logical because violence increases in cases of drug abuse comorbid with either personality disorders or psychoses.

Violence among patients with major mental disorders is reviewed separately for the behaviors occurring in the community (Chapter 9) and those occurring in psychiatric hospitals (Chapter 10). Major mental disorders include schizophrenia, severe mood disorders, and various other psychotic disorders. These disorders are treated as a group because much of the literature on violence in the community follows this pattern. In reports that do give separate data on diagnostic categories, the diagnostic procedures are not always adequately specified.

Assessment of risk (or prediction) of violent behavior is a central problem in theory and practice. Therefore, this issue is discussed in greater detail than some readers might expect. Recent literature on actuarial prediction frequently presents results of very complicated statistical analyses. These analyses and their limitations are usually not explained because of space limitations; the reader is referred to a specialized mathematical or statistical text. I must admit that I could never understand any of these specialized texts. This was frustrating. I asked my colleague and statistical consultant, Dr. Czobor, for explanations. At the beginning of our discussions, his explanations were as obscure as the specialized texts recommended by the authors. As we progressed, he gradually realized the limits of my education in mathematics. He simplified the explanations, wrote them down, and added illustrations. After several rewrites, he created a text on actuarial prediction (including the Bayes decision) that explained the procedures involved and their limitations, included here as the appendix. Unlike the usual mathematical texts, I understood this explanation. I strongly encourage the reader not to skip this part of the book; if I can understand it, you can, too.

Chapter 11 deals with the psychopharmacology of violence. I considered writing along the lines of receptors affected by the drugs, but most drugs act on multiple receptors, and their mechanism of action is not yet understood to the extent that would permit such a logical presentation. The chapter is therefore written in the traditional style.

In general, the book flows from basic to clinical science. Its organization reflects the current state of knowledge, including the lack of an integrated theory of violent behavior.

Readers may be surprised at the limited coverage of suicide and other self-injurious behaviors. A large amount of clinical evidence and neurobiological data confirms links between inward and outward aggression. However, covering both these aspects of aggression in any depth would have enlarged the scope of the book to the point of making it unfeasible. Many other topics had to be dropped for the same reason.

WRITING STYLE

Readers of the early drafts of several chapters complained that when I gave several opinions on an issue, they were not sure which one I believed. That was because I used the standard writing style for articles in scientific journals, avoiding the first person and resorting to passive voice instead. In a discussion with the editor, we agreed that the standard style could be confusing because I am in the position of a reviewer trying to convey three opinions: 1) the opinion of the author of the article being reviewed, 2) my perception of the consensus opinion of scientists working in a given field, and 3) my own opinion. These three opinions may diverge.

I believe that the reader is entitled to understand which of these opinions is being presented. Using the first person is the logical way to indicate that I am speaking only for myself. Thus, when I write "I think that ..." or "it seems to me ..." or "in my opinion ..." the reader should know that I am expressing my own view, which may or may not be shared by others. To differentiate between the author and the consensus (items 1 and 2 in the previous paragraph), I tend to use the past tense for the authors' results and discussion and the present tense for the consensus.

1

Human Aggression and Criminal Violence

Definitions and Classifications

Everybody knows intuitively what violence is. Unfortunately, intuitions differ. One of the major problems of research into violence and aggression is the definition of the dependent variables. There is a profusion of new data on neurochemistry, psychopharmacology, neurophysiology, and other biological aspects of violent behavior. The definitions of such independent biological variables are typically much clearer than the definitions (and classifications) of the dependent variables measuring violence or aggression. Imagine psychiatric research that has available biological methods of the 1990s but depends on the diagnostic classification and rating scales of the 1940s.

Because aggressive or violent behavior has many different causes, manifestations, and impacts, it is not surprising that experts from many fields have tried to define and classify these phenomena. Zoologists, psychologists, psychiatrists, sociologists, criminologists, law enforcement officials, lawyers, and politicians have all worked hard on this problem. In many cases, experts from one field are unaware of or uninterested in research generated by other disciplines. In other cases, they complain that people from other disciplines have too much control over the important definitions: for example, criminologists complain that they do not control their own dependent variable because the definition of crime (including violent crime) is determined by political-legal acts (Gottfredson and Hirschi 1990, p. 3). The definitions and classifications are sometimes driven by pragmatic political considerations rather than by scientific research. This multidisciplinary effort has left us with an array of definitions and classification systems pertaining to aggression, violence, and violent crime.

In this chapter, I state definitions adopted for the purposes of this book and review the definitions and classification systems that either are useful in understanding research in the neurobiology of violence or may hold promise for the future.

Instruments for the assessment of hostility and for counting aggressive incidents are reviewed. An analogous review of methods for counting crime is provided.

DEFINITIONS USED IN THIS BOOK

Various definitions of aggression are available. I adopted Moyer's definition because it applies to animals and humans, excludes aggression against self, is linked to a typology of animal aggression (Chapter 2), and is widely known. The definition is "overt behavior involving intent to inflict noxious stimulation or to behave destructively toward another organism" (Moyer 1976, p. 2). This definition appears to exclude aggression against inanimate objects; however, Moyer later adds the following (p. 3): "Destructive behavior toward inanimate objects is only considered aggressive if frustration or aversive stimulation is involved." Frustration is then defined as a "condition that blocks or prevents the fulfillment of intent." Moyer correctly states that the intentions of animals remain unknowable and that this portion of the definition accordingly applies only to humans. Unfortunately, human intent is not an easy concept to understand or define.

Several other points about this definition of aggression need clarification. First, the aggressive behavior must be overt. Aggressive fantasies, dreams, plans, or other forms of covert aggression do not meet the definition. Second, the overt behavior may involve physical aggression, verbal aggression, or both. Third, the definition does not include self-injurious behaviors such as self-mutilation or suicide. This exclusion does not imply denial of psychological and biochemical commonalities between self-injurious behaviors and outward aggression; the decision to exclude self-injurious behaviors was intended to achieve greater clarity.

This definition largely ignores the context of aggression as a subtype of competition and thus disregards its positive role as a mechanism serving evolution. The narrow definition I adopted reflects this book's focus on humans.

Hostility is a term with multiple meanings. In addition to overt aggression, it may include temper tantrums, irritability, refusal to cooperate, jealousy, suspicion, and many other attitudes and behaviors (Buss and Durkee 1957). In general, the term is applied to human rather than animal behavior. I use the term primarily to describe unfriendly human attitudes. This usage conforms with much of the literature.

Violence denotes aggression among humans. It is not used to describe animal behavior; however, human behavior can be described as either violent or aggressive. The term *aggression* tends to be used more frequently in biomedical or psychological research, whereas *violence* (or *violent crime*) is more commonly used in criminology, sociology, law, and public policy. This interchangeable usage (depending on context) of the terms *aggression* and *violence* is not generally accepted. For example, Valzelli (1981) proposed that violence is an abnormal form of aggression: "violence might be interpreted as the extreme pathology of irritable and perhaps competitive aggression more than an irrational exasperation with other kinds of aggression" (p. 124). However, I think that such definitions are too vague for practical use and perhaps even for the development of testable hypotheses. Thus, in this book, the two terms have the same meaning; their use is largely governed by their context. The term *violence* is used in this book's title to convey my primary interest in human (rather than animal) aggression.

Problems in the Definitions of Human Aggression

The principal problems revolve around intentionality. The concept of *intent* was introduced into these definitions to exclude harmful actions occurring accidentally. However, mental disorders may distort, reduce, or abolish the capacity to form an intent.

We will deal with mental disorders, and the problem of intent will be with us much of the time. For example, I write about aggressive behavior during alcoholic intoxication, although the capacity of an intoxicated person to form an intent is uncertain. The definition of aggression hinging on a person's intent is not useful for such cases, but there is no easy solution to this problem.

In addition to the fuzziness of the term *intent,* the definitions of human aggression are further weakened by problems in deciding what verbal expressions are aggressive and by acts of omission that may have noxious consequences (e.g., failure to adequately feed a helpless patient). An extensive critique of older definitions of aggression was published elsewhere (Megargee 1982, pp. 82–86).

There is even a lack of agreement about the advisability of using the terms *aggression* and *violence* in reference to humans. It was suggested that *aggression* may carry an inappropriately positive connotation (in the context of socially desirable competitive or assertive behaviors) and that *violence* may appear restrictive because of its forensic implications. The term *destructive* has been proposed to replace *aggressive* and *violent* (Eichelman and Hartwig 1990). A definition of destructive behavior was offered: "Behavior which results in partial or complete injury to the physical or psychological integrity of a person or object" (p. 289). This definition was provided for the purpose of psychiatric nosology of destructive behavior (see "Incident Pattern Scales" below). It was not concerned with the intent of the person inflicting the injury and therefore did not address the issue of accidental (unintended) harm.

At this point, the reader has probably come to the conclusion that defining aggression, violence, or destructive behavior (or even trying to decide which terms are worth defining) is a frustrating exercise. There is no perfect definition. The "I can tell it when I see it" dictum used by a judge to define pornography has an instant appeal to common sense. Furthermore, its validity is universal: without any modification, it can be readily used to define aggression, violence, or anything else. The problem with this approach is that it gives no help in questionable or marginal cases. It is in these cases that people using common sense (and no definition) tend to disagree with each other.

ASSESSMENT INSTRUMENTS

Assessment Instruments for Aggressiveness and Hostility

Assessment instruments describe a relatively permanent *personality trait* (aggressiveness, hostility, impulsiveness, or propensity for violent behavior). They may be used as independent variables in the studies predicting violent behavior.

Before specific instruments for this purpose were developed, aggression (or hostility) was assessed by use of general scales such as the Minnesota Multiphasic Personality Inventory (MMPI) or by clinical descriptions. A classification system for criminal offenders was designed by use of the MMPI (Megargee and Bohn 1977). The use of MMPI subscales has been extensive (G. I. Brown et al. 1990; Kristianson 1974; Lothstein and Jones 1978; Rogers and Seman 1983; Valzelli et al. 1967), and it will probably continue.

The *specific trait inventories or scales* usually contain items that capture feelings (such as anger, resentment, or suspicion), behaviors (history of physical and verbal assaults), or a combination of the two. In principle, the subject is the main source of historical information used by these scales. Thus, these instruments are very dependent on the subjects' cooperation, memory, intelligence, and general mental competence.

The *Buss-Durkee Hostility Inventory* (BDHI) (Buss and Durkee 1957) represents this type of instrument. First tested with college students, this self-administered inventory has been widely used in psychiatric and prisoner populations. The BDHI has seven hostility items (or subscales): Assault, Indirect Hostility, Irritability, Negativism, Resentment, Suspicion, and Verbal Hostility. An additional item measures guilt. The items are clearly geared toward trait features, and idioms are used. Some examples are "I have known people who pushed me so hard that we came to blows" (Assault) and "I tend to be on my guard with people who are somewhat more friendly than I expected" (Suspicion). Psychiatric patients sometimes find it difficult to understand the erudite wording of this inventory. The Irritability subscale alone (G.I. Brown et al. 1990) and the combination of the Irritability and Assault subscales (Coccaro et al. 1991) were related to deviant serotoninergic function (see Chapter 3). The use of the BDHI is reviewed elsewhere (G.I. Brown et al. 1990).

The *Brown-Goodwin Inventory* detailing lifetime history of aggression was constructed in the context of a classical study of aggression and cerebrospinal fluid amine metabolites (G.L. Brown et al. 1979). Because the subjects in that study were soldiers, a particular emphasis was placed on aggressive responses to authority. The inventory covered nine categories: 1) temper tantrums, 2) nonspecific fighting, 3) specific assaults on other people or property, 4) school discipline, 5) relationship with supervisors, 6) antisocial behavior not involving police, 7) antisocial behavior involving police, 8) military disciplinary problems not involving the military judicial system, and 9) difficulty with the military judicial system. Each of these nine items was scored at one of five frequency levels ranging from 0 (never) to 4 (many or multiple). The inventory had very high interrater reliability.

The *Life History of Aggression* (LHA) (Coccaro et al. 1997b) is a trait measure developed by modifying the Brown-Goodwin Inventory (see above). It has high interrater and test-retest reliability, as well as acceptable concurrent validity.

The *Albert Einstein College of Medicine Past Feelings and Acts of Violence Scale* is a 12-item instrument that was used in psychiatric inpatients (Plutchik et al. 1989), violent self-referred patients, prisoners, patients with temporal lobe epilepsy, and college students (Plutchik and Van Praag 1990). Violent self-referred patients had the highest scores on this scale; this finding was interpreted by the authors as support for the scale's validity. In general, however, there has not been much systematic effort to validate the trait inventories or scales by obtaining information from sources other than the subjects themselves. Such sources might include family members, significant others, various caregivers, and records generated by the criminal justice system (see "Criminal Violence" below).

Assessment Instruments for Aggressive Incidents

Unlike assessment methods for aggressive traits, which have been available for more than three decades, the instruments for the assessment of aggressive events (incidents) were not developed until the mid-1980s. The lack of incident scales has delayed the development of research on human aggression because these scales are necessary for studies of anti-aggressive effects of new treatments, for studies focusing on prediction of violent behavior (as a dependent variable), and for policy decisions regarding patient management, ward staffing, and institutional administration. Some of these instruments were designed to capture a *single recent aggressive incident*. More recently, another type of instrument that describes the *incident pattern and frequency* has emerged.

Single-Incident Scales

Most scales for rating violent incidents were designed for use with psychiatric patients. Information is provided primarily or solely by the staff; administration of these instruments does not require the subjects' cooperation. Several such scales were developed and were used in their authors' projects (Brizer et al. 1987; Palmstierna and Wistedt 1987; Wistedt et al. 1990).

The *Overt Aggression Scale* (OAS) (Yudofsky et al. 1986) has been widely accepted, used, and modified by others. The OAS, designed for use in psychiatric hospitals, recognizes four types of aggressive behavior: verbal aggression, physical aggression against self, physical aggression against objects, and physical aggression against other people. There are four degrees of severity for each aggression type; each degree is defined or illustrated by anchor points. The scale also lists staff interventions. The interrater reliability of the scale has been published (Yudofsky et al. 1986). The version of the scale shown in Figure 1–1 (Silver and Yudofsky 1991) has weighted scores for each of the severity levels of the four types of aggression and for the staff interventions; these improvements enable the user to compute a meaningful "total aggression score" (the sum of the weighted scores for aggressive behaviors and interventions) for each event.

Similar psychometric improvements of the original OAS were introduced (apparently independently) by another group, who called their scale the *Modified Overt Aggression Scale* (MOAS) (Kay et al. 1988). Another group has also adapted the OAS (see "Incident Pattern Scales" below); confusingly, they also called their version the Modified Overt Aggression Scale, complete with the acronym MOAS (Knoedler 1989).

OVERT AGGRESSION SCALE (OAS)
Stuart Yudofsky, M.D., Jonathan Silver, M.D., Wynn Jackson, M.D., and Jean Endicott, Ph.D.

IDENTIFYING DATA

Name of Patient	Name of Rater
Sex of Patient: 1 Male 2 Female	Date / / (month/day/year) Shift: 1 Night 2 Day 3 Evening

No aggressive incidents (verbal or physical) against self, others, or objects during the shift.   (check here)

AGGRESSIVE BEHAVIOR (check all that apply)

VERBAL AGGRESSION	PHYSICAL AGGRESSION AGAINST SELF
❏ Makes loud noises,, shouts angrily ❏ Yells mild personal insults (e.g., "You're stupid!") ❏ Curses viciously, uses foul language in anger, makes moderate threats to others or self ❏ Makes clear threats of violence toward others or self (e.g., "I'm going to kill you") or requests to help to control self	❏ Picks or scratches skin, hits self, pulls hair (with no or minor injury only) ❏ Bangs head, hits fist into objects, throws self onto floor or into objects (hurts self without serious injury) ❏ Small cuts or bruises, minor burns ❏ Mutilates self, makes deep cuts, bites that bleed, internal injury, fracture, loss of consciousness, loss of teeth

PHYSICAL AGGRESSION AGAINST OBJECTS	PHYSICAL AGGRESSION AGAINST OTHER PEOPLE
❏ Slams door, scatters clothing, makes a mess ❏ Throws objects down, kicks furniture without breaking it, marks the wall ❏ Breaks objects, smashes windows ❏ Sets fires, throws objects dangerously	❏ Makes threatening gesture, swings at people, grabs at clothes ❏ Strikes, kicks, pushes, pulls hair (without injury to them) ❏ Attacks others causing mild-moderate physical injury (bruises, sprains, welts) ❏ Attacks others causing severe physical injury (broken bones, deep lacerations, internal injury)
Time incident began: ___:___ A.M./ P.M.	Duration of incident: ___:___ (hours/minutes)

INTERVENTION (check all that apply)

❏ None ❏ Talking to patient ❏ Closer observation ❏ Holding patient	❏ Immediate medication given by mouth ❏ Immediate medication given by injection ❏ Isolation without seclusion (time-out) ❏ Seclusion	❏ Use of restraints ❏ Injury requires immediate medical treatment for patient ❏ Injury requires immediate treatment for other person

COMMENTS

Figure 1–1. The Overt Aggression Scale.

Source. Reprinted from Silver JM, Yudofsky SC: "The Overt Aggression Scale: Overview and Guiding Principles." *Journal of Neuropsychiatry and Clinical Neurosciences* 3:S22–S29, 1991. Used with permission.

Several other scales to measure aggressive behavior have been described (Hallsteinsen et al. 1998; Nijman et al. 1999; Palmstierna et al. 1999).

Incident Pattern Scales

Incidents of aggressive behavior sometimes occur in clusters. Certain patients, particularly the mentally retarded, have aggressive incidents many times a day for weeks or months. Under these conditions, it is unrealistic to expect the staff to fill in the appropriate OAS form every time an incident occurs. Therefore, a retrospective adaptation of the OAS was done to capture the aggressive incidents occurring over a period of 1 week (Knoedler 1989; Ratey and Gutheil 1991; Sorgi et al. 1991). The form has several columns to indicate the frequency of the aggressive behavior. The obvious advantage of this form is that it is completed just once each week for each patient, no matter how many incidents occurred. The disadvantage, I think, is that the staff members who fill out the form may not have witnessed the incidents personally, and even if they did, their recall of the incidents may not be very good. This retrospective adaptation of the OAS is called the *Modified Overt Aggression Scale* (MOAS)—the same name and acronym used by a different group for the modification described in the preceding paragraph (Kay et al. 1988). An elaborate instrument has been developed to capture overall characteristics of a person's aggressive ("destructive") behavior; it is primarily intended for use in psychiatric patients (Eichelman and Hartwig 1990). Two single-incident scales and two incident pattern scales were administered to 199 consecutively admitted psychiatric patients; the scale total scores were strongly intercorrelated, confirming concurrent validity. Interrater reliability was positively related to the severity of the aggressive incidents (Steinert et al. 2000).

The incident pattern and frequency scales are analogous to typical scales measuring change in psychopathology that occurred over a standard period, such as 1 week. Such scales have been used in psychopharmacologic studies for several decades.

Another method of capturing aggressive incidents is to rely on *standard official documentation* provided by hospitals or prisons. These documents are generated to comply with various mandates and policy requirements.

DETECTING AND REPORTING VIOLENT INCIDENTS IN PSYCHIATRIC HOSPITALS

In psychiatric hospitals, three levels of documentation yield information on violent incidents: individual *patient charts; ward journal reports* (a log of ward events completed by aides or nurses at the end of each 8-hour tour of duty); and official *incident reports,* which are written at the ward and collected centrally. Much of the literature on inpatient violence is based on these official reports of violent incidents (fights or assaults). It is therefore important to critically examine the validity of such official reports.

Early data suggested that official documents underreport incidents (Lion et al. 1981).

We compared the official incident reports with patient charts and ward journals to estimate official underreporting of physical assaults. In our definition, assault required physical contact between patients, such as hitting, kicking, pushing, biting, hair pulling, scratching, or strangling. We found that a realistic minimal estimate of the incidence of physical assaults in young male schizophrenic patients is 1.5 times that reflected by official incident reports. The unreported incidents were primarily those that resulted in no injuries.

To determine whether the ward journal underreports violent events, we independently assessed the incidents by direct observations and by interviewing staff members at the end of each shift on which the investigators were not present on the ward. This was done for a period of 4 months. We found that only 63% of violent incidents occurring on the ward were entered into the ward journal (Brizer et al. 1987).

Direct visual observation is inferior to videotaping in two respects: an observer cannot watch all patients simultaneously all the time, and violent events sometimes develop too fast to be captured in detail by an observer. Realizing that we might have missed some incidents that were not seen or mentioned in interviews, we installed video cameras and continuously recorded the action in the dayroom of a 15-bed state hospital ward specializing in the management of violent behavior (Brizer et al. 1988; Crowner et al. 1991). This method has detected brief exchanges of slaps, kicks, pushes, or punches; fewer than 50% of these exchanges were reported in any of the documents mentioned above. In addition, the videotaping drew our attention to low-hostility "playful wrestling" among patients; it is not clear whether these events are precursors of real violence. The videotaping method enabled us to carefully review the events immediately preceding each violent incident. Watching the tapes repeatedly in slow motion revealed the role of akathisia in assailants and victims (Crowner et al. 1990) and the cues (e.g., threats and provocations) emitted by the participants immediately before a fight.

In summary, I have described five methods used to detect and to report violence in psychiatric patients: continuous videotaping, direct visual observation, interviewing staff members immediately after the end of their shift, studying charts and ward journals, and reviewing official incident reports. Continuous videotaping captures most events and gives the most detailed information; there is a gradually increasing loss of information as one progresses from videotaping to the official incident report. The loss of information is greatest for the assaults that result in no injuries or only very minor ones.

CRIMINAL VIOLENCE

Who Should Read This, and Why

Research on violence is scattered across many fields. Biologists, psychiatrists, neurologists, psychologists, and other specialists use the results of criminological research or at least some data on crime without realizing that they have left their own areas of expertise. Most people assume they understand crime; as two criminologists observed, "there is scarcely any topic ... on which people have more confident opinions" (J. Q. Wilson and Herrnstein 1986, pp. 24–25). Therefore, this section on criminal violence was written to introduce noncriminologists to the topic of crime.

Some clinicians may believe that the following section on criminal violence is strangely juxtaposed to the preceding segment dealing primarily with violence in psychiatric inpatients. However, these topics share important features. There are similarities between violent behavior in the hospital and violent behavior in the community, and between "criminal" and "noncriminal" violence. Much of the violent behavior exhibited by psychiatric inpatients would be punishable by law if perpetrated in the community by offenders who are not mentally ill. A main difference between violence committed by psychiatric patients and that committed by nonpatients is its differential treatment by the criminal justice system. Police and prosecutors largely assume (sometimes tacitly) that psychiatric patients are incapable of criminal intent or that the intent may be hopelessly difficult to prove. In the United States, violent suspects who look mentally ill to the police may not be arrested and charged (see "Detecting and Reporting Crime" below), and, until recently, psychiatric inpatients were almost never arrested in the hospital. However, serious violence or drug dealing on the hospital grounds may lead to arrest, which is sometimes followed by prosecution (Volavka et al. 1995). Most patients who are arrested in a hospital have a history of prior arrests; overall, these arrestees more closely resemble the population of criminal offenders in the community than the population of psychiatric inpatients.

On the other hand, the prevalence of serious mental disorders among jail inmates is several times higher than that in the general population (Abram and Teplin 1991; Grinfeld 1992; Teplin 1990). Thus, the distinctions between criminal and noncriminal violence are imposed by interactions between the criminal justice and mental health systems. These interactions (and the distinctions between the two types of violence) are somewhat arbitrary and should not obscure the basic behavioral similarities between aggressive behavior by patients and that by nonpatients.

A history of *violent crime predicts inpatient violent behavior* (Convit et al.

1988a, 1988b). This finding, if confirmed, reinforces the conceptual similarity between violent behavior in the hospital and that in the community. In this context, the history of self-reported criminal acts (and of arrests and convictions) is clearly relevant to a mental status examination and should not be ignored.

Much research on violence relies on *arrest and conviction records*. This reliance is almost inevitable, because such data, collected by the criminal justice system, provide information on the violent behavior of large populations that would otherwise be prohibitively expensive to obtain. However, proper interpretation of these data requires some insight into the workings of the criminal justice system.

Finally, from the *public policy* standpoint, violent crime is by far the most important form of aggressive behavior. For these and other reasons, the reader needs to know about crime, criminal violence, and the criminal justice system. The following section would bore professional criminologists, who are therefore advised to skip it. It primarily describes the American criminal justice system. Many of the features of the American system are similar to those of systems operating in Canada and in Western European countries; however, some differences exist. These differences are beyond the scope of this book.

Crime and Criminality: Definitions

Crime is an "intentional violation of the criminal law, committed without defense or excuse and penalized by the state" (Nettler 1978, p. 33).

The violation must be *intentional*. Criminal intent cannot be formed without mental competence (or "capacity"). Such competence is absent in children. Furthermore, competence may be diminished or abolished by mental disorders. This is the basis of the insanity defense—a legal concept that is currently under scrutiny in the United States (Phillips et al. 1988; Wettstein et al. 1991).

An act becomes a crime only if it violates a *criminal law*. Different societies have different laws at different times, but certain acts, such as murder and robbery, are universally considered crimes and were probably considered wrongs before the first law was formulated. Human beings share a moral sense that begins developing in early childhood and is universal across cultures (J.Q. Wilson 1993, p. 141).

Crime is a law violation occurring *without defense or excuse*. The defenses or excuses include diminished competence, legally recognized justification for an action that otherwise would be considered a crime (e.g., killing in self-defense), and acting under duress (when a person is forced into criminal action by a threat).

Violent Crime

Murder (and nonnegligent manslaughter), robbery, aggravated assault, and forcible rape are the principal offenses listed as violent crimes by the U.S. Department of Justice (Maguire et al. 1993, p. 358). In this book, reference to violent crime encompasses these four offenses. The most frequent of these is aggravated assault:

> [Aggravated assault is] an unlawful attack by one person upon another for the purpose of inflicting severe or aggravated bodily injury. This type of assault usually is accompanied by the use of a weapon or by means likely to produce death or great bodily harm. Simple assault is excluded. (Maguire et al. 1993, p. 711)

Simple assaults are those in which no weapon is used and no serious injury results. Legal definitions of the other offenses can be found elsewhere (Maguire et al. 1993, pp. 710–711). The definitions are very broad, and they do not capture very well the degree of severity (or gravity) of each crime. Arson, extortion, kidnapping, riot, hit and run (a traffic offense), and child abuse are additional offenses sometimes considered to be violent crimes (Megargee 1982, pp. 168–170).

A rating scale for measuring the seriousness of crimes was constructed by criminologists Sellin and Wolfgang (Sellin and Wolfgang 1964; Wolfgang et al. 1985). These authors developed relative weights for various crimes by asking judges, police officers, and students to rank-order the crimes according to perceived severity. The S-W Index (named for the authors) is computed for each criminal event; the index is based on all the offenses that occurred during that event.

Criminality

Crime is an individual event that occurs when a person possessing certain characteristics (propensity) concludes that there is an opportunity, and acts to break a law. Criminality is an individual's propensity to commit crimes. Some criminologists argue that this propensity is largely based on inadequate *self-control* (Gottfredson and Hirschi 1990, pp. 87–94) or impaired *impulse control* (J. Q. Wilson and Herrnstein 1986, pp. 435–437). A lack of control emboldens these individuals not only to commit crimes but also to do things that, although not illegal, are deviant: they abuse alcohol, skip school, have car accidents, have unwanted pregnancies, and so forth. The reader will note that links among impulsiveness, aggression, and disturbances of the serotoninergic system are being intensively studied by psychiatric researchers; their findings provide a psychobiological basis for the "inadequate self-control or impulse control" theory formulated by criminologists (see Chapters 3 and 7).

Detecting and Reporting Crime

Official Statistics

A nationwide Uniform Crime Reporting program is administered by the Federal Bureau of Investigation (FBI). Certain crimes (including major violent crimes) reported by the victims or discovered by the police are recorded by local and state enforcement agencies. Whenever complaints of crimes are determined to be unfounded, they are eliminated from the count. The remaining offenses ("actual offenses known" or "crimes known to the police") are reported monthly to the FBI. These official statistics have deficiencies (Hindelang et al. 1981, p. 17; Nettler 1978, pp. 58–74). An unknown number of offenses remain undiscovered; if discovered, some remain unreported to the police; if reported, some remain unrecorded. Offense categories are too broad and variable in time and place; thus, dissimilar events are reported in the same category and vice versa. There are no standard detailed procedures for reporting multiple offenses and multiple victims in the same incident or criminal operation. The official statistics are based to a large extent on reports by local police, who may vary in their biases and their enthusiasm for record keeping. One of the possible forms of bias is the racial profiling practiced by some local police departments in the United States. For example, some troopers patrolling the New Jersey Turnpike were illegally targeting black and Hispanic drivers for traffic stops. The stops were ostensibly for speeding or minor violations such as broken lights, but the police searched the cars for drugs. This practice biases the arrest statistics because it probably leads to an underestimation of the rates of drug offenses among white drivers.

In addition to the crimes known to the police, many other indicators of violent (and other) crime are also reported. One of those reports gives the number of crimes "cleared" (usually by arrest). The clearance rate is the proportion of crimes known to the police resulting in an arrest of a suspect. Unlike the reports on known crimes, the arrest reports provide information on the personal characteristics of the suspects.

In 1998, the clearance rates for violent crimes were as follows: murder, 69%; aggravated assault, 58%; forcible rape, 50%; and robbery, 28%. The rate for property crime was 17% (Pastore and Maguire 2000, p. 369). These clearance rates are valid for the general population but not necessarily for offenders with a mental disorder. Mentally healthy perpetrators avoid capture (and arrest) by leaving the crime scene; it is possible that at least some offenders with a mental disorder are too confused, disorganized, or delusional to do that. Interviews with prisoners concerning the circumstances of their arrest indicated that the majority of mentally ill offenders were in fact arrested at the crime scene, and more than a quarter of schizophrenic patients reported themselves to the police (Robertson 1988).

Arrests made by police are generally reported, and to that extent, arrest records are prone to fewer errors than are the records of crimes. However, in the United States, the police have considerable discretionary power in deciding *whether to arrest* and *what to charge*. That discretionary power is perhaps less important in case of a very serious crime (J. Q. Wilson and Herrnstein 1986, p. 36); if the police have a body and a suspect with a weapon, there is usually no choice but to arrest and charge the suspect with murder or manslaughter. However, suspects in many lesser crimes do not get arrested; instead, the police decide on an alternative disposition. The decision to arrest may depend on the suspect's age, race, mental and physical status, and history of offenses. It may also depend on the police officer's training, experience, race, and bias. It is possible that the police (who are largely white) overarrest suspects who are poor and nonwhite and underarrest those who are affluent and white. The decision to arrest is also affected by the situation; when the police are overwhelmed or outnumbered (for example, during riots), they may choose to retreat rather than arrest perpetrators committing crimes right in front of them.

The discretionary power to adopt alternatives to arrest is typically exercised when suspects are juvenile or appear confused (in which case they may be taken to a hospital emergency room rather than to the police station). Only 3 of 115 mentally ill patients who exhibited violent behavior leading to hospitalization were arrested (Lagos et al. 1977). On the other hand, the label of mental disorder may have an opposite effect, increasing the officers' inclination to arrest (Teplin 1984).

In general, even if an arrest is made, the charge may not fully reflect the severity of the criminal behavior. For example, police are sometimes reluctant to charge a husband who has been beating his wife with assault; if an arrest is made, it may be for a lesser offense such as disorderly conduct (Teplin 1985).

Arrest statistics thus *underestimate* the "true" crime rate and provide a *biased* description both of offender characteristics and of the type of criminal behaviors actually occurring. These deficiencies of the arrest statistics are difficult to estimate or correct unless researchers (presumably unbiased) directly observe individual encounters between the police and the citizens. Such observations were in fact collected (Teplin 1985), and I discuss them in detail in another context (see "Violent Behavior Among Identified Psychiatric Patients Estimated From Arrest Rates" in Chapter 9).

After arrest for a violent offense, all offenders are not necessarily prosecuted. Among those who are, the arrest, prosecution, and conviction all might have been for the same offense (e.g., offense *X*). However, in another case, the arrest could have been for offense *X*, but prosecution and conviction could have been for offense *Y*. Or the arrest, prosecution, and conviction offenses could have been, respectively, *X*, *Y*, and *Z*. In many instances, the offense for which the person is convicted is lesser than the offense charged. Such reductions are common after the accused person agrees to plead guilty to the lesser offense (plea bargaining).

The next stage after the conviction is *sentencing*. Not everybody convicted of violent crime (even murder) is incarcerated. The seriousness of the crime, the offender's prior record and perceived dangerousness, and other factors affect sentencing. At each stage of the criminal justice system, the quality of the legal defense plays a role. The quality of legal services is related to their cost, and characteristically, the offender's wealth affects his or her fate. Court-assigned lawyers are free but are sometimes inexperienced and overworked.

At each stage of the offenders' progress through the criminal justice system, the information about their offenses is adapted. The initial police report of the offense and the arrest record give the most immediate and detailed information. At each subsequent stage, the information is increasingly diluted and distorted, and eventually the offender's computerized record of his or her criminal history may be limited to a list of coded offenses for which he or she was arrested and convicted. Such lists are sometimes called "rap sheets." Due to plea bargaining and other factors, such lists may be quite misleading. Nevertheless, much of the published research on the neurobiology of violent crime uses information from such lists as the primary dependent variable. Many workers in this area did not use even these crude estimates of criminal history. Instead, the offense that led to the current incarceration ("instant offense") was used to classify offenders. A similar approach was taken in the classification of offenses (and offenders) as "impulsive" or "nonimpulsive" (see Chapter 7).

Population Surveys

In view of the deficiencies inherent in the official statistics described above, additional methods for measuring crime are used. The most important of these methods are population surveys. There are two main types of population surveys: surveys of households to estimate the unreported proportion of victimizations and surveys of the general population to estimate (by self-reports) the proportion and characteristics of persons committing crimes.

Victimization. The U.S. National Crime Survey Program selects a sample of households for a series of seven interviews taking place at 6-month intervals. Information is elicited on crimes committed against any member of the household. The information includes the type of victimization, whether the incident was reported to the police, relationship to the offender (for violent crime), and perceived gender and race of the offender. A main intent of victimization surveys is to reveal the "dark figure" of crime (Nettler 1978, p. 87): the crime unreported to the police and therefore unrecorded in most statistics. In the United States in 1998, the dark figure was 61% (Pastore and Maguire 2000, p. 194). According to the victims, only 38% of crimes (46% of violent crimes) were reported to the police. In general, the information obtained in victimization surveys about the victims, the criminals, and the patterns of crime incidence is not strikingly different from the picture presented by the official statistics. The main difference between these two sources of information is the much greater volume of crime reported in the victimization surveys.

Self-reported criminal activity. Victimization surveys provide only a limited amount of information about the characteristics of offenders and no information about the proportion of persons committing crimes. Such data can be estimated by asking people to confess. Anonymous or nonanonymous self-reports can take the form of questionnaires, interviews, or sorting cards bearing the names of crimes. External validation of the self-report can be provided by official statistics, and various methods of self-reporting have yielded different validity estimates depending on respondents' characteristics (Hindelang et al. 1981). Other methods that may be used to validate self-reports include interviewing the subjects' peers and administering polygraph tests on the subjects.

We tested the validity of self-reports of arrest by psychiatric inpatients, most of whom had chronic schizophrenia (Convit et al. 1990b). Comparison with official arrest records demonstrated a moderate level of agreement; surprisingly, patients reported more arrests to us than were officially recorded.

Direct Observations of Criminal Activity

Many people have accidentally observed a violent crime, but systematic observations are rare because perpetrators prefer privacy. Shoplifting is frequently recorded on video cameras. Researchers studying youthful urban gangs have observed approximately 10 thefts for every court appearance on theft charges (Nettler 1978, p. 77).

Crime Rates of Individuals

Typical aggregate crime statistics are published in the form of per capita crime rates. For example, the rate of aggravated assault known to the police in the United States in 1998 was 360 per 100,000 inhabitants, and the arrest rate for this offense was 194 per 100,000 (Pastore and Maguire 2000, pp. 266, 339). Similar statistics are available for individual states. These statistics tell us about violent crime in a geographic area and are useful for studying trends over time. However, they do not inform us about violent criminal behavior of individuals—a main focus of the neurobiology of violence.

The total number of crimes committed depends on how many persons commit crimes and on how frequently they commit them. Thus, the crime rate is the product of two proportions:

$$\frac{\text{crimes}}{100,000} = \frac{\text{criminals}}{100,000} \times \frac{\text{crimes}}{\text{criminal}}$$

The proportion of criminals (defined as persons committing at least one crime in a specified period) is called *prevalence,* and the frequency of crimes (the number of crimes committed per year by the average criminal) is called *incidence* (J. Q. Wilson and Herrnstein 1986, p. 30). Another source gives a slightly different definition of incidence (Gottfredson and Hirschi 1990, p. 240). Incidence and prevalence can be computed from arrest reports, self-reports, or direct observations. Incidence distinguishes ordinary offenders from career criminals.

SUMMARY AND CONCLUSIONS

Aggression, hostility, and violence have been defined. These definitions have flaws; perfect definitions are impossible. The concept of intent is particularly difficult to define.

Assessment instruments for aggressiveness and hostility (such as the Buss-Durkee scale) have been reviewed. Instruments for counting and classification of individual incidents of overt aggression have been evaluated, as well as the newly emerging instruments to describe incident patterns and their frequency.

Methods for detection of violent incidents in psychiatric hospitals underreport aggression. The official incident reports show maximal underreporting, whereas video recording is closest to the true incidence of violent incidents.

Crime and criminality have been defined. Official statistical indicators include rates of crimes known to the police, arrest rates, prosecution and conviction rates, and incarceration rates. These indicators are complemented by population surveys assessing either victimization or self-reported criminal activity. Aggregate statistics measuring local crime rates have been compared with indicators measuring crime rates in individuals. Prevalence and incidence have been defined.

2

Aggression Among Animals

Aggression is one manifestation of competition, the active demand by two or more individuals for a common limited resource (E. O. Wilson 1976, p. 243) such as food, reproduction (access to mating), or territory. Individuals may compete by aggression or other strategies such as scrambling—in other words, appropriating resources before the others get to them. Scrambling obviates the need to fight or to otherwise interact with others. Observers of aggression in rodents noticed that it was linked to other behaviors that, although nonaggressive, could not be conceptually separated from fighting. Therefore, the term *agonistic behavior* was coined to include not only aggression but also conciliation, retreat, and other defensive activity occurring in the context of fighting (Scott and Fredericson 1951).

Animal aggression encompasses many different behaviors besides overt physical fighting. It may be manifested, for example, by fighting rituals and threats. The purposes served by these behaviors vary among species (including humans). Given these heterogeneities, it is understandable that no generally accepted definition of aggression exists. Definitions are discussed in Chapter 1.

Because literature on animal aggression is vast, I only outline the features that will, I hope, help the reader to understand subsequent chapters dealing with humans, and I limit my review to studies of mammals, with an emphasis on primates.

Although animal experimenters in the late 1960s published data linking the serotoninergic system to aggression, the first analogous human studies were not published until 1979 (G. L. Brown et al. 1979). This 10-year gap suggests that clinicians' awareness of animal literature could be improved.

TYPES OF AGGRESSION IN ANIMALS IN THEIR NATURAL HABITAT

Aggression has evolved, within the framework of competition, as a set of contingency plans for a set of stimulus conditions. Certain stimuli elicit specific types of aggression. These stimuli and the aggressive responses can be studied by observing animals relatively undisturbed in their natural habitat or in the laboratory. Animals in their natural habitat engage in various forms of aggression; several systems have been developed to describe and classify these forms. One such system describes seven kinds of aggression (Moyer 1976); it has influenced subsequent research and is outlined below.

Predatory Aggression

Predatory aggression aims at killing and (sometimes) consuming the animal's natural prey; the prey is an animal of different species than the predator (interspecies aggression). Predatory attack is elicited by the appearance of prey, is facilitated by food deprivation, and is inhibited by fear. In general, there is no difference between males and females in this type of aggression. The prey's defense (antipredatory aggression) is sometimes classified in this group. The predatory attack is usually quiet; there is no display of threatening behavior. Thus, the purpose, the patterns, the tactics, and sometimes even the weapons set predatory aggression clearly apart from other types of aggression.

Intermale Aggression

Intermale aggression, unlike predatory aggression, is directed against (male) individuals of the same species (intraspecies aggression). In a majority of mammalian species, the male is more aggressive than the female under most conditions, and the most frequent target of aggression is a male of the same species (conspecific). These gender differences in patterns of aggression become apparent before maturity in many species, including primates.

Intermale aggression may result in death of one of the contestants, but that is not its primary aim. Competition for access to females underlies much of intermale aggression, and the resolution of such contests does not require death of the defeated participant.

The aggressive encounter may be ritualized; it usually results in a demonstration of superiority of one individual over another. Such a demonstration is usually accomplished without serious injury to either contestant. Intermale aggression may be defused or prevented by submissive behavior or by escape. After several aggressive contacts between a given pair of males, the subordinate animal avoids repeated defeats by submissive posturing in response to anticipatory fighting postures and threats by the dominant male: a dominance-submission relationship is created. A series of such relationships in an established colony or group of animals contributes to the hierarchical social order, which can thus be maintained with a minimal number of actual fights.

Fear-Induced Aggression

Fear-induced aggression is one response available to the defensive animal that is unable to escape from a threat. Other possible responses in this situation include freezing or submissive posturing. Before fighting back, the cornered animal usually tries to escape.

Maternal Aggression

Maternal aggression against intruders approaching the young has been documented in many vertebrates. The aggression typically occurs during the lactation period, but females of some species become very aggressive during the last days of pregnancy. Maternal aggression is typically fierce, as attested by the accounts of hikers who were attacked by grizzly bear sows and lived to tell the tale.

Irritable Aggression

Irritable aggression can be elicited by a variety of internal and external stimuli. Males show this type of aggression somewhat more frequently than females. In certain species, some irritable aggression in females shows cyclic patterns, being driven by reproductive rhythms. In general, irritable aggression can be elicited by frustration, pain, or deprivation of food, water, sleep, or social contact. Unlike other types of aggression, the target of the attack is quite nonspecific. It can be any organism or even an inanimate object.

Sex-Related Aggression

Males sometimes threaten or attack females for the purpose of mating with them (aggressive courtship). Furthermore, actual mating behavior of males in some species includes movements that look like aggression, but in most cases, the females sustain no injuries or only minor ones.

Instrumental Aggression

Instrumental aggression is elicited by the experimenter's manipulations of the animal's environment and accordingly is discussed below under "Paradigms for the Study of Animal Aggression in the Laboratory."

Territorial Aggression

Territorial aggression has been abandoned by Moyer as a useful construct because it consists of elements of other forms of aggression. However, other researchers list territorial aggression in a separate class by itself (E. O. Wilson 1976).

Territorial animals spend most of their time within their home range. Within that range, there is an area that the animals will defend against intruders (mostly conspecifics). That defended area is called the animals' *territory*. Territoriality is widespread among mammals, including primates.

Most of the time, defense of a territory may be accomplished without actual fights. Many animals deposit scents that mark their territory; for example, dogs spray trees or fire hydrants with their urine. These marks inform conspecifics of the animal's recent presence and perhaps warn them off (the evidence for this warning function is ambiguous). Furthermore, some animals emit calls that may similarly warn others. These warnings, combined with the experience of previous physical encounters with the defenders, keep intruders at bay for long periods. For example, in 2,500 hours of watching a territorial species (indri monkey), only six meetings between troops were observed (Jolly 1985, p. 143). When an intrusion occurs, intruders are confronted by animals defending their territory. The defenders display threatening behavior; the intruder may retreat or display similar behavior. This threatening behavior may lead to a standoff, which is then resolved by physical fights. Such fights are usually won by the defenders.

Each of the activities that may serve territorial defense has been observed among primates. Long-term observations in several primate species suggest that the defense is successful, resulting in the defenders' exclusive use of approximately 90% of their home range (Jolly 1985, pp. 143–144).

In summary, animal aggression occurring in the natural habitat can be classified into two main types: 1) predatory aggression and 2) other types of aggression, including intermale, fear-induced, maternal, irritable, sex-related, and territorial aggression. The classification is imperfect; there are some overlaps among classes. However, the classification is helpful in several ways. First, it provides a framework for animal studies of underlying biological mechanisms; for example, many laboratory paradigms aim at emulating certain types or classes of naturally occurring aggression (see "Paradigms for the Study of Animal Aggression in the Laboratory" below).

Second, I think that the classification and description of animal aggression is relevant for the understanding of human violence. For example, most readers have probably witnessed a competition or a fight between two men (or boys) for a woman. A comparison of that experience with the previously described intermale aggression will perhaps convince most readers that some important characteristics of this subtype of aggressive behavior are shared by humans and other species.

Of course, there are human violent behaviors (for example, urban riots) that appear to have no clear analog or antecedent among animals. That, however, does not mean that all human aggression is specific for our species or that studying animal aggression is irrelevant to understanding humans.

PARADIGMS FOR THE STUDY OF ANIMAL AGGRESSION IN THE LABORATORY

The laboratory situation allows controlled emulation of the naturally occurring stimuli eliciting aggression; furthermore, new stimulus paradigms (e.g., brain stimulation) can be introduced. Laboratory studies of aggression are important because they provide information about the biological and social underpinning of this behavior. Understanding the underlying biology is a prerequisite for the development of psychopharmacologic treatments for aggression; testing such treatments in animals constitutes a large part of the laboratory research into aggression. For example, the development of antiaggressive drugs requires considerable testing of behavioral effects in animals. I now review some of the major paradigms used to study aggression.

Predatory Aggression

Rats killing mice (muricide) has been a traditional paradigm to study predatory aggression in the laboratory (Karli 1956), although there are some doubts about the predatory nature of the behavior (Miczek 1987, p. 203). One of the problems is that the mouse is not the rat's usual prey. Not all rats will kill mice; some will not do so even after food deprivation. Muricidal aggression can be *induced* in rats that normally do not exhibit this behavior (i.e., in nonmuricidal rats) by social isolation, administration of various drugs or diets (see "Serotonin" below), or surgical interventions such as the removal of olfactory bulbs. Conversely, muricidal behavior can be *blocked* by drugs.

Maternal Aggression

Lactating rats will attack male or female intruders, and this paradigm has been used for the study of drug effects on aggression (Olivier et al. 1985). The obvious advantage of this paradigm is that it offers an opportunity to study aggression in females, who are otherwise generally more placid than males.

Frustration- or Extinction-Induced Aggression

As mentioned above, frustration may elicit irritable aggression. After a period of rewarding (reinforcing) a behavioral response, animals are frustrated when the reward is omitted (extinction), and irritable aggression may ensue. It is also possible to reinforce a behavioral response intermittently (rather than omitting the reinforcement completely and permanently). These paradigms allow the experimenters to generate carefully graduated levels of frustration (and aggression) in their subjects.

First studied in birds, extinction-induced aggression has been demonstrated in mammals, including primates. Rats trained to press a bar to obtain food will attack another rat during the second or third minute after the reinforcement is omitted (T. Thompson and Bloom 1966). Squirrel monkeys were trained to press a bar to receive food. The number of bar presses required to receive a portion of food was then increased; the monkeys responded by biting a rubber hose provided for this purpose. A similar response was obtained when the food reward was discontinued (Hutchinson et al. 1968).

Isolation-Induced Aggression

Social deprivation elicits predictable aggressive behavior in many animal species. One of the most frequently used paradigms for the study of aggression is to isolate an adult male mouse for a period and subsequently observe its interactions with another mouse that is introduced for this purpose. The isolate usually threatens and attacks the other mouse; however, a proportion of isolated mice will show defensive postures instead of attacking ("timid" mice) (Krsiak 1975). Isolation-induced aggression in mice has been used to test antiaggressive effects of antidepressants (Delini-Stula and Vassout 1981), anxiolytics (Garattini and Valzelli 1981), and "serenics," a class of drugs with specific antiaggressive effects (Olivier et al. 1990). Interestingly, elevations of plasma testosterone levels and of testis weights were elicited by isolating rodents. Relationships between aggression and testosterone levels exist (see "Hormones and Aggression" below).

The effects of long-term social deprivation on aggression in monkeys are complex. The aggression elicited in monkeys in this way is of the irritable type (see "Irritable Aggression" above). It does not occur as a response to a specific stimulus, and the targets are variable. The effects of social deprivation depend on the subject's age at the time of deprivation.

Rhesus monkeys were separated at birth from their mothers, and each was placed in an isolated chamber for 6 months; they saw no living creature during that period. Food, water, and cleaning were all provided by remote control (Harlow and Harlow 1967). After this period of isolation, they were placed in cages housing monkeys that had been raised with others. The isolates first responded with overwhelming fearful reactions. However, over a period of several years, the isolates began to attack other monkeys. These attacks were indiscriminate: the targets were sometimes large adult males against whom the isolates had no chance of winning; and they were sometimes juveniles, which are usually not attacked by normal monkeys of the isolates' age. It appears that if monkeys are deprived of the opportunity to learn social skills (including the meaning of various social signals) during their first 6 months, they may not be able to develop adaptive strategies to avoid aggression. Thus, they may not respond appropriately (by submissive gestures) to threats by larger peers, or they may not inhibit their own aggression in response to submissive behavior by juveniles (Moyer 1976, pp. 197–198). Various types of social deprivation (much less severe than those imposed by Harlow and Harlow) are now used to study behavioral and biochemical effects of anomalous rearing (Higley et al. 1991).

Pain-Induced Aggression

Administration of painful stimuli may result in aggression of the irritable type (see "Irritable Aggression" above). The typical laboratory paradigm calls for repetitive electric pulses administered through the bars of a grid floor of a cage containing two rats. When the foot shock is administered, the rats assume an upright posture facing each other, their forepaws move up and down as if they were boxing, and they vocalize. The number of times this posture is assumed depends on the stimulus intensity, the animals' strain and age, and variables that may be introduced by the experimenter. This paradigm has been used to study the effects of drugs and neurotransmitters on aggression (Sheard 1981).

There are many problems with the paradigm. The posture assumed by the rats is a defensive one. It is thus not clear that this paradigm presents a good model of aggression. Furthermore, the drugs or other variables under study may affect pain perception; thus, antiaggressive effects of a drug may be distorted by its analgesic effect in this paradigm. The stress of this experimental situation may have a direct effect on aggression; it may also alter pain perception. These problems make it difficult to interpret the results obtained with this paradigm.

Aggression Modulated by Brain Stimulation

Electrical or chemical stimulation targeted at relatively small brain areas may elicit motor fragments of aggressive behavior or complete acts of aggression that cannot be distinguished phenomenologically from spontaneous aggressive acts. Much work was done in the cat. Electrical stimulation of the medial hypothalamus resulted in a defensive display involving piloerection, hissing, baring of teeth, and readiness to attack if provoked (Hess and Brugger 1943). This behavioral complex has been varyingly labeled as affective aggression, rage, or defensive attack. The stimulation of the lateral hypothalamus, lateral preoptic area, pontine tegmentum, and other areas elicited a predatory attack characterized by quiet killing of the prey without signs of autonomic arousal (D.A. Smith and Flynn 1979; Wasman and Flynn 1962). These aggressive behaviors can be elicited by stimulating some points, but stimulation of other points within these structures evokes only uncoordinated fragments of aggressive behaviors, or it has no obvious effect.

Much electrical brain stimulation of the monkey has been performed by Delgado and his group (Delgado 1963). The aggressive behaviors elicited in primates are variable and complex. The environmental situation modulates the effect of electrical stimulation. For example, a gibbon receiving identical stimulation of the central gray matter under four environmental conditions exhibited different responses: when under restraint, the animal responded to the stimulation by making threatening gestures; stimulated while alone in a cage, he jumped around but did not attack or bite anything; stimulated in a cage colony where he was the dominant male, he selected a low-ranking gibbon and attacked him; when free in a gibbon colony established on an isolated island, the gibbon ran away and hid in the bushes (Delgado 1981).

Thus, responses evoked by brain stimulation depend on the species, the test conditions, and the stimulation site. I am not sure how reliably the responses exhibited by Delgado's gibbon could be replicated.

Aggression Modulated by Brain Lesions

Most of the information on the effects of experimental brain lesions on aggression has been obtained by studying the rat; many of these studies were reviewed elsewhere (Albert and Walsh 1982). In general, the brain structures that modulate aggression can be identified by changes in aggressive (or, more generally, agonistic) behavior after their removal. These structures include the lateral septum, the median and dorsal raphe nuclei, the olfactory bulbs, the amygdala, and the median hypothalamus. Specific types of agonistic behavior (defense, predatory mouse killing, and nonpredatory attack on a conspecific) may be inhibited by activating specific combinations of some the structures enumerated above. Extensive functional interconnections among these structures suggest their complex interactions in the inhibition or modulation of agonistic behavior. When lesions are made in several of these structures in the same animal, the lesions appear to have additive effects on agonistic behavior. Evidence from experiments involving lesions of the median and dorsal raphe nuclei suggests that serotoninergic neurons inhibit mouse killing. The median raphe neurons supply much of the serotoninergic innervation of the limbic system, whereas the dorsal raphe neurons project more diffusely to the neostriatum, the thalamus, and the cerebral and cerebellar cortices (Kandel et al. 2000, p. 1214). The importance of the limbic system in the regulation of aggression has been demonstrated in other species, including humans (Eichelman 1983; Mark and Ervin 1970); I return to this issue later.

Ablation experiments in the monkey are relatively rare. The classic study used 16 rhesus monkeys whose temporal lobes were removed bilaterally (Kluver and Bucy 1939). The main purpose of the experiment was to study visual agnosia. However, the experimenters also noted "emotional changes" in that the animals lost their capacity to express anger or fear by facial expression and vocalization. Furthermore, physical attacks were eliminated; the animals would no longer engage even in defensive fighting.

Three rhesus monkeys who appeared dominant in their group were subjected to bilateral amygdalectomy (Rosvold et al. 1954). Two of these monkeys lost their dominant positions, although they appeared more aggressive or fearless in their behavior toward the experimenters after the operation. These observations were made in caged animals.

The effects of bilateral lesions of uncinate cortex and amygdaloid nuclei were studied in free-ranging rhesus monkeys who were, before the operation, members of an established social group (Dicks et al. 1969). This experiment provided an opportunity to observe the effects of the lesions on social interactions under natural conditions. Operated subjects ($n=2$) showed social indifference, lost their ability to display the normal aggressive and submissive gestures, were attacked and expelled by their group, and soon died. Subsequent operations in five monkeys were therefore limited to the amygdala. One of these subjects inappropriately attacked the dominant monkey in his group, was chased away, and soon died. Another one also died after leaving his group. Three subjects (who were somewhat younger) gradually regained their social skills and survived.

The results suggest that temporal lobe structures, particularly the amygdala, play a complex role in the modulation of aggression in primates. Removal of the amygdala does not have a universal "taming" effect. Instead, it disrupts the ability of the animal to conform its aggressive (or submissive) behavior to the established social norms of its group. Normal function of the amygdala is thus necessary for the animal's selection of aggressive (or submissive) behaviors appropriate for a given social situation.

Dorsolateral frontal lobe lesions in rhesus monkeys resulted in a diminished occurrence of threats and a concomitant increase of aggression (M.H. Miller 1976). Orbitofrontal lesions in vervet monkeys were not followed by any change in the rate of aggressive behavior expressed toward conspecifics. However, the operated animals threatened a human observer more frequently postoperatively than they had done preoperatively (Raleigh et al. 1979).

NEUROTRANSMITTERS, RECEPTORS, AND AGGRESSION AMONG ANIMALS

Serotonin

Evidence supporting the importance of serotonin in the inhibitory control of aggression has been growing steadily since the 1960s. Some of that evidence was obtained by experimental manipulations of the serotoninergic system in rodents. The serotoninergic system was suppressed by a dietary reduction of tryptophan (a serotonin precursor), by drugs eliciting relatively selective axonal degeneration of serotonin-containing neurons, or by blocking tryptophan hydroxylase—the rate-limiting enzyme for serotonin synthesis—with p-chlorophenylalanine (PCPA). Each of these three manipulations has increased muricidal behavior of the rat (Applegate 1980; Gibbons et al. 1978, 1979).

Furthermore, mice showing isolation-induced aggression (see "Isolation-Induced Aggression" above) had a decrease in brain tryptophan (B.L. Miller et al. 1979). Similarly, social isolation reduced brain serotonin turnover in mice, and this effect could be observed only in those strains that react to isolation with aggression (Valzelli and Bernasconi 1979). Thus, it appears that the effects of the animal's environment (isolation) produce a neurochemical change that elicits (or disinhibits) aggressive behavior.

Increased aggressiveness and lowering of brain serotonin levels were observed in the adult offspring of mice given alcohol during gestation (Krsiak et al. 1977). The behavioral results of this experiment are shown in Figure 2–1. Interestingly, increased locomotion was also observed in the offspring; this observation led the authors to speculate about the possibility of prenatal alcohol exposure causing hyperactivity in humans.

Behavioral effects observed by Krsiak et al. (1977) were confirmed; prenatal alcohol exposure elevated juvenile play fighting and postpubertal aggression in rats (Royalty 1990). Prenatal exposure to alcohol elicited additional delayed effects on the brain in various experimental paradigms. The exposure impaired spatial memory in the rat (Gianoulakis 1990), suggesting a hippocampal dysfunction. Hippocampal cell density was reduced in rats exposed prenatally or postnatally to alcohol (Wigal and Amsel 1990). Long-term behavioral effects of prenatal exposure in rats were reviewed elsewhere (E.P. Riley 1990). The common findings include increased motor activity, gait abnormalities, deficits in various learning tasks, and deficits in maternal behavior of prenatally exposed females toward pups. These animal findings suggest that the hyperactivity and learning disorders observed in humans exposed prenatally to alcohol may be adequately explained without invoking effects of the postnatal rearing environment. Prenatal exposure of rodents to paroxetine (Coleman et al. 1999) and to diazepam, phenobarbital, haloperidol and fluoxetine (Singh et al. 1998) also results in increased aggression.

However, we cannot be quite certain that the postnatal rearing environment has no effect. The behavior of the prenatally exposed offspring may influence the mother's responsiveness. This influence was demonstrated only for the first 9 postpartum days in the rat (Ness and Franchina

ACTIVITIES

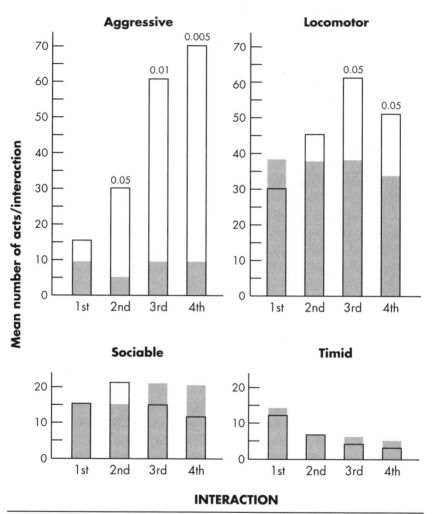

Figure 2–1. Behavior of adult male offspring (*n*=14) of alcohol-treated female mice and of control offspring (*n*=14, *shaded columns*) in paired interactions with nonaggressive intact male mice. Interactions (*n*=4) were repeated at weekly intervals. Numbers below columns indicate sequence of interactions. Numbers above columns indicate levels of significance (Mann-Whitney *U* test, two tailed).

Source. Adapted from Krsiak M, Elis J, Poschlova N, et al.: "Increased Aggressiveness and Lower Brain Serotonin Levels in Offspring of Mice Given Alcohol During Gestation." *Journal of Studies on Alcohol* 38:1696–1704, 1977. Copyright 1977 by Journal of Studies on Alcohol, Inc., Rutgers Center of Alcohol Studies, New Brunswick, NJ 08903. Used with permission.

1990). One can, however, imagine similar effects of child behavior on the mother confounding studies in humans.

Serotoninergic effects on aggression have been demonstrated in non-human primates. Plasma tryptophan levels (and presumably brain tryptophan levels) of captive vervet monkeys were manipulated by feeding them amino acid mixtures that were tryptophan free, were nutritionally balanced, or contained excess tryptophan (Chamberlain et al. 1987). The effects of these mixtures on aggression were observed under two separate conditions: no competition (spontaneous aggression) and competition for food (competitive aggression). The results are presented in Figure 2–2.

Reduction of plasma tryptophan levels resulted in significant increases in the number of spontaneous and competitive aggressive events in the males (but not in the females); the competitive condition yielded more aggressive events than the spontaneous one. Tryptophan elevation suppressed competitive aggression in males and females; this suppression was not due to a general sedative effect of tryptophan because locomotion was not affected. These results indicate that serotoninergic effects on aggression are particularly pronounced in males and that the effects are greater if the animal is aroused or stressed. I return later to the role of stress (see "Cortisol-Releasing Factor, Adrenocorticotropic Hormone, and Corticosteroids" below).

Antiaggressive effects of tryptophan in the vervet monkey were augmented by the concurrent administration of fluoxetine, a relatively selective inhibitor of serotonin reuptake. Fluoxetine alone suppressed aggressive behavior; this effect was dose dependent. The effective dose was 1 or 2 mg/kg; 0.5 mg/kg was ineffective. These data were obtained in an experiment testing many treatment regimens (some of which I do not review here); each regimen lasted for 6 days (Raleigh 1987). The antiaggressive effects of tryptophan and fluoxetine were similar despite their differences in structure and metabolism. This similarity provides additional evidence suggesting that a serotoninergic mechanism is involved in the antiaggressive effects of these substances. Note that these results were obtained in a species closely related to humans, with doses of fluoxetine similar to those administered to depressed patients. Thus, these results are relevant for human psychopharmacology; I return to fluoxetine when I discuss antidepressants (see "Antidepressants" section in Chapter 11).

Additional evidence for a role of the serotoninergic system in aggression was obtained in 28 free-ranging male rhesus monkeys (Higley et al. 1992). The monkeys' aggressivity was estimated primarily by examining the wounds and scars presumably received in fights; limited direct obser-

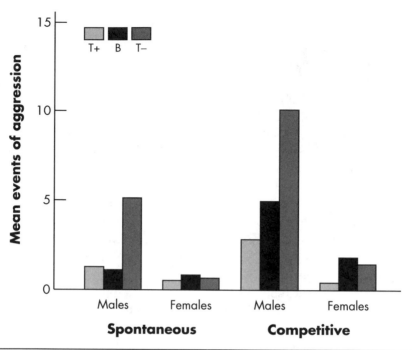

Figure 2–2. Spontaneous and competitive aggression in vervet monkeys after various amino acid mixtures. T+=tryptophan supplemented. B=nutritionally balanced. T–=tryptophan free.

Source. Reprinted from Chamberlain B, Ervin FR, Pihl RO, et al.: "The Effect of Raising or Lowering Tryptophan Levels on Aggression in Vervet Monkeys." *Pharmacology, Biochemistry, and Behavior* 28:503–510, 1987. Copyright 1987 Pergamon Press Ltd. Used with permission.

vation of aggressive behavior was possible. Cerebrospinal fluid (CSF) and blood samples were obtained after the monkeys were trapped and anesthetized. The ratings for aggressivity were inversely related to the CSF concentration of 5-hydroxyindoleacetic acid (5-HIAA), a metabolite of serotonin; the relationship was strikingly similar to that observed in humans (G.L. Brown et al. 1979) (Figure 2–3).

The rate of mortality was ascertained over a 4-year period after obtaining blood and cisternal CSF samples from an expanded sample ($N=49$) of free-ranging, 2-year-old male rhesus monkeys. Four years later, 6 of the 49 subjects were known to be dead and an additional 5 had been missing for more than 2 years and were presumed dead; these subjects had low CSF 5-HIAA concentrations. None of the subjects from the quartile with the highest CSF 5-HIAA concentrations were dead or missing. Direct observations of aggressive behavior showed that dead or missing

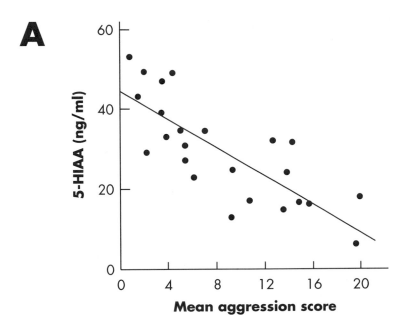

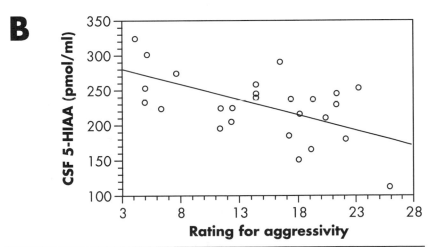

Figure 2–3. Aggression and cerebrospinal fluid 5-hydroxyindoleacetic acid (CSF 5-HIAA) in young men with personality disorders (*A*) and in young vervet monkeys (*B*).

Sources. *Panel A* reprinted from Brown GL, Goodwin FK, Ballenger JC, et al.: "Aggression in Humans Correlates With Cerebrospinal Fluid Amine Metabolites." *Psychiatry Research* 1:131–139, 1979. Used with permission.
Panel B reprinted from Higley JD, Mehlman PT, Taub DM, et al.: "Cerebrospinal Fluid Monoamine and Adrenal Correlates of Aggression in Free-Ranging Rhesus Monkeys." *Archives of General Psychiatry* 49:436–441, 1992. Used with permission.

subjects had initiated escalated aggression (Higley et al. 1996). These findings suggest that low CSF 5-HIAA concentration quantified early in life is a powerful biological predictor of future excessive aggression, risk taking, and premature death among male nonhuman primates.

The kind of human aggressivity that is linked to a disturbance of the serotoninergic system is perhaps based on underlying impulsiveness. An animal's inability to delay its response (wait) is similar to impulsiveness in humans. The ability to wait can be measured experimentally, for example, by presenting hungry rats with a choice between immediate access to a small amount of food and delayed access to a large amount. Serotoninergic uptake inhibitors improved the rats' ability to tolerate delay (wait for reward) under such experimental conditions (Soubrie and Bizot 1990).

We may speculate that serotoninergic control of aggression is indirect: an adequate serotoninergic system may enable the organism to wait and develop another (nonaggressive) response to a stimulus that elicits aggression in animals whose serotoninergic system malfunctions.

As mentioned earlier, central serotoninergic system malfunction can be elicited experimentally by surgical or toxic lesions, dietary manipulations, or suppression of tryptophan hydroxylase via PCPA. None of these mechanisms is likely to play a role in the reduced activity of the serotoninergic system described in aggressive animals (or humans) who have not been subjected to such experimental manipulations. These organisms show a relatively permanent (trait) hypofunction of the serotoninergic system. How and when did they develop this trait? The fact that the response of serotonin turnover to social isolation differs among strains (Valzelli and Bernasconi 1979) suggests that the trait may be genetic. Longitudinal prospective experiments in rhesus monkeys demonstrated genetic and environmental contributions to the functions of the central monoamine systems (Higley et al. 1991, 1993). A recent report indicates that a polymorphism (length variation) in the serotonin transporter gene (5-HTTLPR) interacts with rearing environment to modify serotonin function and aggressive behavior in rhesus macaques (Higley et al. 2000). The macaques with the short 5-HTTLPR allele had low CSF 5-HIAA concentrations and were aggressive. However, this was found only in macaques that were reared in peer groups without adult influence. Thus, the phenotypic expression of the short allele was dependent on rearing environment. Relationships between the 5-HTTLPR polymorphism, serotonin transporter availability in the brain, CSF 5-HIAA, and aggression were reported in a study of 11 rhesus monkeys who had experienced parental separation (Heinz et al. 1998). The animals with greater availability of serotonin transporters in the brain stem and with lower

CSF 5-HIAA concentrations were more aggressive. Taken together, the available evidence from animal experiments suggests that genetic and environmental influences shape the long-term functional properties of the serotoninergic system.

Serotonin receptors are involved in the regulation of aggressive behavior, but detailed information is still incomplete. Part of the complexity is due to the fact that there are many serotonin receptors; a total of at least 14 have been identified to date. Male mice whose 5-HT1B gene was experimentally inactivated (knockout mice) and who therefore lack the 5-HT_{1B} receptor showed increased aggressive behavior and more general social disinhibition (Bouwknecht et al. 2001); these observations suggest that the receptor is involved in the inhibitory control of aggressive and impulsive behavior.

The evidence for a role of the serotoninergic system in the control of aggression is very strong, but this neurotransmitter system does not operate independently of the other systems. I provide more information on serotonin than on other transmitters in view of the persuasive evidence for its importance in aggressive behavior in humans (see Chapter 3).

Norepinephrine

Enhancement of central noradrenergic function facilitated aggressive behavior in most animal studies. Acute administration of propranolol, a β-adrenergic blocker, decreased pain-induced aggression in the rat. However, the aggression was increased after withdrawal from propranolol; this increase was attributed to an increased number of cortical β-adrenergic receptors (Hegstrand and Eichelman 1983). Besides pharmacologic means, stressful environmental influences can enhance central noradrenergic function. Repeated immobilization of rats results in an increase in pain-induced aggression, and this increase may last for as long as a month after the stressful experience. Increased activity of tyrosine hydroxylase (the rate-limiting enzyme for norepinephrine synthesis) in the thalamus was linked to this poststress increase in aggression (Lamprecht et al. 1972).

Most of the evidence supports the enhancing role of the noradrenergic system in aggression, but there are reports that appear contradictory or equivocal. Surprisingly, norepinephrine administered intraventricularly decreased pain-induced aggression in the rat (Geyer and Segal 1974). Furthermore, selective depletion of brain norepinephrine with 6-hydroxydopamine increased pain-induced aggression in rats (Thoa et al. 1972). The onset of this increase was several days after the administration of 6-hydroxydopamine; this delay was interpreted to mean development of supersensitivity of the norepinephrine receptors. That interpretation would fit the theory that norepinephrine enhances aggression.

Noradrenergic stimulation may inhibit the release of serotonin in the rat brain (Hahn et al. 1982). It is thus possible that the noradrenergic enhancement of aggression is partially mediated by the serotoninergic system and that a balance between the noradrenergic and serotoninergic activity in the central nervous system is important for the modulation of aggressive behavior.

Dopamine

Multiple dopamine receptor subtypes have been identified (Kandel et al. 2000, pp. 1199–1200); most effects described in the literature on aggression are apparently attributable to the D_2 subtypes. Central dopamine agonists increase aggressive behavior. Rodent aggression was enhanced by L-dopa (Lammers and van Rossum 1968) and by the dopamine agonist apomorphine (Senault 1970). Intraventricular administration of dopamine increased pain-induced aggression in rats (Geyer and Segal 1974); the opposite effect was noted for norepinephrine in the same experiment (see previous section).

Many effects of amphetamine, especially those concerning motor activity, are mediated by dopamine receptors and modulated by opioid receptors (Winslow and Miczek 1988b). Amphetamine has complex effects on aggression; the mechanism of these effects is unclear. The same doses of amphetamine *decreased* aggressive behavior in mice that were aggressive at baseline (Krsiak 1979) but *increased* that behavior in nonaggressive mice (Krsiak 1975). Furthermore, there are differential dose effects on various elements of agonistic behavior. Low doses of amphetamine increased attacks, whereas high doses elicited defensive behavior (Miczek 1987, p. 267). The narcotic antagonist naltrexone had variable effects on amphetamine-induced modifications of aggressive behavior (Winslow and Miczek 1988b); these results suggest that such behavior is not consistently modulated by endogenous opioids (see "Endogenous Opioid Peptides" below).

On the other hand, amphetamine, L-dopa, cocaine, and apomorphine exacerbated aggressive behavior elicited by withdrawing mice from morphine (Kantak and Miczek 1988). It is possible that opiate administration stimulates opiate receptors, which inhibit release of dopamine from adjacent presynaptic dopamine nerve terminals. This release inhibition results in supersensitivity of the postsynaptic dopamine receptors. Withdrawing the opiate lifts the suppression of the presynaptic dopamine release; this in turn results in dopamine (and, more generally, catecholamine) overstimulation. This overstimulation underlies the opiate withdrawal syndrome, including the aggressive behavior that is an integral part of that syndrome in rodents. Therefore, substances that further stimulate catecholamine receptors aggravate the syndrome (Kantak and Miczek 1988; Lal et al. 1971). Dopamine antagonists suppressed aggression (Yen et al. 1959), but the doses required for the antiaggressive action in various paradigms were generally so high that they elicited sedation and impairment of locomotor activity (Miczek 1987, pp. 206–209).

Catechol-O-methyltransferase (COMT) and monoamine oxidases (MAO-A and MAO-B) are the principal enzymes involved in the inactivation of catecholamines such as norepinephrine, epinephrine, and dopamine (see Chapter 3). Based on the preceding discussion, it seems reasonable to hypothesize that these enzymes could be involved in the regulation of aggressive behavior: low activity of these enzymes would be expected to increase the likelihood of aggression. Indeed, studies of mice whose COMT gene (Gogos et al. 1998) or MAO-A gene (Cases et al. 1995) was experimentally inactivated (knockout mice) provided support for this hypothesis. The effects on aggression were sexually dimorphic, being limited to males.

γ-Aminobutyric Acid

Potentiation of the γ-aminobutyric acid (GABA) central activity generally decreased pain-induced and predatory aggression, whereas decrease of GABA activity had opposite effects (Haug et al. 1980; Puglisi-Allegra 1980; Simler et al. 1983). GABA has at least three binding sites in the brain: the $GABA_A$ and $GABA_B$ receptors and the GABA transporter. Most of the known effects are attributed to $GABA_A$. The $GABA_A$ receptor complex can interact with several compounds. In addition to the GABA site, it contains sites for benzodiazepine agonists, benzodiazepine antagonists, and barbiturates. Central GABA activity is enhanced by benzodiazepines, and benzodiazepine treatment was reported to reduce aggression in various experimental paradigms (Christmas and Maxwell 1970; Randall et al. 1960; Valzelli 1973). These "taming" effects of benzodiazepines, however, are not always elicited. Chronic treatment with chlordiazepoxide increased aggression among mice (Fox et al. 1970). More recent investigations have discovered bidirectional effects of benzodiazepines on aggression (see "Benzodiazepines" section in Chapter 11).

Endogenous Opioid Peptides

After the discovery of opiate receptors and their endogenous ligands, an effort was made to determine the role of this system in the modulation of aggressive behavior. That effort was spurred on by the knowledge that morphine, an exogenous ligand, had reduced aggressive behavior in animals under most experimental conditions. It was logical to theorize that endogenous opioid peptides (i.e., endorphins) functioned as the body's own analgesics, sedatives, and antiaggressive agents. Thus, the opiate antagonists naloxone and naltrexone were hypothesized to increase aggressive behavior. Tests of these hypotheses generated complex results. Low doses of naloxone (0.1 mg/kg ip) increased defensive behavior in rats, whereas very high doses (4–10 mg/kg ip) had the opposite effect (McGivern et al. 1981; Rodgers 1982). The opiate antagonist naltrexone had no effect on aggressive behavior in squirrel monkeys (Winslow et al. 1983).

Certain endogenous opioid peptides are available for administration to animals. β-Endorphin given subcutaneously reduced pain-elicited aggression in rats (Tazi et al. 1983); this effect depended on the baseline level of fighting (Tazi et al. 1985). Met-enkephalin given intraventricularly decreased isolation-induced aggression in mice (Poshivalov 1982). These and similar results are fragmentary, and it is difficult to draw firm conclusions from them.

When a mouse is attacked and defeated by another mouse, it develops analgesia. The analgesia can be blocked by pretreatment with narcotic antagonists, and it shows cross-tolerance with morphine (Miczek et al. 1982); these properties demonstrate that the analgesia is mediated by endogenous opioids. It appears that this defeat-induced analgesia is mediated primarily by opioids that are released and act within the central nervous system (M.L. Thompson et al. 1988).

The role of opioid receptors in aggression during morphine withdrawal has been mentioned previously (see "Dopamine" above).

HORMONES AND AGGRESSION

Testosterone and Other Androgens

Adult male mammals of most species fight about access to females for mating. This conflict underlies much intermale aggression (see "Intermale Aggression" above). It is closely related to testosterone levels when the competition for mates is direct (such as when males fight for access to a female). If the competition is indirect, for example, when mediated by competition for status, the relationship between fighting and testosterone is less clear (Huntingford and Turner 1987, p. 104).

The initiation of serious intermale fighting does not occur before puberty in the rat and in many other species; the appearance of such fighting in developing mice was linked to increasing testosterone levels (Moyer 1976, p. 240). This is the *activational* effect of testosterone.

In most mammalian species, castration of adult males resulted in reduced aggression, and testosterone replacement reversed this effect (Huntingford and Turner 1987, p. 107). During mating season, sharp increases in plasma testosterone levels co-occurred with increases in intermale fighting in deer and other species (Huntingford and Turner 1987, p. 105). Social isolation of male mice increased aggressive behavior and plasma levels of testosterone and testis weight (Sayegh et al. 1990). Taken together, these observations suggest a causal link between testosterone and fighting and perhaps between male gender (and the Y chromosome) and fighting.

The role of the Y chromosome in aggression may be mediated by 1) the chromosome's effect on the responsiveness of target organs (including the brain) to circulating testosterone; 2) its effect on testosterone biotransformation (which may again be regional, specifically affecting the brain or its parts); or 3) its modulation of the "organizing" effects (see "Prenatal Exposure to Androgens" below) of testosterone on the development of the brain (Carlier et al. 1990). (However, another hypothesis suggested a serotoninergic mechanism for the possible role of the Y chromosome in aggression [Roy et al. 1990]).

Testosterone may increase the readiness to fight, and fighting experience may in turn elevate plasma testosterone levels. These levels remain high in the victor and fall in the loser of the fight. In several primate species, testosterone levels are higher in the dominant males than they are in the subordinate males (Baldwin 1992, p. 91; Huntingford and Turner 1987, p. 116; Winslow and Miczek 1988a). These differences may lead to reproductive incapacitation of weak competitors without exposing them to continuous hopeless fights with dominant males.

Testosterone may enhance the effects of alcohol on aggression. In the dominant squirrel monkeys during the mating season (when testosterone levels are naturally elevated), low doses of alcohol (0.1–0.3 g/kg) increased the frequency of aggressive behaviors such as threats and grasps. This effect was absent outside of the mating season, and it could not be demonstrated in subordinate monkeys (Winslow and Miczek 1988a). Furthermore, exogenous testosterone increased the sensitivity of subordinate monkeys to an alcohol-produced increase of aggressive behaviors (Winslow et al. 1988). The issue is complex because alcohol reduced plasma levels of testosterone in monkeys (Winslow and Miczek 1988a) and in humans (J.H. Mendelson et al. 1978). Nevertheless, it is tempting to speculate that some young adult human males might be sensitized by their naturally high levels of testosterone to the aggression-facilitating effects of alcohol; the plasma level of testosterone at the moment when an aggressive event occurs may be less relevant than the sensitization. Unfortunately, experiments testing similar hypotheses in humans have not produced supporting evidence (see Chapter 3).

In general, the effects of testosterone on aggressive behavior vary with the animal's experience and the situational context. These factors, demonstrable in rodents, are particularly pronounced in primates. As we have seen, a monkey's position in the social hierarchy (dominance or subordination) codetermines the effects of testosterone.

Prenatal Exposure to Androgens

Fetal androgens affect the development of the central nervous system and gender-specific responses of adult individuals. These effects are called *organizational* (as opposed to the activational effects described previously). The male fetus supplies its own testicular androgens. In the case of female fetuses, the androgens may come from adjacent male fetuses. Each of the female mouse fetuses located in the uterus between two male fetuses had unusually high testosterone blood levels. As adults, after ovariectomy, such female mice showed more pronounced aggressive behavior elicited by testosterone than other adult female mice that had been located in the uterus between other females (Vom Saal 1983). Conversely, male fetuses that had been located in utero between two females developed into adults that were less sensitive to the aggression-enhancing effects of testosterone.

Adult male mice that had been castrated immediately after birth were less sensitive to the aggression-enhancing effect of testosterone treatment than were their adult counterparts that had been castrated just before puberty (Barkley and Goldman 1977).

In an exceptional species, prenatal and perinatal androgens may affect aggressiveness immediately after birth. Newborn spotted hyenas (females and males) have very high levels of androgens. Females are born masculinized—both anatomically and behaviorally—due to fetal exposure to these hormones, and neonates of both sexes have erupted front teeth. Litters are usually twins. Siblings start fighting immediately after birth, and one of the same-sex siblings may not survive (Frank et al. 1991). This siblicidal behavior subsides within several weeks after birth. The prenatal and neonatal high levels of androgens are compatible with organizational or activational effects on aggression.

Progesterone and Estrogen

Aggressiveness varies as a function of the estrus cycle in females of many mammalian species. However, there is no uniformity as to the specific part of the cycle where aggressiveness peaks. In some species, such as the rhesus monkey, it reaches its zenith around estrus (Floody 1983, p. 59); in others, such as rats and hamsters, it reaches its nadir at that time (Huntingford and Turner 1987, p. 101). It seems that female monkeys are attacked by males when they are in estrus but by females when they are near menstruation (Floody 1983, p. 60). These observations, however, were not replicated in all primate species.

A great deal of attention has been paid to the behavior of nonhuman primate females around estrus, but relatively less is known about their perimenstrual behavior. From day 4 before menstruation until menstrual onset, female yellow baboons showed a behavioral syndrome including increased aggressiveness. This and other aspects of the syndrome made it similar to the human premenstrual syndrome (Hausfater and Skoblick 1985). In several primate species, no reliable relationship exists between menstrual cycle and female-initiated aggression. It appears that female aggression in primates is controlled more by social forces such as differences in rank than by the menstrual cycle. A female's position in the social hierarchy does not change with cyclic hormonal fluctuations. Subtle interactions between the social environment and the menstrual cycle might affect aggressive behavior in nonhuman primates.

Prolactin

As mentioned above, maternal aggression is typically observed in lactating females. Maternal aggression in hamsters (but not in mice) can be reduced by drugs suppressing prolactin secretion; this effect can be reversed by injections of prolactin (Huntingford and Turner 1987, p. 103). However, the role of hormones in maternal aggression is indirect and is incompletely understood.

Cortisol-Releasing Factor, Adrenocorticotropic Hormone, and Corticosteroids

Fighting is stressful. It activates the hypothalamic-pituitary-adrenal (HPA) axis and its hormones. The increase in adrenocorticotropic hormone (ACTH) and corticosteroids is greater and lasts longer in the losing rat than in the winning rat (Schuurman 1980). In primates, HPA axis function is related to the social ranking of the animal and to its personality (Sapolsky 1990). Subordinate male baboons had higher levels of cortisol than the dominant males. The subdominant males were hypercortisolemic despite their reduced pituitary sensitivity to a cortisol-releasing factor challenge; this implies that the hyperactivity of the HPA axis was driven by the brain (Sapolsky 1989).

The cortisol levels in a group of dominant males showed relatively permanent within-group differences that were related to the animals' personality or coping style. Low cortisol levels within the dominant group were associated with the following behavioral features: ability to differentiate between a threatening and a neutral presence of another male, likelihood of initiating a fight, likelihood of initiating a fight that he wins, differentiating between winning and losing a fight, and displacing aggression onto a third animal after a fight is lost (Sapolsky and Ray 1989). These behavioral and psychoendocrine traits were apparently beneficial because they were associated with longer tenures in the dominant group (Sapolsky 1990).

The finding of elevated ACTH levels in aggressive rhesus monkeys (Higley et al. 1992) may be related to the method of establishing aggressiveness used in that study. As mentioned above, these authors relied primarily on counting wounds and scars. On that basis, it was difficult to establish who initiated the fights and who won. Perhaps the results reflected residual stress associated with receiving the wounds.

ACTH is secreted concomitantly with β-endorphin (Guillemin et al. 1977). The postdefeat analgesia mediated by endorphins was mentioned previously (see "Endogenous Opioid Peptides" above); β-endorphin may play additional roles in the hierarchical relationships among primates.

SUMMARY AND CONCLUSIONS

Animal aggression has been classified into seven types. The types differ in their functions, targets, triggering stimuli, and underlying biological mechanisms. These mechanisms are usually studied in the laboratory under controlled experimental conditions. The naturally occurring types of aggression can be observed in the laboratory; furthermore, additional paradigms (such as drug administration, brain lesions, or brain stimulation) have been used in laboratory experiments. Over the past 30 years, such experiments have yielded a large amount of information on the neuroanatomical, biochemical, and physiologic mechanisms underlying aggression in mammals. More recent observations in nonhuman primates have revealed complex interactions between biological and social factors governing aggressive behavior.

The structures that modulate aggression in rodents include the lateral septum, the raphe nuclei, the olfactory bulbs, the amygdala, and parts of the hypothalamus. Serotonin is the neurotransmitter most clearly implicated in the inhibitory control of aggression. Potentiation of GABA activity also inhibits aggression. Dopamine and norepinephrine generally enhance aggression, and it is possible that modulation of aggression under normal conditions is implemented by a functional equilibrium between serotonin and the catecholamines.

Testosterone is clearly implicated in aggression, and its effects, particularly in primates, interact with social factors. Hormones of the HPA axis play an important and—at least in male baboons—very intricate role in the regulation of aggression.

In anatomically intact animals not treated with drugs or other substances, social factors such as dominance appear to be more important than biochemical factors in regulating aggression. This preponderance of social factors is more apparent in primates than in lower species. Social factors influence levels of neurotransmitters and hormones; these substances in turn affect the animal's behavior and thus its social standing.

The role of biological factors in the regulation of aggression can be increased by experimental interventions such as inducement of brain lesions or administration of drugs. Experiments using these techniques may provide animal models of human brain disorders associated with increased aggressivity. Such models are suitable for the development of pharmacologic treatments and perhaps for the ultimate prevention of human disorders linked with aggressivity.

3 | Neurotransmitters, Hormones, and Genes

Many studies link neurotransmitters and hormones to aggression in animals (see Chapter 2). In this chapter, I review the evidence in humans.

SEROTONIN

Serotonin (5-hydroxytryptamine, 5-HT) exhibits inhibitory control over aggression in a large number of animal species; the evidence for rodents has been available since the late 1960s. The role of the serotoninergic system in human violent behavior apparently was not tested methodically until the late 1970s. The research approaches can be divided into four groups:

1. Studies of the cerebrospinal fluid (CSF) levels of 5-hydroxyindole-acetic acid (5-HIAA)
2. Studies of tryptophan content in plasma and of serotonin uptake in platelets
3. Neuroendocrine challenges of central serotonin receptors
4. Molecular genetic studies

Cerebrospinal Fluid Studies

Levels of 5-HIAA, a principal serotonin metabolite, were simultaneously measured at autopsy in the cortex and the CSF in 48 individuals; they were significantly correlated (r=0.78, P<0.001) (M. Stanley et al. 1985). The CSF 5-HIAA level is believed to reflect presynaptic serotoninergic activity in the brain (Coccaro 1989). Reduced CSF levels of 5-HIAA thus indicate a reduction in central serotoninergic activity.

Low levels of CSF 5-HIAA were discovered in depressed patients who had a history of violent (but not nonviolent) suicide attempts (Asberg et al. 1976). Psychological links between inward and outward aggression have been known to psychiatrists since Freud. Biological links were discovered by investigators at the National Institute of Mental Health (NIMH), who reported that lifetime aggressiveness was negatively related to the CSF levels of 5-HIAA (G. L. Brown et al. 1979) (Figure 2–3). The Brown-Goodwin Inventory for lifetime aggressiveness is described in Chapter 1 (see "Assessment Instruments for Aggressiveness and Hostility" section). There was an association between aggressiveness and a history of suicidal behavior.

This trivariate relationship between low CSF 5-HIAA, suicidal behavior, and aggressiveness has been confirmed in a sample of Finnish prisoners who had a history of alcohol abuse and were incarcerated for murder or attempted murder (Linnoila et al. 1983). These offenders showed unusual cruelty to their victims. The murderers whose offense was classified as impulsive ($n=27$) had lower CSF 5-HIAA levels than the other offenders ($n=9$). The lowest levels were found in the impulsive offenders who had a history of suicide attempt. Furthermore, the recidivistic offenders had CSF 5-HIAA levels 22% lower than those who committed only one violent crime. Taken together, these findings led to the proposition that *impulsiveness* was the common factor on which the trivariate relationship was based (Linnoila et al. 1983). Relations between serotoninergic functioning, impulsiveness, suicide, and aggression were later integrated into a neurobiological model (Mann 1998; Mann et al. 1999). Impulsiveness and its definition are discussed in detail in Chapter 7.

A somewhat similar study compared 16 convicted murderers, 22 suicide attempters, and 39 control subjects (Lidberg et al. 1985b). Fifteen of the 16 murderers were considered impulsive (criteria undefined). The CSF 5-HIAA levels of suicide attempters were lower than those of control subjects. The murderers' levels were similar to those of the control subjects; however, a small subgroup ($n=5$) whose victims were their sexual partners had particularly low levels of CSF 5-HIAA. Perhaps these offenses were committed in a state of extreme emotional turmoil. That turmoil state could not have directly affected the measured CSF composition because the lumbar punctures were performed at least 40 days after admission to the forensic unit, but this subgroup might have been more impulsive (as a trait) than the others. I do not think that this Swedish report (Lidberg et al. 1985b) can be interpreted as a confirmation of the findings in Finnish offenders (Linnoila et al. 1983).

The trivariate relationship between suicide, aggression, and low CSF

5-HIAA was supported by observations in three severely depressed patients who killed their children and attempted suicide (Lidberg et al. 1984). However, history of adult aggressive behavior was related to low CSF 5-HIAA levels in patients *without* a history of suicide attempt (B. Stanley et al. 2000).

The relationship between low CSF 5-HIAA and aggression was observed in various other populations, including children and adolescents diagnosed with attention-deficit disorder, oppositional disorder, or conduct disorder (Kruesi et al. 1990).

Additional evidence suggesting a serotoninergic dysfunction in violent patients was provided in a French study of six XYY males. A decrease in central serotonin (but not dopamine) turnover was demonstrated by studies of CSF before and after administration of probenecid (Bioulac et al. 1980). It is possible that the serotoninergic dysfunction was related to the chromosomal abnormality. This possibility has not been explored in other studies of XYY samples, although one of the subjects who had very low CSF 5-HIAA in another study (Linnoila et al. 1983) was an XYY male. Violent behavior among XYY males is discussed later in this chapter. It is interesting that four of the six XYY males in the French study were arsonists (Bioulac et al. 1980). Intrusive thoughts about violence and fear of acting on these thoughts were reported to preoccupy two patients diagnosed with obsessive-compulsive disorder who had low CSF 5-HIAA levels (Leckman et al. 1990). Overt aggression did not occur in these two patients. The authors suggested that violent ideation alone (in the absence of its behavioral expression) may be associated with a serotoninergic disturbance.

A group of 20 Finnish male arsonists who set fires impulsively had reduced levels of CSF 5-HIAA in comparison with violent offenders and with nonviolent control subjects (Virkkunen et al. 1987). Furthermore, the majority of the arsonists showed an abnormally low blood glucose nadir after an oral glucose challenge. The role of serum glucose in the neurobiology of violence is discussed separately (see "Insulin" below).

Impulsiveness was not clearly defined (except that the arson was not committed for profit). The violent offenders were drawn from a sample reported earlier (Linnoila et al. 1983) to match the arsonists for age, height, and sex. It is not clear how many of these violent offenders were deemed impulsive. One of the advantages of these studies (Linnoila et al. 1983; Virkkunen et al. 1987) was that their imprisoned subjects had no access to illicit drugs or alcohol, either of which might have otherwise distorted the results. The relationship between reduced levels of CSF 5-HIAA and impulsive offending was replicated in a different sample by the same research group (Virkkunen et al. 1994).

The offenders whose CSF findings were reported earlier (Linnoila et al. 1983; Virkkunen et al. 1987) were followed up for 3 years after their release from prison (Virkkunen et al. 1989b). The criminal register of Finland was searched for violent offenses or arson committed by these subjects during the follow-up period. Low CSF 5-HIAA and a low glucose nadir after a glucose challenge (see "Insulin" below) predicted recidivistic offending in this sample. Both measures were obtained while the subjects were still in prison. Linear discriminant analysis with these two measures as independent variables correctly classified 46% of the recidivists (6 of 13) and 95% of the nonrecidivists. When the 5-HIAA values were entered alone, all subjects were classified as nonrecidivists; when the 5-HIAA value was the second variable to be entered (after the glucose nadir), it slightly improved the accuracy of the prediction. Thus, the researchers concluded, "the 5-HIAA concentration by itself cannot be regarded as a predictor variable for recidivism" (Virkkunen et al. 1989b, p. 602). Most of the predictive power was due to the glucose nadir values.

Unfortunately, the glucose nadir failed to predict violent recidivism in a larger sample (DeJong et al. 1992). The sample consisted of 248 murderers and 100 arsonists. It included the 58 subjects from the previous study by the same group of investigators (Virkkunen et al. 1989b). Because the second sample included the first one, and because other variables (e.g., impulsiveness, personality disorder) were entered into the prediction equations jointly with the glucose nadir variable, the second study cannot be viewed as an attempt to replicate the first one. Nevertheless, I can assume that a proper attempt to replicate the earlier glucose nadir results (Virkkunen et al. 1989b) would have failed. This is particularly regrettable because, as mentioned above, the glucose nadir results provided most of the predictive power (Virkkunen et al. 1989b). Taken together, these Finnish-American studies illustrate the need for cross-validation of actuarial predictions.

The relationship between low levels of CSF 5-HIAA and aggression could not be replicated in a small study of schizophrenic patients (Kunz et al. 1995). It is possible that aggression in schizophrenia is mediated by a neurochemical pathway involving primarily catecholamines rather than serotonin (see below).

All reports reviewed in this section so far share the same paradigm: they test hypotheses concerning relationships between the CSF 5-HIAA level and some type of deviant behavior exhibited by the study subjects. A different paradigm was used in a study of newborns (Constantino et al. 1997). CSF 5-HIAA was assayed in 193 newborns in whom lumbar punctures were performed for clinical reasons unrelated to research. Parents were interviewed, and a statistically significant relationship between low

CSF 5-HIAA and family history of antisocial personality disorder was observed. The relationship was modest; family history of antisocial personality disorder accounted for less than 5% of the variance in CSF 5-HIAA levels. Nevertheless, this finding lends some support to the notion that a serotonin system dysfunction mediates genetic liability to deviant behavior. If there is a causal relationship between serotonin dysfunction and deviant behavior, this study suggests that the dysfunction is likely to be a cause rather than a consequence of the behavior.

Tryptophan and Serotonin in Plasma

Tryptophan, the serotonin precursor, is discussed extensively in Chapter 2. Reductions in tryptophan levels in the blood increased aggressive behavior (and vice versa) in many species, including nonhuman primates. Tryptophan competes with other large neutral amino acids (leucine, isoleucine, phenylalanine, tyrosine, and valine) for a carrier mechanism transporting these amino acids to the brain (Fernstrom and Wurtman 1972). Thus, the plasma ratio of tryptophan to these competing amino acids is important for the tryptophan influx into the brain.

Low tryptophan ratios were detected in the plasma of hospitalized fasting alcoholic patients who had no access to alcohol for at least 7 days and who reported a history of "incarceration for assaultive behavior against people or property" (L. Branchey et al. 1984, p. 221). These "assaultive" patients ($n=7$) were a subgroup of a sample composed of 43 patients. Aggression and low tryptophan ratios co-occurred with depression, lending additional support for the trivariate relationship discussed above in the section on CSF 5-HIAA.

Similarly to the results of the animal experiments described in Chapter 2, plasma tryptophan levels in humans can be elevated by dietary enrichment. Short-term administration of tryptophan elicited drowsiness in healthy adults (Spinweber et al. 1983; Yuwiler et al. 1981), but neither elevation nor reduction of plasma tryptophan affected aggressiveness as measured in a laboratory experiment with healthy adult male subjects (S. E. Smith et al. 1986). However, in two small studies some beneficial effects of tryptophan treatment in aggressive psychiatric patients were reported (Morand et al. 1983; Volavka et al. 1990).

The relation between plasma tryptophan and aggression remains controversial. In a sample of 89 Swedish male offenders, plasma levels of tryptophan were *elevated* in violent criminals in comparison with healthy control subjects, and the levels of homicide offenders were *higher* than those of nonviolent criminals (Eriksson and Lidberg 1997). These findings are counterintuitive because they appear to be inconsistent with the findings of low CSF 5-HIAA in impulsive violent persons described above. However, they are consistent with the finding of an association between high whole blood serotonin level and violent behavior in a New Zealand birth cohort (Moffitt et al. 1998). The association was limited to males. There was an interaction between the subjects' rearing environment, serotonin level, and violence: the association between high serotonin level and violent behavior was particularly strong in the subset of subjects who grew up in conflicted families ("family members sometimes hit each other"). Thus, the relation between serotonin and violence was apparently modified by environmental effects (witnessing violence or perhaps being subjected to it as a child), and/or by a propensity to violence that was genetically transmitted.

Platelet Uptake of Serotonin

The kinetics and other properties of the blood platelet serotonin uptake closely resemble presynaptic serotonin uptake in neuronal preparations. This peripheral measure is therefore thought to represent presynaptic serotonin function in the central nervous system.

Male outpatients ($n=15$) who complained of loss of control and violent outbursts were compared with matched healthy control subjects (C.S. Brown et al. 1989). None of the subjects were psychotic or epileptic; personality disorders were apparently not diagnosed. Platelet serotonin uptake was lower in the outpatients, and it was inversely related to impulsiveness as measured by the Barratt scale (Barratt 1985a). Thus, this study provided indirect support for a reduced central presynaptic serotoninergic function in impulsive aggression.

Neuroendocrine Challenges

Until recently, direct observational methods to study serotoninergic receptors (aggregate or subtypes) in vivo have not been available. Neuroendocrine challenges offer an opportunity to indirectly study central serotoninergic activity. Fenfluramine releases presynaptic stores of serotonin, blocks serotonin reuptake, and stimulates postsynaptic serotonin receptors. This enhancement of central serotoninergic activity is reflected by elevations of plasma prolactin levels. As demonstrated in healthy volunteers, these elevations are dose dependent and can be blocked by metergoline, a $5\text{-HT}_1/5\text{-HT}_2$ receptor antagonist (Quattrone et al. 1983). Thus, the magnitude of the increase in the plasma prolactin level after a single dose of fenfluramine (fenfluramine challenge) is a measure of central serotonin activity.

A study (Coccaro et al. 1989) using fenfluramine challenge included patients with major affective disorder (n=25), patients with personality disorders (n=20), and healthy control subjects (n=18). All subjects were male. The results are presented in Figure 3–1.

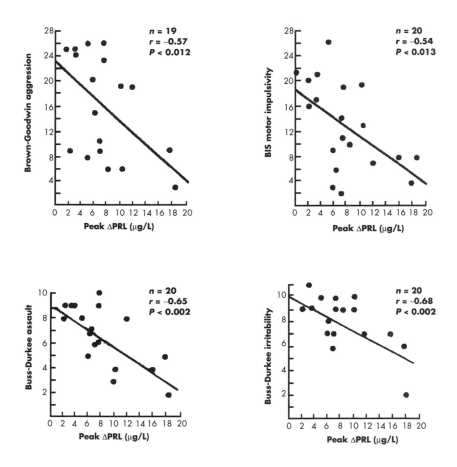

Figure 3–1. Peak prolactin responses (ΔPRL) to fenfluramine correlated with scores from the Brown-Goodwin scale (*top left*), Barratt Impulsiveness Scale (BIS) (motor impulsiveness subscale) (*top right*), Buss-Durkee Hostility Inventory (assault subscale) (*bottom left*), and Buss-Durkee Hostility Inventory (irritability subscale) (*bottom right*).

Source. Adapted from Coccaro EF, Siever LJ, Klar HM, et al.: "Serotonergic Studies in Patients With Affective and Personality Disorders." *Archives of General Psychiatry* 46:587–599, 1989. Used with permission.

In the group with personality disorders (but not in the affective disorder group), the prolactin response was inversely proportional to aggressiveness as measured by the Brown-Goodwin scale (G.L. Brown et al. 1979) (see Chapter 1) and by the "Assault" and "Irritability" items of the Buss-Durkee scale (Buss and Durkee 1957) (see Chapter 1) and was also inversely proportional to impulsiveness as measured by the Barratt scale (Barratt 1985a). Reduced prolactin response was also related to the history of suicide attempts and alcohol abuse. These results imply a hypofunction of the central serotoninergic system in persons prone to impulsive actions, including suicide attempts, alcohol abuse, and aggression. An extension of this study brought the total number of subjects up to 54 (21 with borderline personality disorder, 33 with other personality disorders), and the original results were further supported (Trestman et al. 1992).

A serotoninergic hypofunction in aggressive patients with personality disorders was confirmed and localized by a study that used positron emission tomography to provide a brain map of the effects of a fenfluramine challenge (Siever et al. 1999). Six impulsive-aggressive patients with personality disorders (four males, two females) and five healthy males were evaluated for changes in regional glucose metabolism after administration of fenfluramine or placebo. Volunteers demonstrated increases in glucose metabolism in orbital frontal cortex and adjacent ventral medial frontal cortex, cingulate cortex, and inferior parietal cortex, whereas impulsive-aggressive patients showed no significant increases in glucose metabolism in any region after fenfluramine administration. Compared with volunteers, patients showed significantly blunted metabolic responses in orbital frontal cortex, adjacent ventral medial cortex, and cingulate cortex, but not in inferior parietal lobe.

A modest negative correlation was detected between a composite index of aggression history and impulsivity, and prolactin response to fenfluramine in a community sample of male subjects ($N=75$) (Manuck et al. 2000). Similar relation between prolactin response and impulsiveness was found in another sample of healthy volunteers (Evans et al. 2000). Consistent with those findings, a blunted prolactin response to fenfluramine was detected in patients with major depression and anger attacks (Fava et al. 2000).

However, essentially opposite results of a fenfluramine challenge were reported in 24 male drug abusers (Fishbein et al. 1989b). Prolactin response was maximal in subjects who were particularly impulsive and aggressive. Impulsiveness and aggressiveness were determined by a combination of scales, one of which (the Buss-Durkee) was also used by the group reporting opposite results (Coccaro et al. 1989). It is possible that the substances these patients abused affected their prolactin response. Unfortunately, specific substances abused by these patients were not reported.

Similar to the results of Fishbein et al. (1989b), increasing degrees of aggressive behavior were *positively* correlated with the prolactin response to fenfluramine challenge in a sample of 34 boys (average age, 10 years) who were younger brothers of convicted delinquents (Pine et al. 1997). It appears that the children's age interacts with the relationship between the prolactin response to fenfluramine challenge and aggressiveness: young aggressive boys had a significantly greater prolactin response to fenfluramine than young nonaggressive boys, but that difference could not be detected in an older age group (Halperin et al. 1997). In a study of disruptive boys, prolactin response was largely unrelated to ratings of aggression. Furthermore, age was not associated with prolactin response and had no effect on the relationship between prolactin response and aggression. Thus, this study provided no evidence for a relationship between central 5-HT function and aggression in disruptive boys (Schulz et al. 2001). Similar negative results were reported in adolescents with alcohol use disorder (Soloff et al. 2000).

Furthermore, an *elevated* prolactin response to fenfluramine was found in patients with Alzheimer's disease who were aggressive (Herrmann et al. 1998) or agitated (Mintzer et al. 1998). The reason for this finding is unclear.

If central serotoninergic activity reduces aggressive behavior, then the enhancement of that activity by the administration of fenfluramine should have antiaggressive effects. This hypothesis was tested formally in 10 male parolees with antisocial personality disorder whose aggressive and impulsive responses were measured using the Point Subtraction Aggression Paradigm (PSAP), a laboratory test of aggression (Cherek and Lane 1999). Fenfluramine challenges produced significant dose-dependent decreases in aggressive and impulsive responses.

Taken together, the results of these fenfluramine challenge studies suggest that a hypofunction of the central serotoninergic system, preliminarily localized in the orbitofrontal, ventral medial, and cingulate cortices, may be linked to impulsive aggression. However, this hypofunction could not be demonstrated in all studies, and negative or even opposite results were reported in small samples of children, adult drug abusers, and Alzheimer's disease patients.

Fenfluramine has been withdrawn from the market because of a rare adverse effect; several other agents are used for similar neuroendocrine challenges of the central serotoninergic system. One of them is *m*-chlorophenylpiperazine (m-CPP), a postsynaptic serotonin agonist (and a metabolite of the antidepressant trazodone). Similarly to results of the fenfluramine challenge, serum prolactin levels are elevated after the administration of m-CPP; reduced prolactin response (response blunting) reflects a reduction of serotoninergic function. Fifteen men with the diagnosis of antisocial personality disorder and substance abuse received an m-CPP challenge; so did 12 control subjects (Moss et al. 1990). The results indicated blunting of prolactin response in the antisocial subjects. Psychological assessments suggested that the blunting was associated with assaultiveness and dysphoria but not with impulsivity.

Another challenge method uses prolactin response to buspirone, a 5-HT_{1A} receptor agonist. Prolactin response to buspirone was negatively related to aggressiveness (Coccaro et al. 1990). Thyrotropin-releasing hormone (TRH) stimulates secretion of both thyrotropin and prolactin. Blunted prolactin response to TRH was reported in unipolar patients with anger attacks. The attacks were alleviated and the prolactin response was increased after treatment with fluoxetine, a relatively selective inhibitor of serotonin uptake (Fava et al. 1993; J.F. Rosenbaum et al. 1993).

The origin and the nature of the serotoninergic dysfunction I discussed previously remain to be clarified. The dysfunction may be genetically transmitted. Experiments in rhesus monkeys demonstrated genetic and rearing environmental contributions to the functions of the central serotoninergic system (Higley et al. 1991, 1993) (see Chapter 2). Brain injury may have contributory effects (Van Woerkom et al. 1977). It is possible that the dysfunction is linked to alcohol consumption and to glucose metabolism (see "Insulin" below). However, the exact nature of these relationships is not completely understood.

In summary, CSF 5-HIAA, plasma tryptophan, platelet serotonin uptake, and neuroendocrine challenges suggest that an unspecified central dysfunction of the serotoninergic system is linked to impulsive behavior, and perhaps antisocial behavior. Impulsive aggression and violent suicide are subtypes of such behavior. The dysfunction of the serotoninergic system is relatively stable in the sense that it can be detected long after (or before) any impulsive behavior: it is a trait rather than a state.

These links between the serotoninergic system and aggression have not been confirmed in all populations tested. They may be specific for certain populations (perhaps for alcoholic persons) and for certain subtypes of aggression. Impulsive aggression is not clearly defined. Furthermore, the origins of the serotoninergic dysfunction, as well as its exact nature, remain unknown. It is not clear which serotonin receptor subtypes in which areas of the brain are involved.

Despite these uncertainties, the recent expansion of our knowledge about serotonin and aggression is promising. The trait nature of the serotonin dysfunction could be an advantage for the potential detection of a propensity for impulsive violent behavior and perhaps for the prediction of dangerousness. Furthermore, detailed information about serotonin function in aggression may open the door to the development of specific antiaggression treatments. One of the new avenues for drug discovery is the evolving area of pharmacogenetics that is based on improved understanding of the molecular bases of phenotypic variation.

Molecular Genetic Studies

As shown in the preceding text, serotonin function is related to aggression. Furthermore, aggressive behavior is heritable (see Chapter 5). Thus, genes that code for proteins involved in serotoninergic activity are candidates for roles in the regulation of aggressive behavior. Studies of these genes have become feasible relatively recently, and the results are somewhat preliminary. So far, the studies have focused on the gene coding for tryptophan hydroxylase (TPH), serotonin transporter (5-HTT), and several serotonin receptor subtypes.

TPH is the rate-limiting enzyme in serotonin synthesis. Two bi-allelic polymorphisms have been identified on intron 7 of the TPH gene. By convention, the two alleles in this polymorphism are designated L and U alleles. Although no functional significance has been demonstrated for these polymorphisms, the L allele has been associated with reduced CSF 5-HIAA level and a history of suicide (Nielsen et al. 1998). In male subjects with personality disorders, the LL genotype was associated with higher scores for impulsive aggression on the Buss-Durkee Hostility Inventory (BDHI) (Buss and Durkee 1957; New et al. 1998). A similar trend for an association between the L allele and aggressiveness was found in male patients diagnosed with schizophrenia or schizoaffective disorder (Nolan et al. 2000). However, an opposite association (i.e., with the alternate U allele) was found for aggressiveness in a large sample of healthy subjects (Manuck et al. 1999). Consistent with this association, the prolactin response to fenfluramine challenge was blunted among (male) subjects in this sample having any U allele.

Thus, it is possible that mentally healthy and mentally disordered subjects differ in their association between the TPH polymorphism and aggression. Discrepant results among association studies may be due to confounding effects of population stratification (aggressive and nonaggressive subjects may have been drawn from genetically different groups that coincidentally also differ in the frequencies of L and U alleles). Furthermore, it bears repeating that neither the TPH intron 7 polymorphism, nor any other polymorphism in linkage disequilibrium with it, has any known functional significance. Until such functional significance is demonstrated, reports of behavioral association with the intron 7 polymorphism should be viewed with caution.

The 5-HTT protein mediates presynaptic reuptake of serotonin and thus terminates serotoninergic neurotransmission. The gene that codes for the 5-HTT protein contains a polymorphism with two common alleles differentiated by length. The longer allele is designated L; the short allele, S. This is a functional polymorphism; the L allele has higher transcriptional activity (it produces more 5-HTT protein) than the S allele. An association between this polymorphism and personality traits has been reported (Lesch et al. 1996; Mazzanti et al. 1998), but the finding was not replicated (Gelernter et al. 1998). Rhesus macaques have a homologous 5-HTT polymorphism, and animals with the S allele are persistently aggressive (Higley et al. 2000).

Type 2 (but not type 1) alcoholism is associated with impulsive violent behavior; a serotoninergic dysfunction is probably an underlying mechanism of this disorder (see Chapter 8). The contribution of the 5-HTT polymorphism to that dysfunction was studied in 114 type 1 nonviolent alcoholic individuals, 51 impulsive violent recidivistic offenders with type 2 alcoholism, and 54 healthy control subjects (Hallikainen et al. 1999). All subjects were male. All subjects with alcoholism were examined in a forensic hospital where they were sent after committing a serious impulsive violent offense (41% committed at least one attempted murder). The results are summarized in Table 3–1.

The frequency of S allele was higher among subjects with type 2 alcoholism than among subjects with type 1 alcoholism (χ^2=4.86, P=0.028) and among healthy control subjects (χ^2=8.24, P=0.004). The odds ratio for SS genotype versus LL genotype was 3.90 (95% confidence interval, 1.37–11.11; P=0.011) when subjects with type 2 alcoholism were compared with healthy control subjects. The results indicate that the 5-HTT promoter polymorphism is associated with type 1 alcoholism that involves antisocial personality disorder and impulsive, habitually violent behavior. Like any association study, this one is limited by the possibility of a confounding effect of population stratification. This limitation, however, is mitigated by the fact that all subjects were white Caucasians of Finnish origin—a relatively homogeneous population.

These results obtained in Finnish alcoholic subjects may not generalize to other populations. No association between aggressive behavior and 5-HTT polymorphism was detected in a sample of New York patients with personality disorders (New et al. 2000) or in a New York sample of schizophrenic individuals (Saito et al. 1999).

Table 3–1. Serotonin transporter genotypes and allele frequencies in alcoholics (type 1 and 2) and healthy control subjects

| Group | Genotype | | | Allele | |
	LL	LS	SS	L	S
Type 1 alcoholism (*n*=114)	50 (44%)	37 (32%)	27 (24%)	60%	40%
Type 2 alcoholism (*n*=51)	15 (30%)	18 (35%)	18 (35%)	47%	53%
Control (*n*=54)	26 (48%)	20 (37%)	8 (15%)	67%	33%

Source. Adapted from Hallikainen T, Saito T, Lachman HM, et al.: "Association Between Low Activity Serotonin Transporter Promoter Genotype and Early Onset Alcoholism With Habitual Impulsive Violent Behavior." *Molecular Psychiatry* 4:385–388, 1999. Copyright 1999 by Nature Publishing Group. Used with permission.

The serotonin 1B receptor gene polymorphism (5-HTR1B G861C) was linked to "antisocial alcoholism" (apparently type 2) defined by the co-occurrence of the diagnosis of alcoholism with the diagnoses of antisocial personality disorder or intermittent explosive disorder (Lappalainen et al. 1998). The linkage was demonstrated by family studies in two populations—one in Finland (n=640) and one derived from a Southwestern American Indian tribe (n=418). The allele 5-HTR1B 861C had a higher frequency in the antisocial alcoholic individuals in both populations. This study has many strengths, including a family-based design, replication in two unrelated populations, and a large number of subjects. The study was not designed specifically to study aggression, and the diagnosis of antisocial personality using the DSM-III-R criteria adopted by the authors can be made without evidence of any act of overt physical aggression; the problems with this diagnosis are discussed in Chapter 7. Because of the method of diagnosis, it is not known how many of the antisocial alcoholic subjects committed any violent acts.

In another study, a HTR1B polymorphism was associated with higher impulsive aggression score on the BDHI in New York patients with personality disorders (New et al. 1999). However, it was the 861G allele that was associated with aggression. This result appears inconsistent with the large study discussed above (Lappalainen et al. 1998); of course, the populations and the measures of aggression used in these two studies were different. In any event, the role of this receptor in the inhibitory control of aggression has been demonstrated in 5HTR1B knockout mice (Bouwknecht et al. 2001) (see Chapter 2).

NOREPINEPHRINE

The animal literature on norepinephrine and aggression is somewhat more equivocal than that on serotonin; nevertheless, certain types of stress-related aggression are associated with increased activity of the norepinephrine system (see Chapter 2). Human studies of norepinephrine have been less extensive than the studies of serotonin reviewed above. The norepinephrine and serotonin studies generally used similar methods and were conducted jointly.

CSF Studies

Similar to the relationship between 5-HIAA and central serotoninergic function, the CSF levels of 3-methoxy-4-hydroxyphenylglycol (MHPG), a major central metabolite of norepinephrine, are believed to reflect the presynaptic activity of the central noradrenergic system. The classic human study that first reported a link between decreased CSF 5-HIAA levels and aggression (G.L. Brown et al. 1979) also provided data on CSF MHPG levels. In contrast to the 5-HIAA levels, the MHPG levels were positively correlated with the Brown-Goodwin scale for lifetime aggression. However, the MHPG finding was not replicated in a later study by the same group (G.L. Brown et al. 1982). Furthermore, CSF MHPG levels did not discriminate among homicide offenders, suicide attempters, and healthy control subjects (Lidberg et al. 1985b); the 5-HIAA results from the same study were reviewed in the previous section on serotonin. In another study, CSF MHPG level was positively correlated with the number of property offenses (not violent) in a subgroup of arsonists (Virkkunen et al. 1987). Arsonists and violent offenders had significantly *lower* levels of CSF MHPG than control subjects; these results were similar to those obtained with CSF 5-HIAA in the same study (Virkkunen et al. 1987) (see "Serotonin" above). The results with CSF MHPG levels were less consistent than those obtained with CSF 5-HIAA.

Peripheral Blood Measures and Neuroendocrine Challenges

Plasma norepinephrine is a measure of peripheral presynaptic noradrenergic function, whereas the growth hormone response to clonidine (a centrally acting α_2 agonist) reflects central noradrenergic postsynaptic activity. These two measures were used in the patients who also received (on a different occasion) the fenfluramine challenge (Trestman et al. 1992). The subjects were patients diagnosed with personality disorders. The growth hormone response to clonidine, as well as the peripheral levels of norepinephrine, correlated with measures of irritability but not with assaultiveness (overt aggression). Measures of overt aggression were associated with a blunted prolactin response to fenfluramine.

In summary, two dimensions of behavior in patients with personality disorders may be conceptualized: 1) a general overreactivity to the environment (hyperarousal or irritability) and 2) a more specific inhibitory effect on aggression. In this model, irritability would be mediated through noradrenergic mechanisms, whereas the inhibitory effects would be serotoninergic. It is possible that the noradrenergic system exerts a modulating influence on the relationship between serotoninergic function and overt aggression. There is some support for this notion in the animal literature mentioned in Chapter 2.

MONOAMINE OXIDASE

Metabolic degradation of serotonin, norepinephrine, and many other endogenous and exogenous monoamines involves monoamine oxidase (MAO). This mitochondrial enzyme is present in many human tissues. It exists in at least two forms, designated type A and type B. Both types are present in the brain; type B is in the platelets. Some of the initial impetus for studying platelet MAO activity was provided by its hypothesized links to the activity of central monoamine neurotransmitters such as dopamine—a transmitter believed to be implicated in the pathogenesis of schizophrenia. Low platelet MAO activity is probably associated with low central serotoninergic activity (perhaps due to common genetic control), but this issue has not been completely clarified; the subject was reviewed elsewhere (Schalling et al. 1988).

Low platelet MAO levels were reported in male student volunteers who had a history of psychosocial problems such as psychiatric contacts or convictions for various offenses. Similar psychosocial problems were found among the relatives of the low-MAO subjects (Buchsbaum et al. 1976). These results suggest that low MAO levels mark a vulnerability to psychiatric disorders.

Encouraged by these results, another group studied platelet MAO activity in a mixed group ($N=37$) of criminal offenders (half of them violent) hospitalized for forensic assessments and in two control groups (Lidberg et al. 1985a). The subgroup of psychopathic subjects diagnosed according to Cleckley's (1976) criteria (see Chapter 7) had lower average MAO activity than the other groups; this difference was significant compared with one of the control groups. The authors hypothesized that their results were related to sensation seeking (Zuckerman 1979) and poor impulse control that probably occurred among their psychopathic subjects. Low MAO activity had been described as a biological correlate of sensation seeking (Zuckerman et al. 1980).

Low platelet MAO activity was associated with impulsivity and aggressivity (but not with sensation seeking), all measured by various rating scales, in a sample of healthy adult men (Schalling et al. 1988).

Impulsive assaultive behavior was reported in eight males affected by an X-linked syndrome that included borderline mental retardation (Brunner et al. 1993a, 1993b). Other behaviors among the affected males included arson, attempted rape, attempted suicide, and exhibitionism. All probands were located in one large Dutch kindred. The locus for this disorder was limited to the area on the X chromosome at the locus of MAO type A. Urinalysis performed in three affected males showed marked elevations in MAO substrates and reductions of MAO products. These results are consistent with MAO deficiency. However, the platelet MAO (type B) activity was normal in all three subjects. Taken together, these findings suggest that the violent behavior of the affected males was caused by a deficiency limited to MAO type A. This point mutation in the gene for MAO A is apparently very rare; nevertheless, the observations of its behavioral effects help us understand the general principles of monoaminergic mechanisms regulating aggressive behavior. The observations are paralleled by reports of increased aggression in MAO A knockout male mice (Cases et al. 1995) (see Chapter 2).

An association between polymorphic variation in the gene for MAO A and interindividual variability in aggressiveness, impulsivity, and central nervous system serotoninergic responsivity was studied in a community sample of 110 men (Manuck et al. 2000). Four variants of the MAO A gene that differ in length and transcriptional activity were genotyped. In the analyses, the two variants with the higher transcriptional activity (alleles 2 and 3) were combined and contrasted with the variants that possess lower transcriptional activity (alleles 1 and 4). All participants had completed standard interview and questionnaire measures of impulsivity, hostility, and lifetime aggression history; 75 subjects received a fenfluramine challenge. Men in the 1/4 allele group (producing less MAO A) scored significantly lower on a composite measure of aggressiveness and impulsivity and showed a higher prolactin response to fenfluramine than men in the 2/3 allele group (producing more MAO A). The co-occurrence of low aggressivity and high prolactin response is consistent with other reports (see section on neuroendocrine challenges in this chapter). However, the association between high MAO A and aggression seems inconsistent with the aggressive behavior observed in the Dutch kindred with MAO A mutation described above (Brunner et al. 1993a, 1993b). It is possible that the mutation affected the neurodevelopment and caused the central serotoninergic system to be abnormal, rendering meaningless any comparison with healthy subjects examined by Manuck and colleagues (2000).

CATECHOL *O*-METHYLTRANSFERASE

Catechol *O*-methyltransferase (COMT) inactivates catecholamines and catechol-containing drugs by catalyzing *S*-adenosyl-L-methionine–dependent methyl conjugation (Axelrod and Tomchick 1958). A common polymorphism in the COMT gene results in a valine to methionine substitution at codon 158. This polymorphism is associated with three- to fourfold differences in the COMT activity between homozygous subjects; heterozygotes have intermediate levels of activity (Lachman et al. 1996). Specifically, the methionine allele results in lower COMT activity.

Interest in the COMT gene as a candidate for a role in mental illness has been kindled by studies of the velocardiofacial (VCF) syndrome (also called Shprintzen's syndrome), a congenital disorder that results in typical facial appearance, cleft palate, cardiac defects, learning disabilities (Shprintzen et al. 1978), and various other mental disorders (Chow et al. 1994; Goldberg et al. 1993; Papolos et al. 1996; Pulver et al. 1994; Shprintzen et al. 1992). Approximately 80%–85% of patients with VCF syndrome have an interstitial deletion on chromosome 22q11 (Morrow et al. 1995). The COMT gene maps to this region; it is deleted in most, if not all, patients with deletional forms of VCF syndrome; and it has been suggested to be a source of the psychiatric manifestations of the illness (Chow et al. 1994).

Subsequent research indicated that COMT polymorphism may be associated with ultrarapid cycling in bipolar disorder (Lachman et al. 1996; Papolos et al. 1998), type 1 alcoholism (Tiihonen et al. 1999) and alcohol consumption among social drinkers (Kauhanen et al. 2000), and obsessive-compulsive disorder (Karayiorgou et al. 1999). Schizophrenia may be related to the COMT polymorphism; the valine allele slightly increased risk for schizophrenia in some family-based studies (Egan et al. 2001; Kunugi et al. 1997; Li et al. 1996), although this was not found in another family-based study (Wei and Hemmings 1999) or in a case-control study (Chen et al. 1999). It appears that the COMT gene polymorphism may have pleiotropic effects (resulting in a variety of phenotypes) on susceptibility and symptomatology of neuropsychiatric disorders.

The COMT polymorphism was reported to be related to cognitive performance and the frontal lobe function (Egan et al. 2001). Specifically, the methionine allele was associated with fewer perseverative errors on the Wisconsin Card Sorting Test, and with lower activation of the dorsolateral prefrontal cortex during a working memory test, than the valine allele. Lower activation (assessed by functional magnetic resonance imaging) was presumed to be a sign of greater functional efficiency. These differences were seen in schizophrenic patients as well as in healthy subjects.

Persistent aggressive behavior is one of the phenotypes that received recent attention. During one of the studies that tested an association between COMT polymorphism and schizophrenia (Strous et al. 1997b), a serendipitous observation was made: the polymorphism, although apparently unrelated to schizophrenia, appeared to be associated with aggressive and antisocial behavior (Strous et al. 1997a). It was the methionine allele (coding for the lower activity of the enzyme) that was observed more frequently in the aggressive patients. This association was replicated in another sample of patients diagnosed with schizophrenia or schizoaffective disorder (Lachman et al. 1998). That study compared patients with a history of multiple assaults with those who had no history of assault. The association appeared to be more clearly expressed in males (Lachman et al. 1998). The patient samples in these two studies (Lachman et al. 1998; Strous et al. 1997a) were collected in the New York metropolitan area; they were ethnically heterogeneous, and the possibility of population stratification confounding the results of these two small association studies has been acknowledged. However, more recently, the methionine allele was also found to be associated with homicidal behavior in schizophrenic (mostly male) patients in Israel (Kotler et al. 1999) and with aggressivity (assessed by the BDHI) in Italian patients with bipolar disorder (Rotondo et al. 1999). Thus, the association between COMT polymorphism and aggression was observed in four association studies using three different human populations, and the ability to generalize from these observations has received some support from the studies of aggressive behavior in COMT knockout mice (Gogos et al. 1998) (see Chapter 2). Interestingly, mice and men showed the same sexual dimorphism—the effect on aggression was more expressed in males.

However, the association between the methionine allele and aggression was not replicated in a large sample of schizophrenia patients in Wales (G. Jones et al. 2001). Unlike some of the positive studies discussed above (Kotler et al. 1999; Lachman et al. 1998), the Welsh patients were not selected for violence.

Thus, provided that the findings reviewed above can be replicated, it appears that the methionine allele is associated with persistent and/or serious aggression in mentally ill subjects, and also with fewer perseverative errors in both mentally ill and healthy subjects, and with lower risk for schizophrenia. Better cognitive performance, better prefrontal functioning, and low risk for schizophrenia can be seen as logically interconnected. However, why is the same allele that is associated with these beneficial features also associated with aggression? To consider this apparent contradiction, one should first realize that some of the patients participating in the studies of aggressive behavior were selected because they showed a lot of it. Persistently aggressive schizophrenic patients differ from their more serene counterparts in many respects, including diffuse neurological impairments (see Chapters 4 and 10). Is it possible that an ability to respond quickly to changed environment, manifested as reduced perseveration in neurologically intact patients, may be transformed into impulsiveness in patients with neurological impairments? Is performance on the Wisconsin Card Sorting Test related to impulsiveness in mentally ill patients, and do aggressive and nonaggressive patients differ in this respect? How does the COMT genotype interact with these relationships? Ongoing research is addressing these and similar questions.

Other transmitters and receptors are discussed in Chapter 11.

HORMONES AND VIOLENCE

Insulin

Hypoglycemia may elicit irritability, aggression, confusion, amnesia, seizures, and eventually unconsciousness. These clinical signs and symptoms are accompanied by electroencephalographic diffuse slowing, sometimes escalating into paroxysmal activity (Dawson and Greville 1963). Hypoglycemic aggression with amnesia may be elicited via an epileptiform mechanism, but the evidence is anecdotal. Fasting hypoglycemia with attendant transitory electroencephalographic epileptiform abnormality was used successfully as a defense in a landmark murder case (Hill and Sargant 1943) (see "Qualitative Assessment of Resting Electroencephalograms" in Chapter 4), and court cases where (postprandial) hypoglycemia was used as a successful defense are still occasionally reported (Brahams 1991). As the popular information and misinformation about postprandial hypoglycemia spread in the United States, lawyers sometimes attempted to use hypoglycemia as a legal defense in situations that do not warrant it (the "Twinkie defense"). The syndrome of violent behavior, electroencephalographic abnormality, and a dysfunction of glucose metabolism received attention in the 1970s (Yaryura-Tobias and Neziroglu 1975), but not much systematic research was done until the 1980s.

Most of the experimental work exploring the role of insulin and glucose in aggression is based on the glucose tolerance test. Fasting subjects are fed a load of glucose (1 g/kg) (Virkkunen and Huttunen 1982). Blood samples are drawn before and then hourly for 5 hours after the glucose ingestion. Insulin is normally secreted in response to the glucose load, and after an initial increase, the blood glucose level decreases below its original fasting level. The lowest level of glucose (glucose nadir) is the principal measure used by researchers in aggression studies. About 50% of the nadirs measured in such studies (which use physically healthy young males as experimental subjects in most cases) are typically within normal limits recognized for clinical purposes by internists.

An anthropologist studying a remote tribal group of native South Americans managed to administer a version of the glucose tolerance test to his subjects and reported what he thought was postprandial hypoglycemia in particularly aggressive group members (Bolton 1976). Hypoglycemia was related not only to overt aggression but also to hostile attitudes and fantasies of these tribespeople. Much of the subsequent work has been done by the same Finnish-American team of researchers that distinguished itself in work on serotonin and aggression (see "Serotonin" above). Habitually violent Finnish offenders with intermittent explosive personality disorder had a significantly lower glucose nadir in the glucose tolerance test than did control subjects. There were also some differences between these groups in the pattern of insulin secretion (Virkkunen 1986a). Hypoglycemia within a group of habitually violent offenders ($N=68$) was associated with reports of aggression under the influence of alcohol, loss of memory of violence, and the father's criminality (Virkkunen 1986b). Similar associations were observed among arsonists (Virkkunen et al. 1987). As mentioned above (see "Serotonin" above), a low glucose nadir predicted recidivistic offending in violent offenders and impulsive fire setters (Virkkunen et al. 1989b), but this result was not replicated in a larger group of similar subjects (DeJong et al. 1992).

A relationship between the glucose nadir and violent crime and impulsivity was not replicated in drug abusers recently admitted for treatment (Fishbein et al. 1992). Perhaps the recently ingested drugs interfered with the glucose tolerance test, obscuring the expected relationship.

In summary, relationships exist among hypoglycemia, violence, and impulsiveness. The relationships are not equally expressed in all types of subjects and in all violent behavior. To better specify these variables, additional studies are needed.

Testosterone and Other Androgens

Many animal studies implicate androgens in aggression (see Chapter 2). These studies demonstrated that levels of circulating androgens are related to measures of aggression in adult animals (activational effects); they also provided evidence for effects of the early (intrauterine) hormone environment (organizational effects). Furthermore, testosterone may enhance the effects of alcohol on aggression in animals. The main topics are the activational and organizational effects of androgens and the effects of antiandrogens.

The activational effects were first studied in relative isolation from other biological variables; some of the later studies addressed these effects in the context of genetic or pharmacologic variables. The typical early design involved a group of aggressive subjects (usually offenders, sometimes sex offenders) and nonaggressive or low-aggressive control subjects. Plasma or saliva levels of testosterone (and sometimes other androgens) were expected to differentiate between the high- and low-aggressiveness groups; the highly aggressive subjects were usually violent criminal offenders selected from a group of prisoners.

Another approach has been to study "normal" subjects (not selected for aggressiveness) and relate their androgen levels to some measures of aggressive attitudes or behaviors. This type of research focused on correlations between current androgen levels and past or present aggressiveness; mediating psychological (but not biological) variables were sometimes considered.

Other research relating androgens to aggression did consider other biological variables. Some studies focused on genetic factors (such as the XYY genotype). Similarly to animal work, interactions among alcohol, testosterone, and aggression have been studied.

The organizational effects were addressed by numerous studies focusing on the consequences of the intrauterine hormone environment for aggressive behavior.

The antiaggressive effects of antiandrogens constitute another (indirect) approach to the study of the role of androgens in aggression. Such effects have been reported in sex offenders and other subjects. Antiandrogens are discussed in Chapter 11.

Activational Effects of Androgens

Subjects Selected for Violent Behavior

Several studies used male prisoners. One study (Kreuz and Rose 1972) found no relationship between plasma testosterone levels and current assaultiveness or the aggressiveness measured by paper-and-pencil tests, including the BDHI, but prisoners who had a history of violent crime committed in adolescence ($n=10$) had higher levels of testosterone at the time of the study (when their average age was 28 years) than the prisoners without such a history ($n=11$). This result was interpreted to indicate a permissive role of testosterone in aggressive behavior during adolescence. There are at least two problems with this interpretation. First, it is not known whether testosterone levels in adolescence were related to those prevailing a decade or so later. Second, the authors chose to classify all escapes from institutions as "aggressive or violent crimes."

This error has distorted their results to an extent that cannot be estimated from their published data. The error also illustrates the importance of proper definitions of dependent variables (measures of aggression and violence) discussed in Chapter 1.

In another study, the testosterone plasma levels of aggressive prisoners ($n=12$) were found to be almost twice as high as those of nonaggressive prisoner control subjects ($n=12$) (Ehrenkranz et al. 1974). The aggressive prisoners were selected because they were imprisoned for violent crimes such as aggravated assault or murder; most continued to be physically aggressive in prison. Scores on psychological rating scales (including the BDHI) were unrelated to testosterone levels. Another study (Bain et al. 1987) failed to confirm differences in androgen levels among forensic patients charged with murder ($n=13$), assault or attempted murder ($n=14$), and property offenses ($n=14$).

Limited information on testosterone levels and their relation to aggression among sex offenders is available. The particularly violent rapists ($n=5$) who inflicted additional physical injury on the victims (e.g., beating the victim during the rape) had higher testosterone levels than the other rapists ($n=47$) and than child molesters ($n=12$) (Rada et al. 1976). This finding was not replicated in another sample of rapists (Rada et al. 1983). Ratings on the BDHI were unrelated to testosterone plasma levels in these sex offenders.

Sadistic sex offenders ($n=20$), nonsadistic sex offenders ($n=14$), and presumably nonviolent prisoner control subjects ($n=15$) were compared on plasma levels of androstenedione, testosterone, sex hormone–binding globulin, free-androgen index, proportion of free testosterone, and several other hormones. This very extensive battery of hormonal assays showed no differences among the groups (Bain et al. 1988).

Repeated samples of plasma testosterone were obtained in male adolescent delinquents ($n=40$) and in control subjects ($n=58$) (Mattsson et al. 1980). The delinquents were classified into several groups according to the degree of violence of their current offense ("instant" offense; see Chapter 1). Several personality inventory scales were administered. Multiple univariate tests were performed to study relationships between personality inventory items and testosterone levels; several statistically significant results of doubtful importance emerged.

Furthermore, the delinquents tended to have higher testosterone levels than the control subjects, and the violent offenders tended to have higher testosterone levels than the nonviolent ones. These results can be interpreted to provide limited support for the early findings concerning the history of adolescent crime discussed above (Kreuz and Rose 1972).

The studies discussed so far used blood assays of testosterone. This method has certain disadvantages. Approximately 98% of the testosterone in the serum is protein bound in a biologically inactive form. Blood sampling is inconvenient. Saliva is easier to collect than blood, and only free testosterone enters the saliva because the large binding molecules do not easily pass through salivary gland cells (Dabbs et al. 1987, p. 174). The ease of saliva collection made it possible to examine the relationship between (free) testosterone and criminal violence in a relatively large sample (*N*=89) of prisoners (Dabbs et al. 1987). The prisoners were divided into two groups (violent versus nonviolent) according to the current offense. The violent group had a slightly higher average level of testosterone; the difference reached the level of statistical significance. The differences between the types of crime committed were maximal at the extremes of the testosterone distribution. Testosterone levels also appeared to be related to behavior in prison; however, these relationships were doubtful because they were detected with multiple univariate tests.

Testosterone levels were measured in saliva in 692 adult male prisoners (Dabbs and Hargrove 1997; Dabbs et al. 1995). Inmates with high testosterone levels were more likely to commit violent crimes in the community and to violate prison rules (particularly the rules involving overt confrontation) than the low-testosterone inmates. The average age of the prisoners was 19.8 years (SD=2.6); the results may not generalize to older populations.

Testosterone is secreted in a pulsatile pattern; thus, assays of this hormone in peripheral blood yield inherently variable results. The testosterone level in the CSF is relatively independent from these fluctuations. Furthermore, free testosterone in the CSF reflects the hormone levels that are directly available at the brain sites. For these reasons, free testosterone in the CSF was measured in a sample of 31 impulsive offenders, 13 nonimpulsive offenders, and 19 control subjects (Virkkunen et al. 1994). The offenders had a history of alcoholism. The offenses were either violent crimes against persons or arson. Among the 31 impulsive offenders, 17 were diagnosed with antisocial personality disorder and 14 with explosive personality disorder. The antisocial subgroup had a higher level of free testosterone than the other subgroups (significantly so in comparison with the control subjects).

Furthermore, CSF testosterone levels were used in a discriminant analysis classifying the subjects as offenders or nonoffender control subjects (Virkkunen et al. 1994). With this procedure, 60% of the subjects were correctly classified, with the offenders showing higher CSF testosterone levels than the control subjects. Arsonists were excluded from the offender group; thus, only the violent offenders were used in the discriminant analysis. The authors interpreted the result of the discriminant analysis as an indication that the high CSF testosterone concentrations were associated with aggressiveness or interpersonal violence. This interpretation is plausible, and it fits with much of the evidence reviewed in this chapter and in Chapter 2. However, it should be noted that aggressiveness was not the only feature differentiating the offender and nonoffender groups. For example, only the offenders were alcoholic. Thus, alternative explanations of the discriminant analysis result are possible.

Testosterone is secreted by the ovaries and the adrenal cortex in *females,* and its levels in females, although lower than those in males, may be related to aggressiveness. This hypothesis was tested in female prisoners, and testosterone levels in saliva were indeed elevated in females whose current offense was an *unprovoked* violent crime, but not in females who had committed a defensive violent crime (e.g., abused women who killed their abusers) (Dabbs et al. 1988). A small study involving violent female neuropsychiatric outpatients demonstrated elevated plasma levels of testosterone compared with those in nonviolent control subjects (Ehlers et al. 1980).

Another study examined how testosterone levels, both alone and interacting with age, were associated with criminal behavior and institutional behavior among 87 female prison inmates. Violent crime was scored from court records. Aggressive institutional behavior was assessed using prison records and interviews with staff members. Testosterone levels were assayed in saliva samples. There were relationships among age, testosterone, criminal behavior, and institutional behavior. Structural equation analysis suggested a causal model in which age leads to lower testosterone, which in turn leads to less violent crime and less aggressive dominance in prison (Dabbs and Hargrove 1997).

In summary, these studies suggest that a history of violent behavior (e.g., violent crime) is associated with a slight but relatively consistent elevation of testosterone levels. This association is probably stronger during adolescence and young adulthood than it is in later life. Correlations between testosterone levels and behavior in prison appeared less consistent, and the correlations with personality inventories were generally weak.

"Normal" Subjects (Not Selected for Violent Behavior)

Adults. The classic study in this area (Persky et al. 1971) used healthy young men ($n=18$), healthy older men ($n=15$), and—somewhat incongruously—hospitalized dysphoric male patients ($n=6$). In addition to the routine plasma testosterone levels, the testosterone production rate was determined. This method called for a priming dose and then an hour-long constant-rate intravenous infusion of radiolabeled testosterone; repeated samples of venous blood were required to determine the metabolic clearance rate of testosterone that was needed to compute the production rate. Several self-administered psychological inventories, including the BDHI (Buss and Durkee 1957), were completed. No measures of overt aggression were available. The testosterone production rates (and, to a slightly lesser extent, the plasma testosterone levels) were strongly and positively related to the BDHI in the younger, but not in the older, group of healthy subjects. Not surprisingly, the testosterone production rate decreased with age.

Attempts to replicate these findings (Persky et al. 1971) yielded mixed results. The negative studies either used a small number of subjects and included determination of the testosterone production rates (Meyer-Bahlburg et al. 1974) or used only the plasma testosterone levels but had large subject samples (Dotson et al. 1975; Monti et al. 1977). Additional negative studies were reviewed elsewhere (Archer 1991).

Several positive studies were reported. Free testosterone was assayed in the saliva and total testosterone and 5α-dihydrotestosterone were determined in the blood of 117 young healthy males who were given a battery of paper-and-pencil tests to measure various aspects of aggressiveness (Christiansen and Knussmann 1987). Numerous (Spearman) correlation coefficients between psychological indices and hormonal values were computed. Those that were statistically significant were clustered around 0.20; the highest one was 0.29. These results indicated a weak positive relationship between androgen levels and some measures of aggressiveness (Christiansen and Knussmann 1987).

In a study of healthy young adults, males ($n=40$) and females ($n=32$) were given an inventory measuring aggressiveness. The inventory, similar to the one used in a study of adolescents discussed below (Olweus et al. 1988), focused on aggressive responses to provocation or threat. Blood samples were assayed for free and total testosterone and for estradiol (Malone et al. 1995). Total testosterone showed the expected (weak) positive relationship to aggressiveness in the males, but there was an unexpected negative relationship in the females. Unexpectedly, estradiol levels correlated with aggressiveness in a pattern similar to that of total testosterone. Approximately 50% of the subjects in this study were homosexual; the effect of sexual preference on relationships among hormones, aggressiveness, and gender was apparently not tested.

Interest in the long-term effects of the administration of testosterone has been kindled by the widespread illicit use of anabolic-androgenic steroids (including testosterone synthetic analogs) for the purpose of improving athletic performance or personal appearance; increased irritability and violent behavior have been recognized as unwanted effects of these substances (see Chapter 8). Several controlled experiments in healthy male volunteers studied the effects of testosterone administration on mood and aggression. Two of these studies used supraphysiological doses (600 mg/week) of testosterone for 6 weeks (Pope et al. 2000) or 10 weeks (Tricker et al. 1996); both studies were placebo controlled and generally well designed. Neither study found effects on angry or aggressive attitudes or behaviors. However, 8 of the 50 subjects became hypomanic in the 6-week study (Pope et al. 2000).

Adolescents.   Normal boys ($N=58$, average age, 16 years) were given a large array of personality inventories and rating scales assessing aggressiveness, impulsiveness, frustration tolerance, anxiety, and extraversion (Olweus et al. 1980). Plasma testosterone levels were associated with self-reports of verbal and physical aggression, particularly the aggression elicited by threats and provocation. Path analysis of the same data suggested that the effects of high levels of testosterone on aggressive responses to threat and provocation were mediated by low frustration tolerance (Olweus et al. 1988).

Relationships between blood levels of eight compounds (luteinizing hormone, follicle-stimulating hormone, testosterone, estradiol, testosterone-estradiol–binding globulin, dehydroepiandrosterone, dehydroepiandrosterone sulfate, and androstenedione) and multiple measures of aggressiveness and other traits were explored in a sample of healthy boys ($n=56$) and girls ($n=52$) (Susman et al. 1987). Multiple zero-order correlation coefficients were obtained. Furthermore, multiple regression equations were computed by use of the eight hormonal levels (plus one derived hormonal measure) as independent variables. The authors' interpretation of their results was that "hormonal levels were related to emotional dispositions and aggressive attributes for boys but not for girls" (p. 1114). The results are complex. It appears that testosterone alone was not related to any measure of aggression. The univariate measures are difficult to interpret because so many were obtained, and the meaning of the multiple regression equations is unclear. The hormone levels used as independent variables in the equations have multiple and complex mutual relationships; these relationships obscure rather than explain the dependent variables.

In summary, studies of androgens in healthy subjects who were not selected for violent behavior yielded inconsistent results. Several reports suggested that a weak relationship may exist between androgen levels and aggressiveness as measured by various paper-and-pencil tests. That relationship may be stronger for the aggressive response to provocation or threat.

XYY and XXY. Links between the Y chromosome, testosterone, and aggression in animals may exist (see Chapter 2). Early observations of several aggressive XYY men inspired a hypothesis that the extra Y chromosome causes increased aggressiveness and that this effect is mediated by increased testosterone secretion. This hypothesis has generated a considerable amount of controversial research.

XYY men were found among institutionalized and delinquent subjects, and several men who committed serious violent crimes were reported to have an extra Y chromosome. These reports, reviewed extensively elsewhere (Owen 1972), led to speculations that an extra Y chromosome conveys an extra dose of masculine aggression. XYY men are generally taller than average, and their height was thought to contribute to their supposed aggressiveness.

Reports linking the XYY genotype to aggression had several weaknesses. The selection of subjects was biased, favoring biological and psychological deviance. Many studies failed to include normal (XY) control subjects. Prevalence of the XYY genotype in the general adult population was not known; therefore, the prevalence data in institutionalized men could not be properly interpreted.

The landmark study (Witkin et al. 1976) identified men representing the top 16% of the height distribution of a Danish birth cohort. Sex chromosome determinations were performed in 4,139 of these tall men; 12 XYYs and 16 XXYs were identified. The remaining men had the normal XY genotype and served as control subjects. Official records of criminal convictions, as well as the results of the intelligence test used by the Danish army to screen recruits, were available to the researchers. The results indicated that the XYY men did have an increased property (nonviolent) crime rate. Their intelligence was low compared with that of the XY control subjects. The crime rates and intelligence test results in XXY males were similar to those in the XYY subsample. This study of official records of XYY and XXY men suggested that low intelligence may be the mediating variable between the extra sex chromosome, breaking a law, and getting arrested. In other words, low intelligence not only increases the likelihood of breaking a law but also reduces the chances of success in evading punishment. For example, one of the arrests occurred after an XYY subject illegally started a fire alarm and then waited around to enjoy the sight of the fire trucks.

In addition to accessing the official Danish records of criminal convictions in all subjects, the researchers examined in detail the XYY and

XXY subjects as well as a subset of matched XY control subjects. These examinations included interviews, hormone blood level assays, and electroencephalograms (EEGs).

There was a significant positive relationship between testosterone levels and criminal convictions among all subjects, including the XY control subjects. During the interviews, the XYY men reported more physical aggression toward their wives than did the XY control subjects (Schiavi et al. 1984). Testosterone levels were not related to these self-reports.

The XYY subjects showed a significant slowing of the average frequency of their electroencephalographic resting alpha activity (Volavka et al. 1977a, 1977b) as well as a reduction of their electroencephalographic response to sine wave light modulated at 10- and 20-Hz frequencies (Volavka et al. 1979). These electroencephalographic findings were interpreted as signs of developmental lag or reduced arousal in the XYY subjects. This sample was too small for a meaningful test of electroencephalographic relationships to crime or violent behavior. However, in other populations, electroencephalographic slowing was an antecedent of property crime (Mednick et al. 1981; Petersen et al. 1982), and it was found in violent offenders (see "Quantitative Assessment of Resting Electroencephalograms" in Chapter 4).

Although the criminal behavior in the XYY Danish men did not appear to be mediated by testosterone (Schiavi et al. 1984), in another report (Blumer and Migeon 1975) improvements in aggressive behavior were described after antiandrogen treatment was administered to four XYY subjects.

In summary, XYY and XXY men are somewhat more likely to be convicted of nonviolent (mostly property) crimes than their XY counterparts. More XYY men than XY control subjects reported that they were physically aggressive toward their wives; their EEGs showed nonspecific features associated with criminal behavior in other populations. The prevalence of the XYY and XXY genotypes is too low for any practical impact on population crime rates.

Alcohol, Testosterone, and Aggression

Testosterone may enhance the effects of alcohol on aggression in animals (see Chapter 2). Several studies addressed this issue in humans. Social drinkers (Dotson et al. 1975) and alcoholic persons (J.H. Mendelson and Mello 1974) were given alcohol; various measures of aggression were taken concurrently with blood sampling for levels of alcohol and testosterone. Alcohol decreased plasma levels of testosterone and increased aggression, but neither the prealcohol levels of testosterone nor their postalcohol suppression was related to the measures of aggression. Thus, these experiments did not support the hypothesis that high levels of testosterone enhance the alcohol-related increase of aggression in humans.

Critique of Activational Effect Studies

The basic assumption behind activational studies is that androgens exert a controlling or modifying effect on aggression. However, the opposite may also be true. The experience of fighting and winning may elevate testosterone levels in animals; the levels are linked to dominance in groups of nonhuman primates (see Chapter 2). Victorious tennis players have elevations in testosterone levels after the match (Mazur and Lamb 1980); additional human studies of this type were reviewed elsewhere (Mazur 1983). Thus, an elevated *testosterone level may be a consequence or a cause of fighting.*

Most of the activational studies used a single sample of plasma for the determination of androgen levels. However, testosterone levels vary across time; *a single specimen is not a reliable reflection of these levels* (Archer 1991).

The measures of aggression used in many studies have questionable validity and reliability. Furthermore, it is not always clear whether they address trait, state, or both. The measures vary widely among studies, making the results difficult to compare. The BDHI was the instrument used in some studies, which has enabled a partial meta-analysis (Archer 1991). It appears that relatively simple measures of aggression based on reliable reports of overt violent behavior (such as crime) are more robustly related to hormonal levels than self-reported scales and inventories. In any event, the *measure of aggression* is usually one of the weaker points in the activational studies.

Finally, these studies generally use many variables but small numbers of subjects. Power analysis is generally not used. The data are usually analyzed by many univariate tests without any correction for test multiplicity. These *errors in experimental design and statistical analyses* render the results difficult to interpret.

Organizational Effects of Androgens

Androgens have organizational effects on the brain during fetal development. These effects have long-term consequences for sexual and aggressive behavior (see "Prenatal Exposure to Androgens" in Chapter 2).

In humans, these organizational effects can be studied by detecting long-term behavioral consequences of excessive fetal exposure to androgens. Two conditions—endocrinopathies such as the adrenogenital syndrome and exposure to hormones with androgenic effects administered to mothers during pregnancy—provide opportunities for such studies.

Adrenogenital Syndrome

Adrenogenital syndrome is usually congenital; the fetus is exposed to excessive amounts of androgen generated in its adrenal gland due to a genetically transmitted metabolic defect. In the female fetus, this androgen exposure results in female pseudohermaphroditism: internal genitalia remain female (unaffected), whereas external genitalia show varying degrees of ambiguity. Surgical adjustment of the external genitalia and long-term cortisone treatment make it possible for these patients to grow up and reproduce as essentially normal females.

On the basis of the animal literature (see Chapter 2), girls with adrenogenital syndrome would be expected to be more aggressive than other girls because of their early exposure to androgen. This was found not to be the case; these girls were not any more likely to start physical fights than control subjects. However, they tended to play and dress like boys (Ehrhardt et al. 1968; Money and Ehrhardt 1972). Boys with adrenogenital syndrome tended to initiate fights more frequently than sibling control subjects (Ehrhardt and Baker 1974).

Prenatal Exposure to Synthetic Hormonal Preparations

Prenatal exposure to synthetic hormonal preparations that used to be prescribed for threatened abortion may lead to the masculinization of female fetuses because of the androgenic effects of these compounds. Females ($n=17$) and males ($n=8$) exposed to progestin in utero were compared with their unexposed sex-matched siblings on a paper-and-pencil test designed to assess the potential for aggressive behavior. The subjects were 6–18 years old at the time of testing. As predicted, the exposed subjects (both females and males) scored higher on this test than the control subjects (Reinisch 1981). Behavioral observations of aggression were not a part of this study.

Effects of prenatal exposure to diethylstilbestrol were tested in adolescent and adult women ($N=30$) compared with unexposed matched control subjects (Ehrhardt et al. 1989). Questionnaires and interviews with the women and their mothers failed to find differences in verbal and physical aggressiveness and in delinquency between the groups. Prenatal exposure to medroxyprogesterone acetate, a compound with antiandrogen effects, was associated with reduced aggressiveness in 11-year-old boys and girls; the antiaggressive effects appeared weak and difficult to interpret in view of the multiple univariate tests performed (Meyer-Bahlburg and Ehrhardt 1982).

In summary, the human studies of the effects of the intrauterine hormone environment on aggression are much less conclusive than the studies in animals. That is not surprising, because most of the experimental observations in animals cannot be directly replicated in humans for practical and ethical reasons and because the determinants of aggressive behavior in humans are more complex than they are in animals. Human studies varied in the types and amounts of hormones to which the fetuses were exposed, in the timing of the exposure, and in the outcome variables. However, it should be noted that the study that showed positive results (Reinisch 1981) was well designed and documented. Because it is now known that the estrogen and progestin treatments during pregnancy had various deleterious effects on the offspring, this study cannot be replicated.

PREMENSTRUAL SYNDROME

Unusual behaviors during menstruation have been observed for many centuries (Ellis and Austin 1971). In the 1930s, literature on "premenstrual tension" began to appear (Frank 1931). This overly narrow term was later replaced by premenstrual syndrome (PMS) because tension is only one of the many manifestations of this disorder (Dalton 1964). The syndrome, however, is not necessarily premenstrual: it extends into early menstruation, and it may occur in women who do not menstruate (e.g., after hysterectomy). The term *premenstrual dysphoric disorder* (American Psychiatric Association 2000) is better defined, but it has not yet replaced the widely used term *PMS*.

The syndrome includes marked affective lability, anger or irritability, anxiety and tension, depression, loss of interest, lack of energy, difficulty in concentrating, changed food intake, changed sleep patterns, breast tenderness or swelling, headaches, joint or muscle pain, feeling of bloating, and weight gain (American Psychiatric Association 2000). Many other physical changes are associated with this syndrome (Dalton 1964); these changes include hypoglycemia, which may account for irritability and perhaps for some of the impulsive or violent behaviors reported to occur in conjunction with PMS. Glucose tolerance tests were performed in a limited number of subjects with PMS, and particularly low nadirs of glucose levels were detected in some of them (Morton et al. 1953). However, another study indicated that the hypoglycemic changes in the patients with PMS were unrelated to any particular phase of their menstrual cycle and that the changes did not co-occur with PMS symptoms (Denicoff et al. 1990).

Multiple hormones are implicated in PMS; its pathophysiology is incompletely understood (Gitlin and Pasnau 1989). Several separate subsyndromes may emerge as the understanding of the underlying mechanisms improves. It would be simplistic to assume a unidirectional relationship between hormones and mental status; abundant evidence in many mammalian species indicates that hormonal secretion is influenced by social and psychological factors and vice versa. Furthermore, PMS has a psychological component that has been experimentally separated from the hormonal status: women who were led to believe that they were premenstrual reported a higher degree of premenstrual-like symptoms than did women who were led to believe that they were intermenstrual (Ruble 1977). Some of the old PMS literature was scientifically inadequate and sexist, implying female inferiority (e.g., Cooke 1945). Unfortunately, such literature has been widely cited. Concerns about possible sexist implications of a mental disorder limited to females led to heated discussions about the very legitimacy of PMS. The fact that PMS is vaguely defined and poorly understood provided additional fuel for such discussions (Hamilton and Gallant 1990).

Premenstrual Syndrome and Crime

Research on PMS and crime usually involves prisoners who are asked at which phase of their menstrual cycle they committed the current ("instant") offense. These data suggest that women commit crimes (*for which they are arrested*) at significantly higher frequencies during premenstrual and menstrual periods than during other parts of their menstrual cycle. This distribution applies to violent crimes (d'Orban and Dalton 1980; Morton et al. 1953) as well as to theft (Dalton 1961). These results do not necessarily imply an uneven distribution of the criminal acts; they may imply an uneven distribution of the probability of apprehension. Depression and lethargy (regular components of PMS) may reduce the capability or motivation of the perpetrators to avoid arrest.

These studies are weakened by their reliance on retrospective self-reports regarding menstrual cycles. The reliability of such self-reports is not known. The suggestibility of PMS discussed above (Ruble 1977) adds concerns about such self-reports.

Nevertheless, these consistent reports (Dalton 1961; d'Orban and

Dalton 1980; Morton et al. 1953), compatible with some anecdotal evidence (Dalton 1975, 1980) and with a considerable amount of older literature cited elsewhere (d'Orban and Dalton 1980; Vanezis 1991), do suggest a connection between the menstrual cycle and crime. It is possible that regular PMS sufferers are more likely to commit crimes than the women who never have that syndrome. That, however, is not clear. The available literature rather implies that women who participate in criminal activity (or in noncriminal violence) are more likely to act during the paramenstrual part of their cycle than at other times.

Despite these doubts, PMS has been used with some success as a defense in criminal cases in Britain (Brahams 1981; Dalton 1980) and in the United States (Sadoff 1988).

Premenstrual Syndrome and Behavior in Institutionalized Women

Girls at a boarding school were found to be more "naughty" during premenstrual and menstrual parts of their cycles than at other times (Dalton 1964, pp. 77–83). No such cyclicity was found in the pattern of boys' infractions. Interestingly, the punishments meted out by the girls' supervisors showed a similar dependence on the supervisors' menstrual cycles: most punishment was given when the *supervisor* was menstruating (Dalton 1964, pp. 77–78). I am not aware of any attempt to replicate these data on punitive supervisors.

Overt aggressive behavior, including physical and verbal attacks, was rated in 45 female prisoners by correction officers unaware of the prisoners' menstrual phase (Ellis and Austin 1971). This behavior was rated over three menstrual cycles. There was an excess of aggressive behavior during the premenstrual and early menstrual phases of the cycle. Somewhat similar results were reported by others (Hands et al. 1974). Compared with the retrospective studies of crime discussed in the previous section, the study of behavior in institutions has certain advantages: the information on menstrual cycle is probably more reliable, and the behaviors of interest can be observed and evaluated.

In summary, PMS (or premenstrual dysphoric disorder) is poorly understood. It seems that women who participate in criminal (or noncriminal) violence are more likely to act during the paramenstrual part of their cycle than at other times. This does not necessarily mean that women who experience PMS are more violent than women who do not. PMS notwithstanding, women are far less violent than men.

SUMMARY AND CONCLUSIONS

Central serotoninergic dysfunction is linked to impulsive violent behavior. The exact nature and the origins of the dysfunction are unclear. Polymorphisms of the genes coding for TPH, 5-HTT, and serotonin receptors such as 5-HT$_{1B}$ may be involved in some forms of the dysfunction. The links between serotonin dysfunction and violence have not been confirmed in all populations tested. Nevertheless, the serotoninergic dysfunction trait could be a marker of propensity for certain types of violent behavior. Furthermore, future antiaggressive treatments may use drug effects on serotoninergic receptors.

General overreactivity to the environment (irritability) is mediated through noradrenergic mechanisms. Polymorphism of the gene that codes for COMT appears to be associated with violent behavior in various psychiatric populations. Variations of the MAO A gene may also be involved in the regulation of aggressive behavior. It is possible that the noradrenergic system modulates the relationship between serotonin and aggression in this way by raising the preparedness of the organism to react aggressively.

Hypoglycemia is associated with impulsive violent behavior, and the link may be mediated via serotoninergic mechanisms and alcohol consumption.

Persons with a history of violent behavior may have slight elevations in testosterone levels, but this effect is not large. The elevation may be a consequence of the behavior or its antecedent. Contrary to early reports, an extra Y chromosome (XYY genotype) is apparently not associated with an increased arrest rate for violent crimes. Effects of the intrauterine hormone environment on the development of aggressive behavior in humans are inconsistent.

PMS may temporarily enhance violent behavior in women who are prone to violence; however, the women who experience the syndrome are not necessarily more violent than those who do not.

4 | Neurological, Neuropsychological, and Brain Imaging Correlates of Violent Behavior

Animal studies have shown that aggressive behavior is modulated by a number of subcortical structures. The roles of the medial and lateral hypothalamus were demonstrated primarily by electrical stimulation of these structures in the cat. Brain lesions in the rat lateral septum, the raphe nuclei, the olfactory bulbs, or the amygdala elicited aggressive or agonistic behavior. Lesions of multiple sites had additive effects on aggression.

Much of the animal data (e.g., that on the amygdala lesions) is relevant for understanding human aggression. Obviously, humans are set apart by the complexity of their central nervous system and by social and psychological influences; it is a truism to state that direct application of animal results to human problems would be simplistic.

Methods used in human studies are largely noninvasive for obvious reasons. They include neurological and neuropsychological tests and examinations. Neurophysiologic techniques such as electroencephalography and evoked potentials have been used in this area for some time. More recent imaging techniques such as positron emission tomography (PET) and magnetic resonance imaging (MRI) in research on violence have begun to yield important insights.

Brain injuries, tumors, and other naturally occurring coarse brain lesions may elicit violent behavior. Information on the roles of various brain structures in aggression can be gleaned from such cases, but its importance is limited: the lesions are usually not limited to one structure; the extent of the lesion is frequently uncertain; control subjects (i.e., people with the same lesions but without violent behavior) are missing; and the lesions affect the patient's behavior and mental status in ways that are not necessarily linked to violence (but that cannot be controlled for).

Surgical procedures permit direct assessment of the role of specific structures in violent behavior. However, operations that might be useful in this respect are limited to a very few cases, and interpretation of the results cannot be generalized to people who do not have the brain disease that necessitated the surgical intervention.

In general, many reports suffer from a sampling bias because subjects who exhibit violent behavior are more likely to receive an evaluation (such as an electroencephalogram) than those who do not. This bias applies to settings such as prisons and forensic units.

This chapter consists of two main parts. First, the effects of brain dysfunctions are examined by use of the methods of neurology and neuropsychology. Second, electrophysiologic methods and studies are reviewed.

NEUROLOGY AND NEUROPSYCHOLOGY

Neurological and neuropsychological methods define the anatomy of the dysfunctions (independently of their origin). Localized or lateralized brain dysfunction and diffuse or multisite brain dysfunction are described in relation to violent behavior. Brain dysfunctions may lead to cognitive deficits; therefore, a review of intelligence in relation to violence is included in this context. Second, violent behavior is discussed in relation to selected disorders: head injuries, encephalitis, and epilepsies.

The logic of this division is flawed; nevertheless, these three bodies of literature have developed along different paths, were written for different (albeit overlapping) readerships, and used somewhat different approaches to the problem of aggression. Division of this chapter along more logical, less traditional lines would not make the data easier to understand.

LOCALIZED OR LATERALIZED BRAIN DYSFUNCTION

Much of the literature on aggression points to a dysfunction of the limbic system (Moyer 1976). The limbic system is a very extensive set of structures extending through parts of the temporal lobes, frontal lobes, thalamus, hypothalamus, septum, and a number of other structures and pathways. The structures are listed in Table 4–1.

Table 4–1. Limbic system structures

Gyrus	Nucleus	Pathway
Subcallosal gyrus	Amygdaloid nucleus	Fornix
Cingulate gyrus	Septal nucleus	Mammillothalamic tract
Parahippocampal gyrus	Hypothalamic nucleus	Mammillotegmental tract
Hippocampal formation	Epithalamic nucleus	Stria terminalis
Dentate gyrus	Anterior thalamic nucleus	Stria medullaris
Indusium griseum	Mammillary bodies	Cingulum
Subiculum	Habenula	Anterior commissure
Entorhinal area	Raphe nucleus	Medial forebrain bundle
Prepiriform cortex	Ventral tegmental area	Lateral and medial longitudinal striae
Olfactory tubercle	Dorsal tegmental nucleus	Dorsal longitudinal fasciculus
	Superior central nucleus	

Source. Adapted from Trimble MR: *Neuropsychiatry.* Chichester, England, Wiley, 1981, p. 15. Copyright 1981 John Wiley and Sons, Ltd. Reprinted by permission of John Wiley and Sons, Ltd.

Temporal Lobes, Thalamus, and Hypothalamus

Links between violence and dysfunction of the temporal lobes, thalamus, and hypothalamus were suggested by several lines of evidence, including clinical observations of naturally occurring lesions and surgical lesions, brain stimulation, and the results of electroencephalography and other imaging methods.

Naturally occurring lesions and dysfunctions of the temporal lobes reported in association with violent behavior were caused by tumors, head injuries (see "Head Injury" below), and sometimes encephalitis such as that occurring with rabies (see "Encephalitis" below). An intracranial (perhaps temporal lobe) tumor was detected at the autopsy of Charles Whitman, the Texas mass murderer who shot people from atop the University of Texas tower. This celebrated case has focused public attention on the temporal lobe as a possible "center for aggression," although the damage to the brain caused by a police bullet made the anatomic localization of the tumor somewhat uncertain.

Although naturally occurring lesions of the temporal lobes may occasionally be associated with violent behavior, this behavior is an exception rather than a rule. Among nine patients with temporal lobe tumors who were selected for the predominance of various psychiatric symptoms in their clinical presentation, only two exhibited some aggressive behavior (Malamud 1967). Presumably, that proportion is even lower in patients with temporal lobe tumors but with no psychiatric problems.

The occasional association between gross lesions of the temporal lobes and violence focused attention on the possibility that functional impairments in that area, perhaps with no detectable structural damage, may increase the propensity to violence. Electroencephalography has provided much support for this notion; I discuss the electroencephalography literature later in more detail.

Computed tomography (CT) and MRI were performed in 23 patients with organic mental syndromes; 14 of these patients had "frequent episodes of violent behavior" (undefined) (Tonkonogy 1991). Five violent patients had local lesions in the anterior-inferior temporal lobe (four on the right side, one on the left).

PET, CT, and electroencephalography were used in a study of four psychiatric inpatients with a history of arrests for violent behavior (Volkow and Tancredi 1987). Regional cerebral blood flow and glucose metabolism were determined. Cerebral blood flow images obtained in four psychiatrically healthy volunteers matched for age, sex, and handedness were used as a reference (control group).

Decreased blood flow in the left temporal area, particularly the left temporal cortex, was discovered in all four psychiatric patients; decreased glucose metabolism was reported in the same areas in two of the patients. Additional abnormalities of blood flow over the frontal lobes were seen in two of the patients. Electroencephalography showed left temporal abnormalities in three of the patients. Results of a CT scan were abnormal in two patients.

In a study similar to that described above (Volkow and Tancredi 1987), seven persons with histories of extremely violent behavior were referred for forensic medical examination because they were considered to have "possible organic brain disease" (Seidenwurm et al. 1997). PET, structural MRI, and quantitative electroencephalography were studied in these violent subjects and in nine comparison subjects without history of violence. Significant reductions of glucose metabolism in comparison with the control subjects were demonstrated in the medial temporal lobes of the violent subjects. These reductions appeared to be symmetrical in the illustrative images; I could find no explicit statement on possible lateral differences. Electroencephalography revealed abnormalities involving temporal areas in four of the violent subjects. Most of the violent subjects had histories of substance abuse and low intelligence.

A study of 372 male patients in a maximum-security mental hospital used CT and electroencephalography (Wong et al. 1994). Patients were divided into three groups according to the violence rating of their preadmission offending. In the most violent group, 20% had focal temporal electrical abnormalities on electroencephalograms (EEGs) (slowing and/or sharp waves), and 41% had structural abnormalities of the temporal lobe on CT (dilated temporal horn and/or reduced size of temporal lobe). The corresponding figures for the least violent group are 2.4% and 6.7%, respectively. Thus, this large study showed that violent offending is associated with temporal lobe abnormalities; lateralization of the abnormalities was not reported in this article.

Tumors of the ventromedial hypothalamus were reported to elicit uncoordinated aggressive behavior and hyperphagia in several patients (Weiger and Bear 1988).

Stimulation and ablation studies of limbic structures in humans yielded results that were more equivocal than those obtained in animals (see "Paradigms for the Study of Animal Aggression in the Laboratory" in Chapter 2). Rage reactions were reported after the amygdala or the hippocampus was stimulated telemetrically via indwelling electrodes in a freely moving patient. Simultaneous EEGs were recorded from indwelling electrodes; some of these recordings were interpreted as paroxysmal discharges in the amygdala coinciding with the rage behaviors (Mark and Ervin 1970). The patient in this well-known case ("Julia") had a long history of violent behavior before the electrodes were implanted. The rage behaviors, however, did not start immediately after the stimulation; this time delay weakened the likelihood of a causal relationship between the electrical stimulation and the patient's rage reactions (Treiman 1991). Another case report of stimulation and subsequent bilateral lesioning of the amygdala in a patient with temporal lobe seizures and rage attacks was reported by the same group (Mark et al. 1975). The seizures and rage attacks stopped after the surgery and did not recur during a 4-year follow-up period. Several other cases of amygdalotomy with various outcomes were described in this communication.

In another study, 18 aggressive patients (16 of whom had epilepsy) underwent amygdalotomy; the procedure resulted in some long-term behavioral improvement "in certain cases in certain situations" (Hitchcock and Cairns 1973, p. 902). This formulation reflects the low quality of the behavioral follow-up and the consequent uncertainty about the true effects of the operation. Six of these patients underwent stimulation and coagulation of the amygdala (bilaterally in five cases) under local anesthesia, and their behavior during these procedures was recorded. Swearing, shouting, threats, or restless destructive behavior occurred during stimulation and coagulation in these patients.

Several other individual cases of aggressive behavior elicited by brain stimulation were reported. However, no aggressive behavior was elicited in hundreds of patients who were electrically stimulated in various parts of their temporal lobes as a part of their evaluation for possible surgical treatment of epilepsy at two large centers specializing in this type of surgery (Treiman 1991, p. 347). These very large samples were apparently not selected for violent behavior. Taken together, these reports (Hitchcock and Cairns 1973; Treiman 1991) suggest that a history of aggressivity may predict aggression during temporal lobe stimulation. It is interesting, however, that the type of aggression elicited by the amygdala stimulation was different from the usual aggressive behaviors exhibited by the patients (Hitchcock and Cairns 1973). The presence of aggressive behavior in the patient's history would thus predict the emergence of some aggression during electric stimulation, but the phenomenology of the emerging aggression remains unpredictable. This unpredictability is perhaps not surprising because the electrical and mechanical stimuli delivered by an electrode are vastly different from natural stimuli reaching the amygdala through its neuronal connections.

Neurosurgeons' estimates of the outcomes of ablation procedures for aggression were summarized (Valenstein 1980). A total of 55 patients operated on in the United States whose results were reported between 1970 and 1980 were included in this summary. The operation sites were the amygdala (n=14), the thalamus (n=18), the hypothalamus (n=4), or multiple targets (n=19).

The therapeutic efficacy of these procedures remains unclear because the results were evaluated with "subjective (or poorly defined) criteria" (Valenstein 1980, p. 158). The operations targeting the amygdala yielded significant behavioral improvements in 4 of the 14 patients; the results were better for the thalamus (12 of the 18 patients improved) and for multiple sites (16 of the 19 patients improved).

The side effects of these operations varied as a function of the brain site and surgical procedure. The thalamic operations had a risk of motor complications (dyskinesias or partial paralysis), whereas the hypothalamic operations were associated with a greater probability of endocrine disorders. The most common psychiatric complication (occurring in 5%–10% of the patients operated on in the 1960s and 1970s) was lethargy or disinhibited impulsive behavior. Both problems were described as transient, but the time course was not clearly defined.

Another series of psychosurgical operations (n=462) was performed by a British neurosurgeon (Turner 1982). Some of these operations were intended to reduce aggressiveness. However, paramedian lobotomies actually caused disinhibition and increased aggression (p. 117). Similar to the American reports, Turner's follow-up procedures were crude and not systematic.

In summary, naturally occurring lesions of the temporal lobes or the hypothalamus may elicit aggressive behavior. However, most of these lesions do not have this effect. Psychosurgical procedures intended to control aggression were performed in a small number of patients. The operations involved primarily the amygdala, the thalamus, or the hypothalamus. The available evaluations of the results of these operations indicate that their risk-to-benefit ratio is unacceptable. However, the surgeons' findings in several patients (Mark and Ervin 1970; Mark et al. 1975) have advanced our understanding of aggression in humans. Electroencephalography studies in large numbers of offenders referred for forensic evaluations or incarcerated in forensic hospitals have revealed temporal lobe abnormalities, and PET studies indicated hypometabolism in these areas in several violent patients. Temporal lobe epilepsy is described in a separate section of this chapter.

Frontal Lobes

Frontal lobes are involved in the executive control, planning, and regulation of behavior. Effects of frontal lobe lesions on personality have been observed since the nineteenth century. Such a case, originally published in 1868, has been reanalyzed using modern methods (Damasio et al. 1994). The patient (Phineas Gage) was a victim of an accident that seriously damaged the frontal areas of his brain. He became impatient, profane, disrespectful, and "obstinate yet capricious and vacillating, devising many plans" that he soon abandoned. This description fits the modern observations of the effects of orbitomedial lesions (see below) as well as the phenomenology of mania.

The long-term consequences of early prefrontal cortex lesions occurring before age 16 months were investigated in two adults (Anderson et al. 1999). The authors compared the two cases with a control group ($N=6$) of patients who acquired similar lesions as adults. Similar to the control subjects, the two patients with early-onset lesions had severely impaired social behavior despite normal basic cognitive abilities, and they showed insensitivity to future consequences of decisions, defective autonomic responses to punishment contingencies, and failure to respond to behavioral interventions. Unlike the other patients with similar lesions acquired in adulthood, both of these patients were occasionally assaultive. In comparison with the control subjects, the two patients showed lower performance on tests of social and moral reasoning. (The presentation of these data is not completely clear in the paper.) In the view of the authors, these data suggested that the learning of complex social conventions and moral rules had been impaired. The observations could be important for the theories of learning law abidance (see Chapter 6); indeed, an accompanying editorial is somewhat provocatively entitled "On the neurology of morals" (Dolan 1999). It will be interesting to see if further research confirms the anatomical and temporal specificity of the function of the orbitofrontal cortex for the development of social and moral behavior in humans (and perhaps in other primates).

Many other observations of the effects of frontal lobe injuries and tumors have been published. Depending on their location within the frontal lobes, lesions may result in two syndromes. Lesions of the *dorsolateral* frontal areas result in apathetic behavior without spontaneously generated activity, whereas *orbitomedial* lesions give rise to impulsive and inappropriate activity executed without any apparent regard for its consequences.

The most authoritative study examining the relationship between frontal lobe lesions and the presence of aggressive and violent behavior was performed in 279 Vietnam War veterans whose symptoms and general behavior were followed up for approximately 15 years after they sustained a penetrating brain wound. Veterans who also served in Vietnam but had not sustained a head injury ($n=57$) were also followed up and served as control subjects; they were matched to the injured veterans for age, education, and time in Vietnam (Grafman et al. 1996). The patients with frontal ventromedial lesions consistently demonstrated more aggressive behavior than did control subjects and patients with lesions in other brain areas. This behavior was manifested more by verbal confrontations rather than by physical assaults, which were reported less frequently. The aggressive behavior was not associated with the total size of the lesion or with the development of seizures. These findings indicate that ventromedial frontal lobe lesions increase the risk of aggressive behavior. The study also explored the long-term effects of the injured veterans' aggressive behavior on their families and close friends. The behavior caused distress, upset household routine, adversely affected veterans' children, and strained the families' financial and other resources.

Prefrontal gray matter volume was reduced in persons diagnosed with antisocial personality disorder in comparison with control subjects (Raine et al. 2000). The subjects with personality disorders had committed more violent crimes than the control subjects, but the specific relationship between violent behavior and gray matter volume was not included in the publication (Raine et al. 2000). Decreases in frontal lobe volume in healthy subjects were associated with Minnesota Multiphasic Personality Inventory scores indicating psychopathic deviance (Matsui et al. 2000).

Much research attempts to link putative dysfunctions of the frontal lobes to violent behavior. Until recently, there were no specific measures of frontal lobe activity—hence the putative nature of the dysfunctions. Many neuropsychological tests tap frontal lobe functions, but these tests are generally not very specific. Electroencephalography can demonstrate frontal slowing, but these slow waves sometimes indicate dysfunctions in distant subcortical areas. PET and single photon emission computed tomography are promising, but research experience in the area of violence has been limited.

PET was used to examine brain function in four violent psychiatric inpatients (Volkow and Tancredi 1987). Dysfunction of the frontal cortex was seen in two of the patients. Another PET study investigated 41 persons tried for homicide and compared them with individually matched nonoffender control subjects (Raine et al. 1997b). Murderers were characterized by reduced glucose metabolism in the prefrontal cortex, superior parietal gyrus, left angular gyrus, and corpus callosum, whereas abnormal asymmetries of activity were also found in the amygdala, thalamus, and medial temporal lobe. In a later reanalysis of these data (Raine et al. 1998a), the rearing environment of the murderers was retrospectively assessed as to the degree of psychosocial deprivation experienced during childhood (physical abuse, neglect, foster home, etc.); these persons were then dichotomously classified as "deprived" or "nondeprived."

As hypothesized, it was the nondeprived murderers who showed maximal reductions of prefrontal glucose metabolism. In this subgroup, the social circumstances likely to elicit deviance are minimized, and therefore biological brain abnormalities are a more likely cause of violent behavior. The differences between the deprived and the nondeprived murderers are illustrated in Figure 4–1.

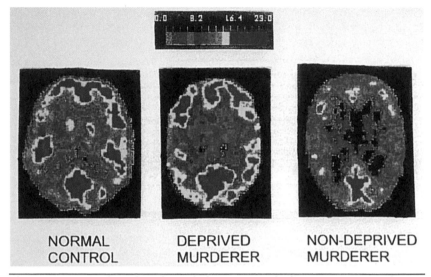

NORMAL CONTROL   **DEPRIVED MURDERER**   **NON-DEPRIVED MURDERER**

Figure 4–1. Reduced prefrontal glucose metabolism (upper part of scan) in one murderer lacking psychosocial deprivation *(right panel)* compared with one murderer with psychosocial deficits *(middle panel)* and one normal control subject *(left panel)*, who both show normal prefrontal activation. Red and yellow indicate areas of highest glucose metabolism, whereas black, brown, and blue indicate areas of lowest activation. The axial slice is taken at 61% of head height above the canthomeatal line.

Source. Reprinted from Raine A, Bihrle S, Buchsbaum M: "Prefrontal Glucose Deficits in Murderers Lacking Psychosocial Deprivation." *Neuropsychiatry, Neuropsychology, and Behavioral Neurology* 11:1–7, 1998. Used with permission.

Preliminary data on magnetic resonance spectroscopy in violent patients are beginning to emerge. A small study indicated that the concentration of *N*-acetyl aspartate (NAA), reflective of neuronal density, was lower in the prefrontal areas of violent patients; furthermore, abnormal phosphate metabolism was detected (Critchley et al. 2000). Similar features were detected in the temporal lobe in the same study. Magnetic resonance spectroscopy may yield various insights about the underlying mechanisms of violent behavior; research in this area is in progress.

Putative frontal dysfunction was tested in 30 young adult criminals by administration of the Trail Making Test (Lezak 1983, p. 556) and a clinical narrative technique (Pontius and Yudowitz 1980). The tests were interpreted to indicate a frontal lobe dysfunction in 10 subjects. A "seizure-like imbalance between frontal lobes and limbic systems" was postulated in a small sample of violent criminals (Pontius 1984), but no empirical measures of frontal lobe function were employed. I think that these authors (Pontius 1984; Pontius and Yudowitz 1980) somewhat overinterpreted their data.

Much neuropsychological work involving violent subjects was published by Yeudall and his group, who used very extensive test batteries (Yeudall 1977, Table 1; Yeudall et al. 1982, Table 1). The results were condensed to show two types of comparisons of the dysfunctions: interhemispheric (left versus right hemisphere) and intrahemispheric (anterior versus posterior).

A battery of neuropsychological tests was used to compare 25 aggressive psychopathic patients with 25 depressed criminal patients. Neuropsychological impairments of both groups were localized in the anterior regions of the brain; the dysfunction was more frequently lateralized to the dominant hemisphere in the aggressive group (Yeudall 1977). Similar results were obtained by the same group of investigators in 86 adult violent offenders (Yeudall and Fromm-Auch 1979).

Neuropsychological impairments specific for the functions of the orbitofrontal and frontal ventromedial cortex were detected in psychopathic prisoners but not in nonpsychopathic control subjects; all subjects were prisoners (Lapierre et al. 1995b). Notably, a smell detection and identification test discriminated between the psychopaths and the control subjects. This is an important finding because the disturbed sense of smell (located probably in the orbitofrontal area) is less likely to be explained by social and cultural factors than many other neuropsychological impairments. A go/no-go task demonstrated the psychopaths' impaired ability to inhibit a response—putatively a function of orbitofrontal ventral frontal cortex. This function is mediated by a serotoninergic mechanism in animals (see Chapter 2) (Soubrie and Bizot 1990) and probably in humans (see Chapter 3), who manifest its impairment by impulsiveness (see Chapter 7).

Frontal brain lesions were reportedly related to documented violent incidents in a sample of 45 neuropsychiatric inpatients (R.W. Heinrichs 1989). The frontal lesions (of various origins) were confirmed through CT. However, "patients were coded as frontally damaged if abnormalities included frontal regions. No differential coding was used for exclusively frontal or exclusively non-frontal lesions" (R.W. Heinrichs 1989, p. 175).

Therefore, I assume that the relationship between lesions and violence in this sample was not specific for frontal lesions.

Electroencephalographic slowing over the frontal and temporal areas was associated with persistent violent behavior in a large sample of criminal offenders (Williams 1969). Similar electroencephalographic slowing over the frontocentral areas was reported in habitually aggressive drug abusers (Fishbein et al. 1989a). These electroencephalographic features recorded over the scalp are generated by underlying cortical neurons, but they may also reflect dysfunctions of deep limbic structures (Williams 1969). I return to electroencephalography later in this chapter.

Although an inhibitory function of the orbitomedial areas of the frontal lobes was hypothesized to suppress inappropriate aggression (Weiger and Bear 1988), the mechanism of this suppression appears vague. A report on patients with head injuries provided a tentative suggestion (Van Woerkom et al. 1977). Two groups of injuries were compared: frontotemporal contusions and diffuse cerebral contusions. The patients with frontotemporal contusions had lower cerebrospinal fluid 5-hydroxyindoleacetic acid (CSF 5-HIAA) levels than the patients with diffuse contusions; a similar trend was seen for CSF homovanillic acid levels. The location and extent of the contusion (frontotemporal or diffuse) were determined by use of clinical symptoms and the spatial distribution of electroencephalographic abnormalities. The patients with frontotemporal contusions were hyperactive or excited (but apparently not aggressive), whereas the other patients had a decreased level of consciousness.

Thus, injuries to the frontal and temporal lobes may reduce serotoninergic presynaptic activity in those areas (and perhaps in other areas of the brain as well). This reduction is then reflected by a decreased CSF 5-HIAA level; injuries to other brain areas may not have this effect. The reduction in serotoninergic activity could lead to impulsive aggression (see Chapter 3).

Because the studies of patients indicate that frontal lobes are involved in the regulation of aggressive behavior, one may hypothesize that imagining scenarios of aggression could be associated with changes of the functional activity in the frontal cortex. This hypothesis was tested by measuring regional cerebral blood flow (rCBF) using PET in healthy volunteers who were imagining scenarios involving emotionally neutral behavior or aggressive behavior (Pietrini et al. 2000). Compared with the imagined neutral scenario, the imagined scenarios involving aggressive behavior were associated with rCBF reductions in the ventromedial prefrontal cortex, suggesting that a functional deactivation of this cortical area occurs when individuals respond to the eliciting of imagined aggressive behavior. These results are consistent with previous findings from animal and human studies showing the involvement of the orbitofrontal cortex in the expression of aggressive behavior.

In summary, the frontal lobes, particularly their orbitomedial areas, are involved in the inhibitory control of inappropriate behaviors. Patients with injuries in these areas may become irritable, short-tempered, hostile, and impulsive. Similar changes may develop as a result of tumors or other naturally occurring lesions of these areas. Serious physical violence, particularly violent crime, is apparently rare in previously nonviolent persons after a lesion limited to the frontal lobes. However, the behavioral changes caused by these lesions have a significant negative impact on patients' families.

Frontal lobe dysfunction was suggested by neuropsychological tests in persons selected for criminal or violent behavior, and the dysfunction may be related to the severity or frequency of violent acts. However, these tests are not entirely specific for frontal lobe dysfunction. Even if one accepts the tests and their results, the correlation between violent behavior and frontal lobe dysfunction says little about causality.

Lateralized Hemispheric Dysfunction

Neuropsychological tests demonstrated impairments lateralized to the dominant hemisphere in a sample of adult aggressive psychopathic patients and violent offenders (Nachshon 1988; Yeudall 1977; Yeudall and Fromm-Auch 1979). However, impairments of the nondominant hemisphere may be involved in impulsive aggression of male adolescents (Nachshon 1983).

Aggressive epileptic patients have predominantly left temporal foci (see "Temporal Lobes, Thalamus, and Hypothalamus" above); no asymmetry in the foci distribution was observed in the nonaggressive patients (Serafetinides 1965). In general, offenders tend to be left-handed more frequently than control subjects (Gabrielli and Mednick 1980); however, psychiatric patients who were not habitually violent were *more* likely to be left-handed than those who were habitually violent (P.J. Taylor et al. 1983).

The number of violent acts observed in psychiatric patients was related to asymmetry of the electroencephalographic delta activity over the frontotemporal regions: the more violence, the more left-sided delta activity (Convit et al. 1991). The relative excess of delta activity suggested a lateralized (left-sided) brain dysfunction. Left-sided focal electroencephalographic abnormalities were also associated with higher number of violent offenses in a large forensic sample (Pillmann et al. 1999). I discuss this further in the section on electroencephalography (see "Electrophysiology" below).

An interesting hypothesis linked the male-female difference in aggressiveness to gender differences in hemispheric functioning: perhaps males are more aggressive because their dominant hemisphere is relatively more vulnerable (Flor-Henry 1976). Literature on hemispheric dysfunction in violent offenders was extensively reviewed elsewhere (Nachshon 1983).

Note that dysfunctions of the dominant hemisphere are not specifically linked to violence. For example, dominant-hemisphere abnormalities in patients with schizophrenia were reported in a large number of studies whose subjects were not selected for violent behavior (Flor-Henry 1983).

In summary, violence tends to be associated with functional impairments of the dominant hemisphere. However, this asymmetry of dysfunctions is not specific for violence.

DYSFUNCTION OF NEURAL CIRCUITRY

The discussion above focuses on individual brain structures. These structures, however, do not function in isolation from each other. The orbitomedial cortex has anatomical connections with the amygdala and the hypothalamus (Weiger and Bear 1988); these connections perhaps subserve functional interactions that control or modulate aggressive behavior (Blumer and Benson 1975). Circuits connecting the orbitoprefrontal cortex, the anterior cingulate cortex, and the amygdala are involved in the regulation of emotions, and dysfunction of that circuitry may facilitate impulsive aggression (Davidson et al. 2000).

In the past, it has been very difficult to test this idea in any direct way. However, a new MRI methodology, diffusion tensor imaging (DTI) (Basser et al. 1994), provides the opportunity to examine white matter microstructure in vivo. DTI provides data on the directionality and coherence of water self-diffusion. The method provides regional measures of diffusion anisotropy, that is, the degree to which diffusion occurs along one direction; it also provides a measure of the mean diffusivity of water. Diffusion anisotropy is influenced by organized structures that preferentially limit the directionality of diffusion. For example, the corpus callosum has very high diffusion anisotropy because its fibers are highly organized. Diffusivity provides a measure of the overall diffusion of water molecules, so that a higher diffusivity implies diminished barriers to that diffusion. In a pilot study of 13 men with schizophrenia, my colleagues, Drs. Matthew Hoptman and Kelvin Lim, have found correlations between higher levels of motor impulsiveness and decreased fractional anisotropy in right inferior frontal regions (Hoptman et al. 2001). This relationship is illustrated in Figure 4–2. They also found strong correlations between higher levels of aggressiveness and increased diffusivity of water in right inferior frontal regions. These inferior frontal regions correspond roughly to orbitofrontal white matter. These preliminary data offer the first evidence that variations in white matter microstructure are related to impulsive and aggressive behavior. These findings, implying impaired organization of the white matter, may represent a structural basis of disturbed brain connections associated with impulsivity and aggression.

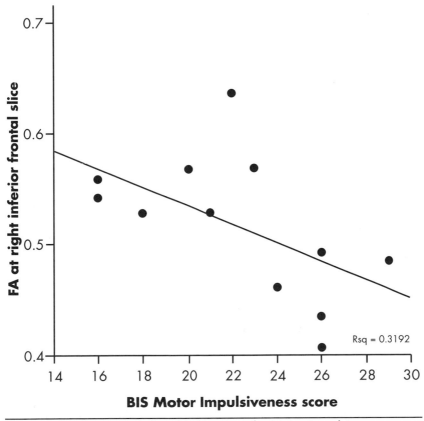

Figure 4–2. Inverse relationship between the Motor Impulsiveness score on the Barratt Impulsiveness Scale (BIS) and fractional anisotropy (FA) in 13 patients with schizophrenia.

DIFFUSE BRAIN DYSFUNCTION

Compared with localized dysfunctions, diffuse dysfunction is somewhat vague. It may reflect lesions in multiple brain structures (multisite lesions), disorder of connecting circuitry, or both. Diffuse brain dysfunction may be operationally defined by results of neuropsychological and neurological batteries that test multiple functions.

Neuropsychological Test Batteries

Neuropsychological test batteries suggested multiple functional brain impairments in violent persons, including adult offenders, juvenile delinquents, and psychiatric patients. The Luria-Nebraska Neuropsychological Battery (Adams et al. 1990) and the Halstead-Reitan Battery were the principal instruments used (Lezak 1983); many additional tests were used by various investigators.

Some of Yeudall's results on lateralization of brain dysfunction were mentioned in the preceding paragraphs (Yeudall 1977; Yeudall and Fromm-Auch 1979). These results were not meant to imply *exclusive* location of brain dysfunction in one hemisphere in any particular group (although such exclusive lateralization did occur in some patients). Many patients showed signs of bilateral dysfunction with a *predominance* of pathology in one hemisphere.

An adolescent birth cohort (n=675) of 13-year-old subjects was examined in New Zealand (Moffitt and Silva 1988). Approximately 15% of the subjects self-reported delinquent acts; 24.7% of the acts were violent (assault), but it is not clear how many persons reported such violent acts.

Verbal, visuospatial integration, and memory deficits detected by a neuropsychological test battery were associated with self-reported delinquency, explaining a modest (2.6%) but statistically significant proportion of the outcome variance (i.e., membership in the delinquent group). This contribution of the neuropsychological tests to the outcome was statistically independent of "family adversity"—a variable created to measure combined effects of low parental education, low parental income, single parent status, large family size, maternal mental health, and poor scores on a measure of family social environment.

The results of this methodologically advanced study are particularly important because these subjects were selected without the biases that usually exist in this type of research, and because they were too young to have experienced the deleterious effects of delinquency such as incarceration, repeated head injuries in fights and traffic accidents, and substance abuse; these factors may confound the results of neuropsychological testing in older subjects. The subjects should be followed up through the age at which they become at risk for violent crime. Longitudinal prospective study of the subjects in this sample promises crucially important results.

Adolescent violent offenders ($n=40$) showed significantly poorer performance on tests of cognitive, perceptual, and psychomotor abilities than did nonviolent offenders ($n=40$) from the same residential treatment school. The group classification was based on unstructured reports of behavior at the school: "Subjects who frequently were seen to attempt to inflict injury ... were classed as violent" (Spellacy 1977, p. 967).

More recently, clear impairments on the Halstead-Reitan Battery were demonstrated in 7 of 14 juveniles condemned to death (Lewis et al. 1988). These impairments were consistent with histories of significant head injuries in these offenders.

Adult violent offenders ($N=86$; ratio of men to women, 75:11) were given an expanded Halstead-Reitan Battery; the findings were abnormal for 89% of the men and 73% of the women (Yeudall and Fromm-Auch 1979). Compared with the control subjects, the violent group had a significantly poorer performance on 24 of the 27 neuropsychological variables. The men showed a greater incidence of dysfunction in the dominant hemisphere, and a clear majority of persons of both genders showed dysfunction of the anterior brain regions (see also "Localized or Lateralized Brain Dysfunction" above).

The differences between the control group and the violent subjects are difficult to interpret. The authors used a "normal control population ... matched for age and handedness" (Yeudall and Fromm-Auch 1979, p. 424). However, the inmates were referred by the courts for a psychiatric examination; presumably, the judges felt that insanity might be an issue. Perhaps nonviolent offenders who were referred for the psychiatric examination because they looked insane would have exhibited the same results on the neuropsychological test battery as the violent ones did.

Another study compared 40 violent and 40 nonviolent prisoners (Spellacy 1978). The two groups were similar in age, socioeconomic class, and ethnic origin. No prisoners with any "diagnosed brain injury" were included (but the author did not specify his diagnostic procedure). A neuropsychological battery testing a broad spectrum of cognitive, language, perceptual, and motor functioning discriminated between the two subject groups. The results indicated that the groups differed in each of these four general areas, and all differences between the groups indicated lower performance in the violent prisoners.

Langevin et al. (1987) used the Halstead-Reitan and Luria-Nebraska batteries and the Wechsler Adult Intelligence Scale–Revised (WAIS-R) to compare 39 violent offenders with 16 nonviolent offenders. The violent versus nonviolent classification was based on the current offense, but the nonviolent offenders' records were screened to exclude those who had a history of violence. All offenders were examined as a part of a pretrial psychiatric examination. The results suggested a trend for impaired performance (and more pathology) among the violent offenders compared with the nonviolent offenders.

Adult schizophrenic patients ($N=37$) in a jail psychiatric unit were given the Luria-Nebraska Neuropsychological Battery, and the patients were classified as "impaired" ($n=12$) or "unimpaired" ($n=25$). The rule for this classification was based on a sum of weighted subtest scores that were not individually reported. It is thus impossible to reconstruct the specific impairments detected; multiple impairments were probably present.

Violent behavior was rated by applying a rating scale for the severity of crimes (Sellin and Wolfgang 1964) to the police and district attorney's reports describing the patients' violent acts (arrests for nonviolent crimes were excluded). The outpatient violent behavior was thus classified as "none" ($n=5$), "mild" ($n=14$), "moderate" ($n=13$), or "severe" ($n=5$). The history of violent acts in the community was associated with neuropsychological impairment ($\chi^2=17.14$, $df=3$, $P<0.001$). Inpatient violence was unrelated to the impairment.

A study of male schizophrenic outpatients ($N=31$) explored relationships between lifelong history of overt physical violence, psychopathology, neuropsychological test performance, and neurological signs (Lapierre et al. 1995a). In this study, the level of neuropsychological impairment was not significantly elevated in patients with a history of violence; unexpectedly, an opposite trend was observed. The authors noted that 42% of their schizophrenia patients had a secondary diagnosis of antisocial personality disorder, but they stated that this comorbidity did not explain their unexpected observations. It is possible that the neuropsychologically more intact outpatients have more interactions with others than those who are more impaired; increased interaction with other people may yield increased opportunity for aggression. In any event, these observations suggest that violent behavior in schizophrenia is a heterogeneous phenomenon that is unlikely to have a single explanation.

Intelligence

Intelligence varies as a function of social, educational, genetic, and many other factors. Some readers may therefore be surprised to see this subject discussed in the context of diffuse or multisite brain dysfunction. The main reason is that an assessment of general intelligence is part of the neuropsychological test batteries that are typically used to define brain dysfunction. Obviously, most of the variation in IQ in the general population is *not* due to any brain dysfunction but rather to the social and other factors mentioned above.

Low intelligence as measured by tests has shown a clear and consistent link to crime (Hirschi and Hindelang 1977). This relationship could not be completely explained by variations in socioeconomic status or other potential confounding variables. Several mechanisms were considered in attempts to explain the relationship between low intelligence and officially reported crime. It was hypothesized that the relationship is spurious because the more intelligent criminals can evade arrest more successfully than the less intelligent ones. However, low intelligence is also associated with self-reported crime (Hindelang et al. 1981). Therefore, the association between low intelligence and crime cannot be attributed to an inability to avoid apprehension.

It is possible that low intelligence, particularly low verbal intelligence, contributes to deviant cognitive styles that favor impulsive uncontrolled behavior without regard for its future consequences. Alternatively, low intelligence may result in academic failure, which in turn decreases the student's attachment to school and impairs his or her socialization. The cascade of events leading from poor academic performance to delinquency has been described (Patterson et al. 1992) (see also Chapter 6).

If low intelligence increases the risk for criminality, then high intelligence may have the opposite (protective) effect. This hypothesis was tested and supported in two samples of subjects who were at high risk for criminal behavior. The first study (Kandel et al. 1988) compared the IQs of four groups of Danish men: those who were at high risk for crime (because their fathers were criminals) but did not become criminals themselves (group a), those who were at high risk and did become criminals (group b), those who were at low risk and did not become criminals (group c), and those who were at low risk but did become criminals (group d). The average IQs of groups a, b, c, and d were 113, 100, 105, and 105, respectively. The average IQ of group a was significantly higher than that of group b, supporting the hypothesis of a protective effect of intelligence. Similar support for a protective effect of high IQ against delinquency was found in a sample of 15-year-old New Zealand boys whose risk was estimated from ratings of antisocial behavior obtained when they were 5 years old (White et al. 1989).

So far, I have dealt with relationships between intelligence and crime in general. I now turn specifically to violent crime. Intelligence tests were frequently administered to violent offenders as a part of neuropsychological assessment. The WAIS-R was administered to 14 juveniles condemned to death for violent crimes; 12 had a full-scale IQ below 90 (Lewis et al. 1988).

Adult violent offenders had lower full-scale IQs than nonviolent offenders (Kahn 1959; Spellacy 1978). A trend for lower IQs in violent offenders was suggested in a small sample (Langevin et al. 1987). On the other hand, there was essentially no difference in IQ between violent offenders and nonoffender (depressive) control subjects (Yeudall 1977, p. 9). Violent offenders may have a selective impairment of verbal IQ compared with performance IQ on the WAIS (Yeudall 1977), but this selectivity was not found in another sample (Spellacy 1978).

Intelligence may mediate the effect of antisocial personality disorder (or psychopathy) on crime. An empirical measure of psychopathy and a culture-free test to estimate intelligence were applied in a sample of 76 white prisoners (Heilbrun 1979). The main finding was that psychopathy was related to violent crime only in the less intelligent prisoners. Interestingly, a rating scale for the impulsiveness of crimes was also administered; the psychopathic prisoners with limited intelligence committed more impulsive crimes than the bright psychopathic prisoners or nonpsychopathic offenders (Heilbrun 1979).

In a follow-up article (Heilbrun 1982), additional modulating variables were introduced: cognitive control, empathy, and self-reinforcement. Interactions between the modulating variables, including intelligence, and psychopathy were explored.

In an attempt to replicate Heilbrun's results, relationships between violence and intelligence were examined in psychopathic and nonpsychopathic prisoners (Hare and McPherson 1984). Psychopathy was associated with higher levels of violence, but no interaction between psychopathy, violence, and intelligence emerged. However, Hare and McPherson differed from Heilbrun on their measures of all variables (psychopathy, violence, and intelligence); this may explain the different results. The concepts of antisocial personality and psychopathy are discussed in Chapter 7.

The studies of intelligence and crime discussed up to this point share a sampling bias because the subjects were prisoners. A recent study of an unselected Swedish birth cohort does not have this bias (Hodgins 1992). The cohort consisted of all 15,117 persons born in Stockholm and living there in 1963. "Intellectually handicapped" members of this cohort ($n=192$) were those placed in special classes for intellectually deficient children and never admitted to a psychiatric ward or institution. Official criminal records were obtained in 1983. Men with an intellectual handicap were 5.5 times more likely (the odds ratio; see "Violence Among Persons With Mental Disorders in Community Samples" in Chapter 9) to have been convicted of violent crime than were men without an intellectual handicap or mental disorder; the analogous odds ratio for women, amazingly, was 24.8.

Neurological Examinations

A neurological examination was administered to 93 subjects in a prison hospital ward (Monroe 1978). Global scores on the examination correlated with various psychopathological features and appeared to validate the construct of "epileptoid" dyscontrol syndrome. This syndrome is one of episodic behavioral disorders (Monroe 1970). These disorders were classified by Monroe into subgroups according to combinations of phenomenological features and activated electroencephalographic theta activity. Today, we would diagnose at least some of these "dyscontrol syndrome" cases as intermittent explosive disorder (see Chapter 7). Monroe's classification and electroencephalographic activation methods are no longer used; however, his pioneering work drew attention to biological bases of violent behavior (Elliott 1984).

Neurological examinations of juvenile homicide offenders yielded abnormal findings such as visual field defects, unilateral Babinski's sign, mild left-sided weakness, clonus, macrocephaly, and multiple "soft" signs (Lewis et al. 1988). The abnormalities were sometimes consistent with the history of head injuries reported by these offenders.

A structured neurological examination was used as a rating scale to yield quantitative data (Convit et al. 1988b). The scale demonstrated multiple neurological impairments in adult assaultive psychiatric patients, particularly in the subgroup of persistent repetitive assaulters who did not respond to treatment (Krakowski et al. 1988a), and in randomly selected male patients in a maximum-security forensic hospital (Martell 1992).

In summary, neuropsychological test batteries and neurological examinations detected multiple and apparently nonspecific impairments of brain functions associated with violence. These impairments were seen in adult and adolescent criminal offenders and in civil (nonprisoner) psychiatric patients. The specific type of impairments varied among studies, but the presence of some impairments of brain function in groups of violent incarcerated persons (although not in each individual) appears to be a robust finding. Lower intelligence is associated with crime—perhaps more so with violent crime.

The origin of these impairments and their role in the maintenance of violent behavior are unclear. One of the possibilities is that some of these impairments reflect head injuries. The injuries might have caused the neuropsychological impairments, and these impairments then led to violent behavior (such as fighting), perhaps through a loss of inhibitory control. In this way, the impairments might have *caused* the fights. However, the impairments might have been *consequences* of injuries suffered in fights, or they might have been *epiphenomena* whose correlation with violence was mediated by a third variable that remained unexplored (e.g., child abuse or prenatal neurodevelopmental problems caused by fetal exposure to various toxins). Deciding among these (and other) possible mechanisms is not possible on the basis of cross-sectional studies; such studies detect correlation rather than causation.

HEAD INJURY

In the preceding sections I discussed cases of head injury with relatively well-established localization. The specific conditions were open injuries of the frontal lobes (Damasio et al. 1994; Grafman et al. 1996; Walsh 1978, p. 117) or contusions of frontotemporal areas (Van Woerkom et al. 1977). However, most reports describing posttraumatic aggressive or irritable behavior deal with diffuse (or inadequately localized) closed head injuries.

Two principal methods are used in the research on diffuse head injuries: aggressive subjects are located and contrasted with nonaggressive ones on the history of head injury (retrospective approach), or subjects who experienced a relatively recent head injury are followed up (prospective approach).

Retrospective Studies

Retrospective studies usually have more detailed and more reliable information on current aggressiveness than on the head injury, which usually occurred many months or years before. An early report indicated that 34 of 100 persons convicted of a felony who were referred for psychiatric evaluation by courts and law enforcement agencies had a history of severe head injury with loss of consciousness (Small 1966). Of these 100 persons, 63 had a history of recidivistic violence; overlap between the violent and head-injured subsets cannot be determined from the data.

Head or face injuries occurred significantly more frequently in 109 delinquent children than in nondelinquent control subjects; the advantage of this study was that the history was obtained from hospital records instead of the usual reliance on the subjects' recall (Lewis and Shanok 1977). Other injuries, accidents, and illnesses were also more frequent in the history of these delinquents. Eight of the 14 juveniles sentenced to death had documented histories of serious head injuries (Lewis et al. 1988).

Head injury with loss of consciousness was reported by 32% of young adult psychiatric patients with a history of aggressive behavior but by only 12% of control subjects (nonaggressive psychiatric patients); this was a significant difference (Felthous 1980).

Interestingly, brain injury increases the risk for schizophrenia (Malaspina et al. 2001), which in turn increases the risk for aggressive behavior (see Chapter 9).

Thus, retrospective studies suggest that head injury may be associated with criminal, perhaps violent, behavior in several different populations. These studies cannot explain the nature of that relationship. As mentioned above, antecedents cannot be distinguished from consequences without prospective studies.

Prospective Studies

Unlike in retrospective studies, which start with a sample of deviant subjects and evaluate the effect of head injuries sustained a long time ago, the subjects in prospective studies come to the researchers' attention at the point when the head injury was sustained (or very shortly thereafter). Prospective studies can be roughly divided into two types: therapeutic and epidemiologic.

Therapeutic studies select patients who became violent within the first days or weeks after the injury; most of these studies focus on short-term treatment and outcome of violent behavior or agitation. Propranolol, haloperidol, lithium, antidepressants, and anxiolytics have been used to treat these states; these treatments are reviewed in the chapter on psychopharmacology (Chapter 11). Epidemiologic studies provide a long-term follow-up of patients with head injuries whose inclusion into the sample is independent of their behavior: they need not be violent to be selected. This approach yields an opportunity to estimate the incidence of violent behavior consequent to the injury.

Epidemiologic Studies

In a representative study of this type, a sample was followed up by a research group over a period of 5 years (Brooks et al. 1986; McKinlay et al. 1981). The patients (final $N=42$) sustained a blunt head injury followed by at least 2 days of posttraumatic amnesia. Caregivers were interviewed repeatedly during the first year and then at 5 years after the injury. The interviewers explicitly asked about changes in the patients' status; this feature of the interview was intended to prevent any confounding of the results by spurious inclusion of deviant behaviors that may have been present before the injury.

During the first year after the injury, 15% of the patients threatened violence and 10% actually became violent. At 5 years, 54% of the patients had issued threats and 20% had exhibited violence. Of all the behaviors surveyed, threats or gestures of violence were "the most frequently reported problem" (Brooks et al. 1986, p. 766). In a 15-year follow-up study of Vietnam War veterans with penetrating brain wounds, approximately 18% of patients with frontal lobe injury threatened to injure certain people, and 15% got into fights (Grafman et al. 1996). (This study is described in more detail in the previous "Frontal Lobes" section).

Thus, violent behavior was observed to emerge after a severe head injury in a proportion of patients, and that proportion was reported to increase at least up to 5 years after the injury. One must consider possible confounding factors to interpret these data. The increased reports of violence might be due to caregivers' sensitization to patients' behaviors or to (false) attribution of patients' usual behavior (predating the accident) to the injury. Even if there was truly an increase in violence, it may not be directly attributable to the effects of the injury on the brain function, but to the patients' frustration in response to the distressing consequences of the injury.

Other longitudinal prospective studies were published (Oddy et al. 1985; Thomsen 1984). These studies did not specifically investigate violent behavior and therefore contain only scattered references to rage, short temper, and irritability. It would be of great interest to study interactions between the patients' preinjury personality and the posttraumatic behavioral changes.

In summary, retrospective studies of psychiatric patients and offenders suggest that a history of head injury may be associated with violent behavior. These studies cannot determine whether the head injury is a cause or a consequence of violent behavior. However, head injuries probably account for some of the neuropsychological, neurological, and electroencephalographic abnormalities encountered among violent subjects.

Prospective studies indicate that severe closed head injuries are frequently followed by agitation and aggressive behavior that require specific intervention in about 30% of the cases (Mysiw et al. 1988). Follow-up in the community of patients with severe head injuries indicates that

10% of the patients exhibit violence at 1 year after the injury, and the incidence of violence continues to rise in subsequent years.

ENCEPHALITIS

Encephalitis can have long-term behavioral consequences, including aggressive behavior, and the localization of pathological changes is variable. Development of such consequences in children was particularly well-known in the past, when adequate treatments for infectious diseases were not yet available.

Lethargic encephalitis (with maximal pathological changes in the substantia nigra and the lenticular nucleus) was known to be followed by personality changes, including the propensity for impulsive aggression (Ford 1960, pp. 434–435; von Engerth and Hoff 1929). Some children, particularly those whose clinical symptoms in the acute phase of lethargic encephalitis were quite minor, became juvenile delinquents and committed serious violent offenses such as murder and robbery (von Engerth and Hoff 1929).

Other types of encephalitis may cause gradual behavioral changes, including the development of aggressive behavior (Greenebaum and Lurie 1948; S. Levy 1959). Incidence estimates for these late effects are apparently not available for any type of encephalitis.

METALLIC TOXINS

There is some evidence that chronic exposure to lead in childhood may result in learning problems and deviant behavior. The exposure might be caused by lead contained in indoor paint in substandard housing and by tap water flowing through lead pipes used in antiquated plumbing systems. In the developed countries, substandard housing units tend to be occupied by people of low socioeconomic status; separating the specific effects of lead from the more general effects of poverty is thus one of the challenges faced by researchers in the field.

Behavioral ratings by teachers and parents, as well as blood levels of lead, were obtained in a sample of 501 British boys and girls ages 6–9 years (Thomson et al. 1989). The authors report that these children lived in a part of town where old lead pipes were used in the plumbing but that the housing units were not substandard. Scores for aggressiveness and antisocial behavior were positively related to blood levels of lead, and this relationship was stronger in boys than in girls. There was a dose-response relationship between behavior ratings and the blood levels of lead; no evidence of a threshold was detected. The relationship, although statistically significant, was modest. These findings suggest that low-level exposure to lead, insufficient to elicit clinical diagnostic signs of lead intoxication, may be associated with aggressive and antisocial behavior. Similar data based on hair analysis were reported in 80 elementary-school children in Wyoming (Marlowe et al. 1985).

Violent incarcerated male criminals had a higher content of lead in their hair than nonviolent prisoner control subjects (Pihl and Ervin 1990). A history of lead intoxication was associated with male juvenile delinquency (Denno 1990). This relationship reached statistical significance (p. 79), but it seems that there were only seven cases of lead intoxication among the 487 males in the sample (pp. 72–73). Furthermore, it is not quite clear how the diagnosis of lead intoxication was made. These findings come from a birth cohort study (Denno 1990) described in Chapter 5.

Taken together, the evidence suggests that lead exposure may be associated with aggressive antisocial behavior. The association is modest. Furthermore, it is not clear whether the association is causal or what the direction of the putative causal relationship would be (hyperactive, aggressive children may act in ways that increase their lead exposure; careless hygiene may be a factor).

Besides lead, there is some (minimal) evidence relating cadmium (Marlowe et al. 1985; Pihl and Ervin 1990) and other metals (Marlowe et al. 1985) to deviant behavior.

EPILEPTIC SEIZURE DISORDERS

Epileptic seizure disorders vary in etiology and manifestations. Most reports on aggression and seizure disorders focused on temporal lobe epilepsy. This subtype, compared with other seizure disorders, is characterized by relatively complicated abnormal behaviors during the seizure (the ictal period) and immediately after it (the postictal period). Some reports on aggression, however, deal with epileptic seizure disorders in general (rather than limiting the topic to any specific subtype). This generalized approach is understandable because most patients with temporal lobe epilepsy experience more than one type of seizure (Rodin et al. 1976). These more general reports deal primarily with behaviors between the seizures (interictal period). Therefore, discussing the links to interictal aggression separately for subtypes of seizure disorders is feasible only to a limited extent. Accordingly, I first discuss temporal lobe epilepsy, describe the observations in the ictal and postictal periods, and then discuss the more general topic of seizure disorders (including temporal lobe epilepsy), dealing mostly with the interictal period.

Temporal Lobe Epilepsy: Ictal and Postictal Periods

Temporal lobe epilepsy denotes seizures arising from the temporal lobe; these seizures mostly have the clinical phenomenology of psychomotor (partial complex) seizures, but some seizures originating from the temporal lobe are actually grand mal. Conversely, some psychomotor seizures originate from areas other than the temporal lobe (e.g., fronto-orbital region). (Niedermeyer 1987, p. 464). Thus, the term *temporal lobe epilepsy* is slightly different in its meaning from the terms *psychomotor seizures* or *partial complex seizures*. The term *partial complex seizures* is now more frequently used than the term temporal lobe seizures, and this usage is more precise because it does not make any assumption about the origin of the seizure. Nevertheless, I chose to continue using the terms temporal lobe and psychomotor seizures to conform to the usage in most of the literature I review here.

A group of 199 patients with temporal lobe electroencephalographic foci had seizures witnessed by trained personnel at a tertiary neurological center. Only 9 exhibited peri-ictal behavior that the authors classified as violent. Seven of these patients merely resisted attempts to restrain them, one beat her chest, and one threw objects (D.W. King and Ajmone Marsan 1977). Thus, no serious violence occurred during or immediately after seizures in these patients seen at a neurological center.

However, different data were reported in incarcerated persons (i.e., persons primarily selected for being violent rather than for being epileptic). A peri-ictal brain dysfunction was implicated in violent criminal behavior in a small proportion of epileptic prisoners (Gunn 1978; Gunn and Fenton 1971), but in as many as 5 of 18 incarcerated juvenile delinquents who had been diagnosed with psychomotor epilepsy (Lewis et al. 1982). These authors (Gunn and Fenton 1971; Lewis et al. 1982) relied primarily on retrospective self-reports by incarcerated subjects to determine whether they had psychomotor seizures during (or immediately before) violent acts. The possibility of amnesia or deliberate distortions makes these self-reports suspect. Furthermore, even if one could be assured that a seizure occurred in close temporal proximity to the violent act, it appears difficult, if not impossible, to determine whether that act was committed during the seizure or in a state of postictal confusion.

These uncertainties were eliminated or greatly reduced when paroxysmal discharges recorded from depth and surface electrodes were seen to co-occur with violent acts of an intensively studied patient (Mark and Ervin 1970).

To resolve the doubts concerning violence during the ictal and postictal periods, concomitant scalp EEGs and videotape recordings of psychomotor seizures were obtained by several groups. An early study with these techniques (Rodin 1973) did not reveal any episodes of serious violence; aggressive behavior could be averted by abandoning attempts to restrain the patient. In a landmark study (Delgado-Escueta et al. 1981), a panel of epileptologists reviewed simultaneous video and electroencephalographic recordings of 33 epileptic attacks (including the immediate postictal period) in 19 patients who were selected for the study from approximately 5,400 patients with epilepsy because of suspected aggression during seizures. Aggressive behavior directed against persons or property was observed during seven complex partial seizures. The severity of the aggression was generally very low; the most serious outburst consisted of shouting and attempts to scratch another person's face. In another video-electroencephalographic study, no violent behavior was observed during seizures in 15 patients (Ramani and Gumnit 1981). Taken together, these three studies found that society had nothing to fear from epileptic patients in either their ictal or their postictal state.

The main strengths of these laboratory studies consist of the electroencephalographic documentation of the seizures and the simultaneous objective behavioral observations. But these very strengths also reduce the ability to generalize the results to nonlaboratory "real-life" conditions in which multiple variables interact with each other. In real life, some of the patients drink alcohol, have access to weapons, and meet people who provoke fights. What a patient does during and after epileptic seizures under such conditions cannot be safely inferred from his or her behavior in an electroencephalography laboratory. Another limitation of these reports (Delgado-Escueta et al. 1981; Ramani and Gumnit 1981; Rodin 1973) resulted from the patient selection. Although the patients in one of the studies (Delgado-Escueta et al. 1981) were selected for suspected aggression *during seizures,* no patients were specifically selected for criminal violence. Therefore, these studies were not designed to test the possibility that seizures increase the likelihood of violent behavior in persons who show a general propensity for aggression. In fact, "extremely dangerous or violent" patients were explicitly excluded from one of the studies (Ramani and Gumnit 1981).

Furthermore, the diagnostic criteria for epilepsy used in the crucial study (Delgado-Escueta et al. 1981) were not explicitly defined. These investigators stated that consecutive and sustained movements organized toward a purpose "are contrary to the nature of epileptic automatism" (p. 715); if such a criterion was used for patient selection, it may have excluded potentially important patients who exhibited violence that somehow appeared purposeful. The reader will recall that some of the retrospective self-reports of seizures linked to criminal acts might have been describing postictal confusion rather than epileptic automatism per se. Thus, it may be possible to reconcile the negative findings (Delgado-Escueta et al. 1981; Ramani and Gumnit 1981; Rodin 1973) and the positive ones (Gunn and Fenton 1971; Lewis et al. 1982): the negative findings perhaps deal with the ictal behaviors, and the positive ones with the postictal behaviors.

Finally, these authors (Delgado-Escueta et al. 1981; Ramani and Gumnit 1981; Rodin 1973) relied on scalp electroencephalographic electrodes to monitor seizure activity. Because clinically relevant subcortical paroxysmal activity is sometimes detectable only through depth electrodes, it is possible that the authors missed electrical paroxysmal features underlying aggressive behavior (Mark 1982).

In summary, the aggressive behavior that may occasionally occur during and immediately after psychomotor seizures is usually trivial, appears purposeless, may reflect confusion, and is probably increased or even induced by attempts to restrain the patient. Exceptionally, serious violence may occur during the ictal and particularly the postictal periods of psychomotor seizures. Such serious violence occurring in close temporal proximity to seizures is extremely rare among unselected patients with psychomotor epilepsy, and it is infrequent even among epileptic patients who are selected for a propensity to violence and other antisocial behavior. The contribution of ictal and postictal aggression toward the population rate of violent crime is negligible despite the notoriety that epilepsy has achieved as a defense in criminal trials. Apparently, the epilepsy defense was mounted in at least 20 homicide cases between 1977 and 1984 in the United States (Pollak 1984); the defense was sometimes successful even in the absence of any clinical or electroencephalographic evidence suggestive of seizure disorder (Beresford 1988).

Temporal Lobe Epilepsy and Other Seizure Disorders: Interictal Period

Most of the reports I have discussed so far did not address the question of interictal violence. This question is even more perplexing than that of ictal and postictal violence. The interictal studies are retrospective. Although some authors tried to estimate the time relationship between seizures and violent acts (Lewis et al. 1982), I doubt that retrospective self-reports can reliably ascertain when the violent acts occurred in relation to seizures because "interictal behavior disturbances may actually reflect unrecognized ictal events" (Engel et al. 1986, p. S3).

To determine whether temporal lobe epilepsy is associated with violence, one would have to study the rates of reliably recorded overt aggressive behavior in representative samples of populations with and without the disease. Such studies have not been done. However, a relationship between epilepsy (any type) and contacts with a criminal justice system was demonstrated by studying close to 100% of the epileptic persons in the population of Iceland (Gudmundsson 1966). Epileptic males were approximately three times as likely to have a criminal offense conviction as were members of the general male population. No description of these offenses was provided.

Separate from the criminal convictions, there was also a record of "offenses against the liquor laws," which apparently occurred in 21% of the males (Gudmundsson 1966, p. 109). I am not sure what these laws were or how the number of offenses against these laws committed by epileptic persons compare with the data for the general population in Iceland. Nevertheless, alcohol abuse may have contributed to the increased rate of criminal convictions in epileptic persons. Most of the other studies used samples of opportunity, and the estimates of prevalence of aggressiveness varied widely, depending on the definitions of aggressiveness and on sampling biases.

A survey of patients with temporal lobe epilepsy seen in London at the departments of neurology, neurosurgery, and electroencephalography reported interictal aggression (undefined) in 7.1% of the sample (Currie et al. 1971). Of 666 patients, 316 (47.5%) were male, with 72 males between 15 and 25 years of age. Thus, young males—the group most likely to exhibit violent behavior—constituted only 10.8% of the entire sample.

A similar prevalence (7.6%) of interictal aggression was reported in another sample of neurology patients with temporal lobe epilepsy seen in the city of Washington ($N=263$, approximately 60% males) (D.W. King and Ajmone Marsan 1977). The aggression was defined as fighting, striking other people, throwing objects, or physically harming oneself.

Because the authors of these two large studies of epilepsy did not use control groups, these prevalences of aggression are difficult to interpret. It is possible that the samples were biased to overestimate the rates of aggression because patients might be more likely to come for treatment if their behavior is not tolerable to their communities, their families, or themselves.

To set these data in a context, I note that the U.S. Epidemiologic Catchment Area Surveys yielded a 1-year prevalence of violent behavior of 2.05% (2.74% for males, 1.11% for females) among respondents without any diagnosable psychiatric disorder (Swanson et al. 1990). Psychiatric disorders were associated with a much higher prevalence of violence. Violent behaviors recorded in this study included striking another person, fighting, or using weapons; elaborate definitions were provided.

Among 31 patients with temporal lobe epilepsy admitted to a psychiatric tertiary care center, 14 were at least minimally violent ("occasional fights or damage to property, no convictions") (Herzberg and Fenwick 1988). Violence was associated with male gender, early onset of seizures, and lower IQ.

Varieties of interictal aggressive behavior in patients presenting at departments of neurology and psychiatry with temporal lobe epilepsy were illustrated by five detailed case reports (Devinsky and Bear 1984). These authors hypothesized vague neurophysiologic mechanisms to explain the patients' aggressive behavior, including the possibility that the orbital prefrontal cortex may be affected by electrical desynchronization spreading from the diseased temporal lobe; this would impair inhibitory control over aggressive behavior. These neurophysiologic hypotheses were criticized for being speculative and reductionistic; the patients' reaction to a chronic and bewildering disease was offered as a parsimonious explanation of their aggression (A.A. Stone 1984).

A.A. Stone's (1984) humanistic explanation is compatible with—rather than contradictory of—proposed neurophysiologic mechanisms. Interictal aggression is a complex phenomenon; it would be surprising if a single cause could be its basis.

Three of five patients described by Devinsky and Bear (1984) had histories of head injury; such injuries (or other damage or dysfunction) may have contributed to the development of aggressive behavior independent of any seizure disorder. Similar inference can be made from findings in 44 patients diagnosed with epilepsy who were referred for psychiatric evaluation because of violent behavior (Mendez et al. 1993). Their seizure characteristics failed to differentiate them from other (nonviolent) epileptic patients, but their comorbid psychiatric diagnoses did. Twenty of these patients met criteria for a schizophrenic disorder, 8 were diagnosed with depression or bipolar disorder, and 25 had mental retardation. The authors concluded that interictal violence was associated with comorbid mental disorders rather than with epilepsy per se. It is of course possible that some of the psychopathology observed and diagnosed as specific and independently occurring mental disorders in fact shared underlying neurophysiologic mechanisms (such as abnormal electrical discharges) with the patients' seizures. Furthermore, it is possible that structural abnormalities that may occur in both schizophrenia and seizure disorders (e.g., those located in the temporal lobes) may give rise to symptoms of either or both disorders.

Summing up the literature on temporal lobe epilepsy and violence, one may conclude that "when appropriate controls are employed, damage or dysfunction in the basal forebrain rather than temporal lobe epilepsy per se appears to be a significant factor in predisposing to psychopathology associated with epilepsy" (Stevens and Hermann 1981, p. 1127).

In a frequently quoted study, patients with temporal lobe epilepsy who were selected for temporal lobectomy were classified as "aggressive" or "nonaggressive"; the classification was apparently based on psychiatric examinations (Serafetinides 1965). The retrospective nature of these examinations made it difficult to clearly describe the aggressive acts. This difficulty led to tautological definitions such as "aggressive behavior ... was taken to mean recurring, unprovoked in the ordinary sense, acts of physical aggression" (Serafetinides 1965, p. 34). Approximately one-third of the patients with temporal lobe epilepsy exhibited overt physical aggressiveness. These patients were not randomly selected from a population with temporal lobe epilepsy; these were the most difficult patients, whose seizures and behavioral problems could not be controlled by medication. Most of the aggressive patients in this study were young boys with an early onset of epilepsy and a left temporal lobe focus (Serafetinides 1965).

Other authors used prison samples to study relationships between violence and epilepsy. An early and much-quoted report of this type described a sample of 105 prisoners charged with murder (Hill and Pond 1952). These prisoners were examined by the authors because they were sent for an electroencephalographic examination by medical prison officers; therefore, a bias toward epilepsy or other neuropsychiatric diseases may be assumed in the selection of this sample. Sixteen cases of clinically confirmed seizure disorders and at least nine additional cases of "blackouts" or alleged epilepsy were identified.

More recent and less biased samples yielded lower estimates, but they did confirm that the prevalence of epilepsy (temporal lobe and other types) among prisoners was much greater than that in the general population. The prevalence of epilepsy (any type) found among adult prisoners in Illinois was 2.4%, which is approximately four times the prevalence in a comparable nonprisoner group (S. Whitman et al. 1984). Similar findings were reported from Britain (Gunn and Fenton 1969).

Two groups reported that epileptic prisoners did not commit more serious or more violent crimes than matched nonepileptic, incarcerated control subjects (Gunn and Bonn 1971; S. Whitman et al. 1984). In one report (S. Whitman et al. 1984), the degree of violence and seriousness of the crime were only rated for the most recent ("instant") offense for which the offender was currently incarcerated; the other report (Gunn and Bonn 1971) reflected more fully the prisoners' criminal careers. The findings did not confirm the hypothesis that epilepsy is related to violence.

Prisoners with temporal lobe epilepsy had a higher overall rate of prior convictions than prisoners with idiopathic (i.e., nonfocal) epilepsy; surprisingly, they had a lower rate of convictions for violent crimes (Gunn and Bonn 1971). Incidentally, no difference in the degree of aggressiveness was reported when an analogous comparison of epilepsy subtypes was performed in a civil (nonprison) sample (Bear et al. 1982, p. 486).

In a study of 97 incarcerated juvenile delinquents, 18 were diagnosed with temporal lobe epilepsy (Lewis et al. 1982). This is a relatively high prevalence of epilepsy compared with estimates in other incarcerated populations (S. Whitman et al. 1984). Perhaps the diagnostic criteria for psychomotor epilepsy used by this group (Lewis et al. 1982, p. 883) were overinclusive, as was suggested by their critics (Ehrenberg et al. 1983; Stevens and Hermann 1981; Virkkunen 1983).

In summary, the prevalence of interictal aggression appears to be independent of the type of epilepsy. The reported prevalence estimates of interictal aggression in epileptic persons vary with the sampling bias. Departments of neurology report lower prevalences of interictal aggression than do departments of psychiatry, with the highest rates reported among incarcerated epileptic persons. The prevalence of aggressive behavior in the population of persons with epileptic seizure disorders is unknown. In my opinion, however, the prevalence is higher than that in the nondiseased general population.

Controlled studies indicate that although prison populations have higher rates of seizure disorders than the general population, the epileptic prisoners do not commit more violent crimes than the nonepileptic prisoners.

Aggressive interictal behavior may be related to damage or dysfunction of the basal forebrain rather than to seizures per se. Left-sided (or dominant-hemisphere) dysfunction may be particularly likely to elicit aggressive behavior. The possibility that anxiety (perhaps secondary to epilepsy) may be a mediating variable in the pathogenesis of interictal aggression remains to be explored. Discrimination and rejection experienced by some epileptic patients aggravate the problems of adaptation to their impairment. These factors may lead to aggressive behavior.

Most studies of aggressive behavior in epileptic persons have identified the same risk factors for violence that are known to affect the nonepileptic population: young age, male gender, deviant rearing environment, low IQ, and low socioeconomic status.

Aggressive behavior in persons with epileptic seizure disorders has particularly complex and heterogeneous causes; interactions among these causative factors remain unclear.

VIOLENCE DURING SLEEP: NOCTURNAL WANDERING

Violence during sleep may occur in persons with various disorders. A sample of 29 subjects with a history of overt physical aggression (21 against others, 8 against self) was studied in detail using sleep electroencephalography, electromyography, and other polysomnographic methods (Guilleminault et al. 1995). It some cases, sleep-disordered breathing or electroencephalographic temporal lobe abnormalities were associated with abnormal arousal. Subjects had incomplete memory of their nocturnal wandering episodes, but they often had vague nightmarish recollections that involved a perceived threat (e.g., the impression of being attacked). The subjects' response to these perceived threats resulted in attacks causing injuries. Carbamazepine appeared to be helpful in preventing the nocturnal wandering and violence.

ELECTROPHYSIOLOGY

Scalp electroencephalographic recordings have been used to study violence since the early 1940s. The only recording method available at that time used oscillographs and pens, which produced the ink-written analog electroencephalographic record on paper. The electroencephalographer would visually scan the paper. This visual assessment of analog electroencephalography is not particularly reliable (Volavka et al. 1971b, 1973) and generally yields only qualitative data. Computer assessment of digitized electroencephalography became generally available in the 1970s. Its main strength lies in the replicable, quantitative assessment of electroencephalographic activity. Standard programs collapse the data from a large number of discrete frequency points into wider conventional bands: for example, delta (0.1–3.5 Hz), theta (4.0–7.5 Hz), alpha (8–13 Hz), and beta (>13 Hz). These primary variables are usually transformed before further use (e.g., E.R. John et al. 1977). Some systems also provide the average frequency (in hertz) within these four bands. These variables are provided for each scalp electrode. A standard system uses 21 electrodes, but larger arrays of electrodes are increasingly common. Programs generate spatial maps of these variables on a projected head surface; these images may be coregistered with those obtained by other methods such as MRI.

The majority of violence-related electroencephalographic studies are confined to the study of resting EEGs. These are usually recorded with the patient in a semireclining position with eyes closed and without any stimulation. There is also a small body of literature on auditory evoked potentials and violence.

Many of the reports reviewed in the following sections on electroencephalography are quite old and technologically primitive, but recent research in this area is scarce. There are other reasons for taking some of this old literature seriously today. Much of this research was surprisingly well conceived, and the questions addressed are still important; the sample sizes are sometimes large; and the EEGs taken before the mass introduction of modern psychopharmacologic treatments (particularly antipsychotics) are valuable because they are not distorted by the effects of these agents.

Because this review is focused on violence, many reports on the relationship of electroencephalography to personality disorders or to deviant behavior in general are not included.

Qualitative Assessment of Resting Electroencephalograms

Children and Adolescents

Abnormal EEGs were associated with aggressive behavior among delinquent boys in various reformatories (Forssman and Frey 1953; Jenkins and Pacella 1943) and among adolescent psychiatric inpatients (Krynicki 1978). Incarcerated adolescent boys who had committed serious violent acts against other persons tended to have more abnormal EEGs than their less violent peers (Lewis et al. 1982). Among 10 juveniles condemned to death for violent crimes, the EEG was definitely abnormal in six and equivocal (possibly abnormal) in the four others (Lewis et al. 1988). However, delinquent adolescents (not selected specifically for violent behavior) did not differ from nondelinquent adolescents on their EEGs (Wiener et al. 1966).

The electroencephalographic abnormalities reported were quite variable, including diffuse or focal slowing, focal sharp waves or spikes, and generalized paroxysmal features. This variability is not surprising, because many electroencephalographic features (including abnormal ones) in children and adolescents are subject to developmental processes that do not progress at the same pace in everybody; furthermore, the ages of the subjects varied from one study to another.

The subjects of the previously described electroencephalographic studies were accused (or convicted) of various offenses; most of them were incarcerated or hospitalized because of their violent behavior. However, there are patients who live in the community and apparently have no contacts with the criminal justice system but who exhibit recurrent aggressive behavior or recurrent bursts of rage, with or without provocation. Such patients are sometimes referred for electroencephalography by their doctors, who are apparently impressed by some of the literature I just reviewed and expect that the EEG might uncover an underlying problem such as epilepsy or brain damage.

Such nonincarcerated patients (N=212) were examined. Approximately 70% ranged in age between 4 and 20 years; the remaining 30% were older. The overall incidence of electroencephalographic abnormality was only 6.7% (T.L. Riley 1979). A similar incidence might be expected in a group of healthy persons used as control subjects in electroencephalographic studies. It should be noted that patients with abnormal neurological examinations, seizures, mental retardation, or any other structural or metabolic brain disorder were excluded. The implication of these findings is that if the patient's violence is not serious enough to require incarceration, and if the patient has no abnormal findings suggestive of brain disease, then the qualitative EEG will probably also not explain his or her violent behavior. The reader will recall a similarly powerful effect of selection bias apparent in the studies of interictal aggression. These results (T.L. Riley 1979) complement the reports of electroencephalographic abnormalities in violent offenders, and this study should not be interpreted as a disconfirmation of those reports.

Adults

An early suggestion of a relationship between violence and brain dysfunction was provided by a widely quoted homicide case reported by Hill and Sargant (1943). This case is cited in Chapter 3 (see "Insulin" in that chapter). The killer had no history of seizures, but there were some clinical signs suggesting a developmental disability. There was also a history of hypoglycemia. He did not eat much during the 12 hours preceding the murder. He remembered the murder but had amnesia for the 7-hour period after it.

His EEG was normal until hypoglycemia was induced. Under this condition, the EEG slowed to 3 Hz with an accompanying clouding of consciousness. The jury was apparently persuaded that the accused was hypoglycemic at the time of the murder and that the electroencephalographic and clinical evidence obtained during the hypoglycemic episodes in the laboratory indicated abnormal brain function. The verdict was "guilty but insane."

Many other descriptions of electroencephalographic abnormalities in forensic patients and other offenders have been published since. This literature has been reviewed elsewhere (Mednick et al. 1982; Volavka 1990); only the reports that are clearly relevant for violence are discussed here.

Hill and Pond (1952) found abnormal EEGs in 52% of 105 homicide offenders. I already mentioned this report and its problem with the biased selection of subjects (see "Temporal Lobe Epilepsy and Other Seizure Disorders: Interictal Period" above). In view of the selection bias, the very high proportion of abnormal EEGs is hardly surprising. However, these authors made an important discovery: electroencephalography is related to the motivation of the killer. The authors devised the following classification system for homicides: incidental killing, clearly motivated killing, apparently motiveless killing, sex murders, and killing by insane persons. This system has logical flaws, but these flaws do not seriously impinge on the basic dichotomy of categories of "clearly motivated" and "apparently motiveless" killings. These categories are abstracted in Table 4–2.

Table 4–2. Electroencephalography and homicide motive

Electroencephalogram	Clear motive	No clear motive
Abnormal	6	14
Normal	22	4

Note. $\chi^2 = 11.96$; $df = 1$; $P < 0.001$.
Source. Adapted from Hill and Pond 1952.

Motiveless homicide was strongly associated with various types of electroencephalographic abnormalities: three EEGs showed some paroxysmal features, but most were described as diffusely abnormal. A typical case in this motiveless group was that of a 23-year-old soldier of dull intelligence who walked into the kitchen and asked for tea. When the cook refused, the soldier swore and shot him. His EEG showed severe diffuse abnormality.

There was no premeditation apparent in this homicide (or the others described in the motiveless group). I would therefore label these crimes as *impulsive*. The reader will recall the previous discussion of intelligence as a mediating variable in impulsive crime by psychopathic persons (see previous "Diffuse Brain Dysfunction" section) and the role of orbitomedial lesions in impulsive aggressive behavior (see previous "Frontal Lobes" section). The electroencephalographic abnormalities in the motiveless homicide offenders represent another aspect of brain dysfunction associated with impulsive aggression.

Several other groups confirmed a high incidence of electroencephalographic abnormalities among homicide offenders incarcerated in prisons or in psychiatric facilities (De Baudouin et al. 1961; Okasha et al. 1975; Sayed et al. 1969) and, to a lesser extent, among baby batterers (S.M. Smith et al. 1973). Similar to the results reported by Hill and Pond (1952), the highest incidence of electroencephalographic abnormalities was found in offenders whose crime was apparently motiveless or had a slight motive (Okasha et al. 1975).

There were, however, several negative reports. Comparisons of EEGs in convicted homicide offenders with those in nonviolent offenders did not reveal any differences in the proportions of abnormal recordings (Langevin et al. 1982a). Posterior temporal slow activity, one of the findings allegedly associated with aggressive behavior (Hill 1952), occurred at similar rates in aggressive and nonaggressive forensic patients (Fenton et al. 1974); however, many subjects were being treated with psychotropic drugs at the time of the electroencephalographic examination. Driver et al. (1974) studied 97 prisoners charged with murder and failed to replicate the earlier electroencephalographic findings (De Baudouin et al. 1961; Hill and Pond 1952; Sayed et al. 1969). The incidence of electroencephalographic abnormality was approximately equal to that in a control group (10%), and only 1 of 23 motiveless killers had an abnormal EEG. This failure to replicate previous findings is important because the sample used by Driver et al. (1974) was large, and the major positive report (Hill and Pond 1952) was written by Driver's predecessors at the same excellent academic institution (Maudsley Hospital, London). The two studies (Driver et al. 1974; Hill and Pond 1952) used identical criteria for the grouping of homicides and classification of EEGs.

The first report (Hill and Pond 1952) was based on alleged offenders seen between 1943 and 1951. The data for the second report (Driver et al. 1974) were collected between 1964 and 1969. It is possible that the criteria for subject selection changed. The first report mentions "a greater concentration ... of individuals suspected of ... brain disease" (Hill and Pond 1952, p. 23), whereas the second report (Driver et al. 1974) does not mention any selection bias.

None of the electroencephalographic studies of alleged homicide offenders mentioned the subjects' criminal careers. Instead, there was an almost exclusive focus on the homicide offense that led to the incarceration. Perhaps the differences among the results of these studies are related to the differences among the proportions of persistently violent subjects included.

The EEGs in persistently violent subjects were reported to be more abnormal than those in persons who commited a solitary violent act. This difference was demonstrated by Williams (1969), who studied EEGs in 333 prisoners accused of violent crimes. These subjects were referred for an electroencephalographic examination by the prison medical officers because of the nature of the crime or because the prison psychiatrist requested it. Therefore, these subjects do not represent a random sample of violent criminals.

Williams (1969) divided the subjects into "habitual aggressives" (n=206) and "others" (n=127). The "others" were more likely to commit a solitary major act of violence (such as murder) than the "habitual" group. Williams gave examples of these solitary crimes; the typical one involved a husband who came home, found a stranger locked in the bedroom with his wife, and killed him. Sixty-five percent of the habitual (persistently violent) group had abnormal EEGs, compared with 24% of the others (χ^2=10.35; df=1; P<0.01). Most of the abnormalities were localized over frontotemporal areas (see "Frontal Lobes" above). Frontal abnormalities were more frequent in the persistently violent group than among those who committed solitary crimes.

When the subjects with epilepsy, mental retardation, or a history of a major head injury were removed, the percentage of abnormal EEGs was only slightly reduced, to 57%, among the "habitual aggressives," but the proportion dropped to 12% among the prisoners who had committed an isolated violent act. The difference in electroencephalographic abnormality between these two groups was highly significant (χ^2=37.5; df=1; P<0.001). Thus, coarse brain disease was not responsible for the electroencephalographic abnormalities associated with persistent aggressiveness.

The selective relationship between *persistent* (but not transient) violent behavior and electroencephalographic abnormality was confirmed in a sample of 222 defendants referred for psychiatric evaluation (Pillmann et al. 1999). Focal abnormalities of the left hemisphere were significantly associated with the number of violent offenses. Temporal lobe electroencephalographic abnormalities (focal slowing and/or sharp waves) were also associated with violence among 262 male patients (mentally abnormal offenders) in a forensic hospital (Wong et al. 1994).

In summary, most of the reports on qualitative electroencephalographic assessment indicated abnormalities in more than 50% of the examined violent offenders. There were no abnormal features specific for violence, but many abnormalities were detected over the temporal lobes. The abnormalities were more likely in persons whose violence lacked a motive and premeditation. Furthermore, the abnormalities were associated with persistent violent behavior rather than with a solitary, albeit major, violent crime. The principal common weakness of these reports is that the subjects were selected for an electroencephalographic examination without explicit criteria; in general, there was a tendency to select persons who had confirmed or suspected neuropsychiatric problems.

These findings have not been uniformly confirmed. The lack of confirmation, I think, is primarily attributable to variable biases in subject selection among studies. Secondary reasons for divergent results probably include variable (unknown) admixtures of impulsive versus premeditated crimes, as well as of persistent versus solitary (or one-time) offenses among the subjects who entered the studies. Another source of variability was concurrent use of psychotropic drugs in the more recent studies; this use was sometimes cursorily admitted, but no attempt was made to account for it. This is disturbing because these drugs are well known to exhibit profound electroencephalographic effects, including slowing of electroencephalographic frequencies and expression of paroxysmal features (similar to those seen in patients with epilepsy). Lastly, the authors often failed to use explicit criteria to define electroencephalographic abnormality. This lack of an explicit definition might reduce the reliability of some of these results, particularly those in children and adolescents.

Quantitative Assessment of Resting Electroencephalograms

Children and Adolescents

Manual measurements of the average frequency of alpha activity were obtained in boys confined to a reformatory (Forssman and Frey 1953). The boys were classified as aggressive or nonaggressive according to "whether the boy had an aggressive-explosive streak in his nature" (p. 70). Their EEGs were classified as containing either low (7–9 Hz) or high (10–12 Hz) alpha frequencies. Low alpha frequency was associated with history of aggression ($\chi^2=9.57$; df=1; $P<0.01$; $N=95$). As was mentioned previously, aggressiveness was also associated with the qualitative assessment of electroencephalographic abnormality in this sample.

In a study of psychiatric inpatients (age range: 12–30 years), hostility measured by various psychological tests was related to the amount of electroencephalographic theta activity (Kennard et al. 1956). A report on six aggressive boys demonstrated that their electroencephalographic frequencies were slower than expected for their ages; the boys' electroencephalographic frequency composition as determined by a computer-assisted analysis would be expected in persons younger than they were (maturational retardation) (Surwillo 1980).

Electroencephalographic frequency composition changes as a function of age, and electroencephalographic abnormality can be expressed in terms of deviation from the electroencephalographic frequency composition expected at a given age (Ahn et al. 1980; Lindsley 1939; Matousek and Petersen 1973; Matousek et al. 1967). The hypothesis that the slowing of the electroencephalographic frequency found in various offenders could be interpreted as a sign of "cortical immaturity" (or developmental retardation) was first offered by researchers studying EEGs in adults (Hill and Watterson 1942). Hill (1944) speculated on "a failure of development in central nervous function, using the Jacksonian concept of 'integration' as the essential process, and postulating a failure of cortical inhibitory control" (Hill 1944, p. 327).

The slowing of the electroencephalographic frequency in adult (or adolescent) offenders could have been caused by many factors other than delayed maturation. The slowing could have been a consequence of violent fights. To test the hypothesis of developmental slowing, one would have to determine the electroencephalographic status of future offenders before they enter the age of risk for criminal offending. Such a test requires recording EEGs in a relatively large sample of children or adolescents, storing the results until the subjects are in their 20s or 30s, determining the subjects' criminality by accessing official records, and establishing whether slowing of the electroencephalographic frequency predated and predicted criminal behavior. In other words, this hypothesis cannot be tested without a longitudinal prospective study.

Three such studies have been published (Mednick et al. 1981; Petersen et al. 1982; Raine et al. 1990b). Each study demonstrated electroencephalographic slowing in future offenders. However, nonviolent offenses (theft and burglary) predominated in these samples; the number of violent offenses was too small to permit meaningful testing of their relationship to electroencephalography.

I hypothesize that brain injuries sustained at various developmental stages contributed to the electroencephalographic slowing found in aggressive offenders. Early brain injuries might have altered the developmental trajectories of various electroencephalographic variables; thus, the maturational and the brain injury hypotheses are not mutually incompatible. In one report on boys in a reformatory (Forssman and Frey 1953), the authors inquired about a history of "cerebral injury" defined as "head injuries with impairment of consciousness, severe rickets, and infections involving central nervous system" (p. 70). Boys who had a history of cerebral injury showed electroencephalographic findings similar to those of boys who were aggressive; unfortunately, the authors did not examine any interactions among these three variables (electroencephalography, injury, and aggression).

The functional importance of the slowing remains unclear. Sleepiness is a possible reason for diffuse electroencephalographic slowing. The arousal hypothesis (see Chapter 6) argues that the avoidance of aggressive behavior must be learned and that a low level of arousal inhibits the learning process (Mednick et al. 1982). Electroencephalographic slowing, low resting heart rate, and low spontaneous fluctuations of skin conductance were demonstrated in a sample of adolescents who later became criminals (Raine et al. 1990b). The coregistration of electroencephalographic slowing with peripheral measures indicating low arousal has strengthened the low-arousal hypothesis of electroencephalographic slowing in criminals.

Alternatively, the slowing may reflect an impairment of cortical function. Such an impairment, particularly one involving the frontal cortex, might result in disinhibition. The behavioral syndromes based on disinhibition include impulsiveness, inability to delay gratification, and antisocial behavior (Gorenstein and Newman 1980).

Adults

Several types and locations of increased theta activity were reported in a mixed population of neuropsychiatric patients, many of whom showed aggressive conduct (Hill 1952). Similar elevations in theta activity, as well as a slowing in alpha activity to 7–8 Hz, were described in a sample of homicide offenders (De Baudouin et al. 1961).

The Buss-Durkee Hostility Inventory (Buss and Durkee 1957) and several other paper-and-pencil tests were used to devise a composite measure of aggressiveness, and EEGs from multiple scalp locations were subjected to computerized power spectra analysis in a sample of 124 drug abusers (Fishbein et al. 1989a). The subjects were drug free for at least 48 hours before data collection. Aggressiveness was associated with increases in the relative amount of delta activity and concomitant reductions in the relative amount of alpha activity. These associations were particularly strong over both central areas, but they were also present over both frontal areas. They remained statistically significant after the effects of substance use and age were accounted for. The associations seemed stronger over the left side, but this lateralization was apparently not tested statistically.

Relationships between electroencephalographic power spectra and violence were studied in 21 right-handed adult male psychiatric inpatients selected for their violent behavior (Convit et al. 1991). The results were similar to those in the previous report (Fishbein et al. 1989a): the level of violence was positively related to the relative amount of delta activity and negatively related to the amount of alpha activity. The relationship was significantly stronger over the left side, particularly frontally (see "Lateralized Hemispheric Dysfunction" above). These results were independent of concurrent antipsychotic medication.

In summary, quantitative assessments found an association between electroencephalographic slowing and violence. In children and adolescents, there was a relative predominance of slow alpha activity (i.e., slowing of the average frequency within the alpha range). Excessive amounts of theta activity in violent youngsters were also reported. Similar phenomena (alpha slowing and excess theta activity) were seen in aggressive adults. Furthermore, adult violence was associated with relative increases in the amount of delta activity and concomitant decreases in alpha activity. These findings may be due to developmental retardation (electroencephalographic immaturity), brain injuries, decreased arousal level, cortical disinhibition, or a combination of these factors. Genetic factors remain unexplored.

Evoked Potentials

Brain stem auditory evoked potentials (BAEPs) are a sequence of seven waves recorded during the first 10–12 ms after a click. These waves originate at various points in the auditory pathway from the distal end of the acoustic nerve (wave I) to the higher brain stem structures (waves VI and VII).

BAEPs (and resting EEGs) were measured in 124 drug abusers; the general structure of the study (Fishbein et al. 1989a) and the electroencephalographic results were described earlier (see "Quantitative Assessment of Resting Electroencephalograms" above). Aggressiveness was associated with longer latencies of waves I, II, and III; these effects were weaker than those described above for the resting electroencephalographic delta and alpha activities. One of the possible interpretations of these longer latencies is a lower arousal state of the aggressive subjects. A similar interpretation is possible for the electroencephalographic slowing found in the same subjects.

Classic auditory evoked potentials (latencies longer than 50 ms) were elicited in a group of highly aggressive boys ($n=6$) and less aggressive control subjects ($n=6$). There was an increased latency of a late negative component (N_2; latency of 294–388 ms) in the highly aggressive group (Dwivedi et al. 1984). Many statistical tests were performed to contrast these very small subject groups, but apparently no correction for this multiplicity was introduced. Therefore, the statistical validity of this finding of increased latency is questionable.

P300, a positive wave with a latency of approximately 300 ms (approximate range, 210–550 ms), is evoked by stimuli resolving the subjects' uncertainty (many other cognitive correlates exist; see Regan 1989, p. 236). Instead of a series of uniform stimuli (the paradigm used to elicit the BAEPs and the classic evoked potentials), the subject receives two varieties of stimuli: frequent stimuli (e.g., 1,000-Hz tones) are randomly interspersed with infrequent stimuli (e.g., 500-Hz tones). The ratio of frequent to infrequent stimuli is usually 4:1. The subject's task is to respond to each infrequent stimulus by a motor response (e.g., pressing a key) or by mentally counting the number of infrequent stimuli. Infrequent stimuli elicit the P300 wave under these conditions. The characteristics of the P300 wave (its latency and amplitude) are related to the subject's cognitive evaluation of the stimuli.

Aggressiveness may be associated with a reduction in P300 amplitude. A group of 51 detoxified alcoholic patients was split into two subsets (with and without a history of aggression). The aggressive alcoholic patients had a significantly smaller P300 amplitude than the nonaggressive ones. Furthermore, the scores on the Buss-Durkee Hostility Inventory (Buss and Durkee 1957) correlated negatively with the P300 amplitude in this sample of alcoholic patients (M.H. Branchey et al. 1988). The aggressive alcoholic patients in this sample who served time in prison for violent acts had alcoholic fathers; the combination of genetic loading and antisocial behavior suggests type 2 alcoholism (Cloninger et al. 1981). It is possible that the reduction in P300 amplitude is related to this form of alcoholism rather than to aggressiveness per se. P300 amplitude reduction may be a marker for alcoholism (or one of its subtypes); this finding was reported in children at risk for the development of alcoholism (Begleiter et al. 1984).

It remains to be seen whether these results can be replicated in aggressive nonalcoholic persons. In general, persons exhibiting antisocial behavior (including 28 "top-security psychopathic prisoners") had *increased* P300 amplitudes (Raine 1988). Unfortunately, no explicit description of violence or aggression in these psychopathic prisoners was provided. Higher amplitude of P300 in these subjects may be associated with increased attention to stimulating events; this increased attention would be a consequence of stimulus seeking or sensation seeking. The potential role of sensation seeking (Zuckerman 1979) in the pathogenesis of antisocial behavior is discussed elsewhere (see "Personality Disorders" in Chapter 7).

Longer latency of P300 was reported in prisoners with a history of violence compared with control subjects (Drake et al. 1988). However, the prisoners were seen because they had "neurologic complaints," whereas the control subjects were not selected according to this bias. There were also associations between the level of violence and the P300 latency within the prisoner group. However, the multiplicity of univariate statistical tests and other problems make generalization of these results difficult.

SUMMARY AND CONCLUSIONS

Naturally occurring lesions of the brain, particularly the temporal lobes and the orbitomedial part of the frontal lobes, may elicit aggressive behavior. MRI and PET studies of violent and antisocial individuals have revealed alterations of the structure and function of the prefrontal cortex. Emerging evidence suggests that the circuitry connecting the orbitomedial part of the frontal lobes with the amygdala and other structures may be dysfunctional in persons who show impulsive violent behavior. Surgical lesions of the amygdala, the thalamus, and the hypothalamus were used to control aggressive behavior in a small number of patients; the dubious benefits were outweighed by the risks. However, interesting information was obtained from depth electrode recordings and stimulation.

Most brain dysfunctions described in violent populations are apparently diffuse (or multisite). The diffuse nature of the dysfunction has been demonstrated by neuropsychological test batteries, neurological examinations, and some surface electroencephalographic studies.

Low intelligence, particularly low verbal intelligence, has been consistently linked to crime in general. More specific links to violent crime probably exist, but the evidence is somewhat equivocal. Protective effects of high intelligence against delinquency were demonstrated in high-risk samples.

Head injuries may be associated with violent behavior. One type of violent behavior may emerge in conjunction with agitation and confusion within days or weeks after the injury and then subside. Another type emerges months or even years later, develops while the sensorium is clear, is characterized by irritability, and is seen as a part of posttraumatic personality change. This change results in significant adverse impacts on the patients' families.

A controversial body of literature examined relationships between aggression and epileptic seizure disorders. The aggressive behavior that may rarely occur during and immediately after seizures is usually trivial, appears purposeless, and can be reduced or avoided by abandoning attempts to restrain the patient. Serious violence under these conditions is extremely rare, but it has been documented in several cases. I think that the contribution of this type of violence to the population crime rates is negligible.

The prevalence of violent behavior between seizures is unknown. Published estimates are distorted by sampling bias and other factors. In my opinion, the evidence suggests that the prevalence is somewhat higher than that in the nondiseased general population. Violent behavior in epileptic persons may be related more to damage to the basal forebrain than to seizures. Many other factors, including the patients' psychological response to this bewildering disease, are probably involved in interictal violence. General risk factors for violent behavior (such as male gender, young age, deviant rearing environment, low intelligence, and low socioeconomic status) are also important in epileptic persons.

Similar to the results of neuropsychological tests, electroencephalographic studies demonstrated diffuse abnormalities associated with violence. However, focal changes over temporal lobes were frequently reported in violent persons. Electroencephalographic abnormalities were particularly pronounced in motiveless, impulsive, violent crime. Furthermore, they were associated with recidivistic (rather than one-time) violence. These findings have not been uniformly confirmed. The differences among the results of electroencephalographic studies are attributable partly to different biases of subject selection.

Quantitative studies demonstrated electroencephalographic slowing in violent subjects. This slowing may be caused by maturational delay, injuries, decreased arousal, and other factors.

A small body of literature on auditory evoked potentials suggests that violent behavior may be associated with deviant processing of sensory input at all levels (from the peripheral nerve to the cortex). These interesting results await replication.

Several common problems and caveats emerge when one attempts to interpret the literature summarized in this chapter. One of them is that of correlation versus causality. As indicated already in the title of the chapter, the observations are predominantly correlational because experiments that could lead us much closer to causes of violent behavior cannot be done in humans. Even in cases when a causal relationship can be inferred, the direction of that relationship is frequently obscure (it cannot be determined whether a phenomenon is a cause or an effect). This is particularly true for retrospective and cross-sectional studies because they do not provide proper information about the timing and sequence of events. Longitudinal prospective studies, particularly those starting in childhood or even during pregnancy, have a much better chance of discriminating between antecedents and consequences.

Specificity of findings is another cause for concern. The dependent variables are nonspecific in the sense that many authors do not define the delinquent or criminal acts they studied; in many cases, it is not clear whether violence was involved. General principles of recognizing aggression and an understanding of the criminal justice system have eluded many authors.

The problems with independent variables are perhaps even worse. First, there are problems with definitions; for example, closed head injuries are difficult to classify meaningfully because the extent and nature of the damage to the brain are variable and are not easily examined. Second, the studies usually do not use control groups, and the selection of subjects is frequently biased. Therefore, the proportions of people with the same neurological problem who do and do not become violent are generally not known. Conversely, the biased selection of violent people who are sent for neurological or electroencephalographic examinations prevents us from estimating the proportion of violent people with neurological problems.

With all these caveats in mind, there are certain inferences one can make about possible neural mechanisms eliciting (or disinhibiting) aggressive behavior in humans. The most simple mechanism would be similar to that seen in animal experiments: a lesion or stimulation of a single structure would increase aggressiveness (of course, in humans it would be a naturally occurring lesion). Limited data of this type are available for the amygdala, but they are too inconsistent. Other candidate structures are the orbitomedial areas of the frontal lobes. Available evidence suggests that under normal conditions this area is involved in the inhibitory control of inappropriate behaviors in general; irritability and impulsiveness may be the consequences of lesions of this area.

However, for every structural lesion eliciting aggression, there are many lesions of the same structure that fail to do so. Having a "center for aggression" would simplify matters, but unfortunately no such center apparently exists in humans.

It seems that diffuse or multisite brain dysfunction may increase aggressiveness via cognitive impairment, which may lead to aggression through several mechanisms: inability to anticipate adverse future consequences of aggression, inability to resolve conflicts verbally, or—in a more complex, indirect way—inability to cope with academic demands at school. School failure starts a series of events that may eventually lead to delinquency and violence.

Failure of inhibitory control may be a concomitant of cognitive impairment, but it may also be observed without cognitive impairment. Some researchers saw the failure of control as a consequence of "cortical immaturity" manifested by electroencephalographic slowing. Alternatively, the slowing (and other psychophysiological features) may be interpreted to indicate low levels of arousal; a theory links such low arousal levels to an inability to learn inhibition of aggressive behavior.

5 Congenital and Demographic Factors

In this chapter, I deal with heritable influences, prenatal and perinatal factors, and the effects of gender, race, and age on violence and crime. The interaction of these effects with mental illness is discussed whenever data are available.

This area of research is controversial. Some of the historical roots of the controversy are discussed in the introduction to this book. An incisive discussion of the controversies and misconceptions surrounding the genetics of crime has been published elsewhere (Raine 1993).

BEHAVIORAL GENETICS

The propensity for aggressive behavior can be seen as a continuous variable that is influenced by genetic and environmental factors. More specifically, the variance of the aggressive behavior (variance of the phenotype, V_p) is equal to the sum of genetic variance (V_g) and environmental variance (V_e):

$$V_p = V_g + V_e$$

The genetic variance can be partitioned into variance due to additive genetic variance (V_a) and dominant genetic variance (V_d).

$$V_g = V_a + V_d$$

Additive genetic variance reflects the extent to which genotypic values add up linearly in their effect on the phenotype, whereas the dominant genetic variance represents influences due to dominance (interactions between alleles at a single locus) and interactions between two or more genes (epistasis). Additive and dominant components of genetic variance are described in more detail elsewhere (Falconer and Mackay 1996, pp. 116–119; Bergeman and Seroczynski 1998)

Twins share a common environment from conception to birth and then during the time that they are reared together; the examples of shared environment include fetal exposure to alcohol due to maternal drinking, parental social class, and exposure to conflicts between parents. Nonshared environment includes, for example, influences of different friends or peer groups. It is important to realize that many biological factors are subsumed under the label "nonshared environment." These include, for example, head injuries, infections, and exposure to various toxins. Shared environmental factors may make twins more similar, whereas the nonshared environment may make them less similar to one another than would be expected from the number of shared genes. Therefore, the environmental variance V_e can be partitioned into shared (V_s) and nonshared (V_n).

$$V_e = V_s + V_n$$

Using the notation defined above, heritability can now be defined. In the broad sense, heritability describes the extent to which an individual's phenotypes are determined by the genotypes (V_g/V_p). Heritability in the narrow sense describes the extent to which phenotypes are determined by genes transmitted from the parents (V_a/V_p). The narrowly defined heritability V_a/V_p thus determines the degree of resemblance between relatives. The response to selection is determined by the narrow heritability V_a/V_p (see Falconer and Mackay 1996, p. 123). Use of V_a/V_p is based on the assumption that all genetic influences are additive. An alternative approach is to assume that all genetic influences are due to dominance (or epistasis). Thus, models can be fitted using either V_a or V_g to estimate the heritability due to either additive or nonadditive genetic variance.

Model-fitting methods based on path analysis have been used to assess environmental and genetic sources of variability. A path diagram is presented in Figure 5–1.

In Figure 5–1, P represents scores on a measure of aggression (P_1 for one twin, P_2 for the other twin). G represents the genotypic variables (additive plus dominant components), E_s and E_n represent, respectively, shared and nonshared environment. The arrows, or paths, are used to define causal relationships. The symbols describing each arrow represent path coefficients. Each of these coefficients estimates the strength of the effect of a causal variable. Twin studies can be used to construct sim-

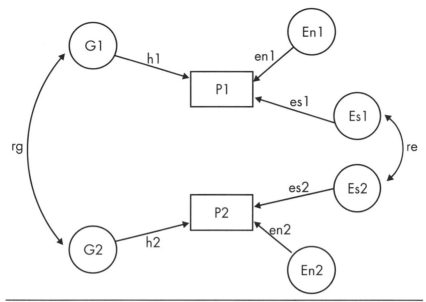

Figure 5–1. Path diagram representing the resemblance between members of a twin or sibling pair.

Source. Reprinted from Bergeman CS, Seroczynski AD: "Genetic and Environmental Influences on Aggression and Impulsivity," in *Neurobiology and Clinical Views on Aggression and Impulsivity.* Edited by Maes M, Coccaro EF. West Sussex, United Kingdom, 1998, p. 67. Copyright 1998 John Wiley and Sons Ltd. Reproduced with permission.

ilar path models to assess relationships between two or more phenotypic variables (e.g., between aggressiveness and impulsivity) for one twin in the pair.

Twin Studies

Twin studies have been traditionally used to partition genetic and environmental causes of various illnesses, and this method has also been utilized to study the causes of deviant behavior.

Monozygotic twins share 100% of their genes with each other. Therefore, the differences between aggressive behavior of monozygotic twins should be due to environmental influences. Dizygotic twins share only 50% (on average) of their genes with each other. Thus, if genes are involved in the propensity for aggressive behavior, monozygotic twins of aggressive probands should be at higher risk for aggressive behavior than the dizygotic twins of aggressive probands. In other words, concordance in monozygotic twins should be higher than in dizygotic twins.

Older twin studies compared monozygotic and dizygotic twin pairs on concordance rates for criminality or delinquency. The studies generally did not provide separate concordance estimates for violent and nonviolent crime, which limits their interpretability for the genetics of violence. Nine of the early studies were reviewed elsewhere (Christiansen 1977). In eight studies with groups of monozygotic and dizygotic twins, pairwise concordance for criminality was greater in monozygotic twins (Christiansen 1977, p. 72). Other twin studies addressed aggressiveness using various personality measures; 24 such studies using male and female subjects of various ages (children, adolescents, or adults) were assessed in a meta-analysis (Miles and Carey 1997). The meta-analysis comprised 17 studies of twins raised together and 3 studies of twins raised apart (plus 4 adoption studies). It revealed that additive heritability and common (shared) environment are responsible for individual differences in aggression. Heritability may account for up to 50% of the variance (Miles and Carey 1997). It appeared that the contribution of shared environment changes as a function of the subject's age. In youth, genes and common environment have approximately equal effects in promoting similarity in aggressiveness. In adulthood, twins tend to have more divergent experiences, and thus the effect of common environment decreases and that of heritability increases.

Recent studies by Coccaro and his colleagues focus on aggression in the context of related traits such as impulsiveness and irritability. These traits, particularly impulsiveness, have definite biological bases (see Chapter 2), and they may underlie certain types of aggression. One of the studies (Coccaro et al. 1993) used data accumulated in a large Swedish sample (up to 500 pairs) of healthy twins separated early in life, and matched twins reared together. One of the premises of this study was that the twins reared together share a family environment, whereas twins reared apart do not. These subjects received a number of personality inventories from which 26 self-reported items were selected because they were related to the constructs of "impulsivity," "motoric impulsiveness," and "aggressiveness." Factor analysis grouped these 26 items into four factors; two of these factors were used to study genetic and environmental influences. Factor I reflected inhibition or lack of aggression and/or assertiveness, and Factor II described behavioral irritability and motoric impulsiveness. Model-fitting analysis revealed an additive genetic influence accounting for 17% of the total variance of Factor I, and nonadditive (dominant) genetic influence accounting for 41% of the total variance of Factor II. The remaining variance was largely accounted for by nonshared environmental influences on both factors.

Two more recent studies by Coccaro and his group analyzed data collected in twin pairs recruited from the Vietnam Era Twin (VET) Registry

(Coccaro et al. 1997a; Seroczynski et al. 1999). This registry consists of 7,375 male-male twin pairs who served in the United States armed forces between 1964 and 1975. The Buss-Durkee Hostility Inventory (BDHI) (Buss and Durkee 1957) and the Barratt Impulsiveness Scale (BIS) (Barratt 1985a) were mailed to 1,208 twins, and data from 182 monozygotic and 118 dizygotic twin pairs were obtained. These scales are discussed elsewhere in this book (the BDHI in Chapter 1; the BIS in Chapter 3), and descriptions are also available elsewhere (Hollander et al. 2000). Four subscales of the BDHI (Direct Assault, Indirect Assault, Verbal Assault, and Irritability) were used to assess the subjects' traits. Model-fitting methods were used to analyze the data. Additive genetic variance accounted for 47% of the individual differences in Direct Assault. The other three BDHI scales showed lower, but significant, heritability of a nonadditive nature. Nonshared environmental influences explained most of the remaining variance. The genetic and environmental sources of covariation between the four BDHI subscales were also studied; a very complicated structure emerged (Coccaro et al. 1997a).

Genetic analyses of the BIS, the BDHI, and their interrelationships were the focus of another study using the same VET set of twins (Seroczynski et al. 1999). Nonadditive genetic variance accounted for 44% of the interindividual variance of the BIS total score. Relations between trait impulsivity and aggression were studied, and a strong relationship between impulsivity (BIS) and the Irritability subscale of the BDHI was observed. Further analyses assessed the genetic and environmental factors mediating that relationship. Impulsivity and irritable aggression shared a large portion of genetic and environmental variance. The close relationship between these two measures is perhaps not surprising in view of the fact that the Irritability subscale addresses constructs like "quick temper" that reflect to some extent impulsiveness. It seemed that overt physical aggression (Direct Assault) was not closely related to impulsivity measured by the BIS. These studies (Coccaro et al. 1997a; Seroczynski et al. 1999) rely on self-reports; the validity of these reports has not been established by collateral information.

Comparing the studies by Coccaro and colleagues (Coccaro et al. 1993, 1997a; Seroczynski et al. 1999) with the results of the meta-analysis described above (Miles and Carey 1997), certain differences may be noted. The model used in the meta-analysis assumed only additive gene action, whereas Coccaro and colleagues used models assuming either additive or dominant heritability. Shared environment accounted for a major part of interindividual aggressivity in the meta-analysis, but not in the Coccaro studies, which demonstrated a major effect of the nonshared environment. Some of the differences between the studies are due to different models with different assumptions. There are also differences in the measures of aggression and the subject selection.

Overall, twin studies support genetic influence on violent and criminal behavior as well as on underlying traits such as impulsiveness and irritability. However, there are some general limitations that should be kept in mind when evaluating twin studies. Monozygotic twins share more environmental influences with each other than dizygotic twins; thus, environmental rather than direct genetic effects might have increased the concordance rates for monozygotic twins. Twins have reciprocal influence on each other. If monozygotic twins influence each other more than do dizygotic twins, then the genetic effects on criminal liability may be overestimated by analyses that ignore such imitative dyadic sibling interactions (Carey 1992). Furthermore, twins have higher rates of complications during pregnancy and birth than do singletons. These complications, interacting with the effects of rearing environment, affect the rates of violent behavior in adulthood, as discussed later in this chapter. Thus, these complications may confound the heritability estimates.

Another factor that may affect these estimates is assortative mating. This is a tendency for persons with a certain phenotype to marry a person who also has that phenotype. Assortative mating may make dizygotic twins more similar to each other, but it will not affect the similarity between monozygotic twins (because they are already genetically identical). This will reduce the differences between monozygotic and dizygotic twins in concordance rates and will thus affect the estimate of heritability. Assortative mating for antisocial behavior and its correlates was studied in a sample of 360 couples from New Zealand (Krueger et al. 1998). Substantial assortative mating was demonstrated for self-reports of antisocial behavior per se and for self-reports of couple members' tendencies to associate with antisocial peers (0.54 on average).

Adoption Studies

If a child is separated soon after birth from the biological parents and placed in an adoptive home, the genetic and environmental effects may be disentangled: the features (e.g., criminality) shared with the biological parents may be considered genetic (or at least congenital), whereas those shared with the adoptive parents are considered environmental in origin. Thus, adoption studies are a powerful method to disentangle genetic and environmental factors.

At least two Scandinavian (Bohman et al. 1982; Mednick et al. 1984) and three American (Cadoret et al. 1990, 1995; Crowe 1972) adoption studies showed concordance between criminal behavior in biological parents and in their adopted-away offspring.

A principal study was based on a cohort of 14,427 nonfamilial adoptions in Denmark (Mednick et al. 1984). A statistically significant correlation was found between the adoptees and their biological parents for convictions of property crimes but not for convictions of violent crimes. The relationship between the convictions of biological parents and those of their adopted-away sons is presented in Figure 5–2. There was no statistically significant correlation between court convictions of adoptees and adoptive parents. In addition, recidivistic property offenses in parents were associated with similar offenses in their biological sons.

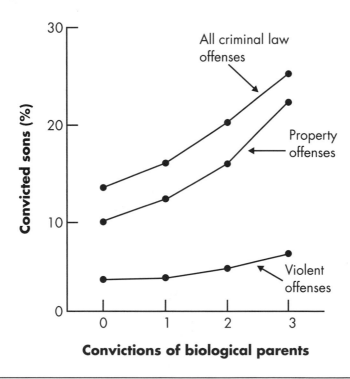

Figure 5–2. Percentage of adoptees convicted of violent and property offenses as a function of the biological parents' conviction.

The report by American and Danish investigators (Mednick et al. 1984) has been criticized for selective placement of the adoptees (Kamin 1985) and for statistical problems (Moses 1985). However, the authors were able to show that the effects of selective placement could not explain the results and that the statistics were valid (Mednick 1985).

The Danish adoptee cohort reported in the comprehensive study (Mednick et al. 1984) was reexamined to determine the role of parental mental disorder in the adoptees' criminal involvement (Moffitt 1987). Substance abuse (mostly alcohol) and personality disorder (but not psychoses) in biological parents were associated with nonviolent criminal behavior of the adopted-away sons. A similar, but nonsignificant, association was found for violent offenses.

These interesting findings cast some doubt on the genetic nature of the criminal propensity transmitted from biological parents to their adopted-away sons in this cohort. The propensity apparently exists, and it is congenital. However, it may have developed during pregnancy or delivery rather than as a direct genetic effect. For example, alcohol use during pregnancy may lead to reduced cognitive performance and increased aggressiveness in the offspring (see the following "Prenatal Exposure to Toxic Substances and Nutritional Deficiency" section). It is thus possible that the increased criminality among the adopted-away offspring of biological mothers who drank during pregnancy can be partly explained by the effects of fetal exposure to alcohol (rather than by direct genetic transmission). A genetic effect, however, may be indirect: alcoholism was perhaps genetically transmitted to the parents.

The studies conducted in the United States are of interest despite their relatively small size. In a study of 286 adult male adoptees, 44 met criteria for antisocial personality disorder (Cadoret et al. 1990). Physical fights were common (69%) among the antisocial probands, but no specific analyses for aggressive or violent behavior were performed in this small sample. Biological parents' criminal convictions and alcohol problems were associated with antisocial personality and alcohol problems in the sons. The interesting aspect of this study is that the environmental effects of the adoptive homes were also considered; alcohol problems or antisocial behavior in the adoptive home was associated with antisocial personality in the adoptees. Furthermore, placement in a lower-socioeconomic-status home was associated with antisocial personality *only if the adoptees' biological parents were criminal*. Although the study was not focused on aggression or violence, it is important in a more general sense because it directly addressed genetic-environmental interactions in the development of antisocial behavior.

A more recent study compared adoptees whose biological parents were diagnosed with antisocial personality disorder or alcoholism (experimental group) with adoptees whose biological parents did not have these diagnoses (control group) (Cadoret et al. 1995). In addition to the parents' diagnoses, the authors established whether the biological mother was drinking alcohol while pregnant with the proband adoptee. There were a total of 95 male and 102 female adoptees, and the age range was 18–47 years. The adoptees and their adoptive parents were interviewed to assess the adoptees' outcomes and the adoptive home environment. Antisocial personality disorder in the biological parents was associated with increased adolescent aggression in the offspring. Furthermore, adverse adoptive home environment interacted with the biological parents' diagnosis: adoptees' childhood and adolescent aggressivity increased with the adverse adoptive home environment in the offspring of antisocial parents (experimental group), but not in the control group (Cadoret et al. 1995, Figures 2 and 3). Prenatal alcohol exposure was associated with antisocial behavior in adult adoptees. In general, combinations of all the independent variables studied as predictors of adoptees' outcomes explained less than 20% of the outcome variance.

Unfortunately, it appears that aggressive behavior in adulthood was not specifically investigated; the adult outcome was characterized as "adult antisocial behavior, the sum of DSM-III adult behavior criterion items for the diagnosis of antisocial personality disorder" (Cadoret et al. 1995, p. 917). Although several of these DSM-III criterion items reflect aggressive behavior (e.g., "repeated physical fights"), it is impossible for the reader to estimate the extent of aggressiveness from the sum of criterion items. Adult antisocial behavior was significantly related to prenatal alcohol exposure.

Thus, the adoption studies provide additional supportive evidence for genetic transmission of antisocial and aggressive behavior. These effects interact with the rearing environment in adoptive homes. In addition to genetic effects, biological mothers may further increase the risk of antisocial behavior in their offspring by drinking during pregnancy.

Adoption studies, however, have inherent problems. The separation of congenital and environmental factors is based on the assumption that the properties of biological parents do not affect the selection of adoptive parents, but such randomization of placements can never be accomplished or even attempted. Placement agencies usually try to match some characteristics of the child with the adoptive family (*selective placement*).

Moreover, the decision to put a child up for adoption is not random, and adoptive parents' behavior may also be affected by the fact that the child is not their biological offspring. This problem can be further aggravated if the adoptive parents are informed by the adoption agency about criminality or alcoholism in the biological family (*parental labeling*). Furthermore, children are adopted at varying ages (thus, varying amounts of environmental experience are shared with at least one biological parent). Finally, the crime rates of adoptees are generally higher than those found in general population (Mednick et al. 1984); in this respect they are not representative, and the ability to generalize the adoption study findings to nonadoptees may therefore be limited. Nevertheless, despite these limitations, adoption studies provide useful information.

In summary, twin and adoption studies indicate genetic influences on nonviolent antisocial and criminal behavior. The issue of genetic influences on violent behavior is less clear. It appears that environmental factors such as prenatal alcohol exposure, pregnancy and delivery complications, and the rearing environment probably interact with genetic influences in the pathogenesis of violent behavior.

The most persuasive evidence for genetic effects on crime was obtained in Scandinavian countries. In comparison with the United States, these countries have much lower crime rates (particularly for violent crime) and much less social inequality. These differences make the Scandinavian populations less suitable for a specific study of violent crime, but more likely to show biological effects on crime in general, because the relative importance of biological compared with social effects on criminal behavior is presumably much greater in Scandinavia than in the United States.

On the other hand, the Scandinavian gene pool is less varied than that in the United States; this reduction in the genetic variance could *reduce* the size of the genetic effects detected in Scandinavia.

PREGNANCY AND PERINATAL FACTORS

Prenatal and perinatal injury to the brain results in many types of neuropsychiatric dysfunction. Effects of the injuries may persist from birth through adulthood. Many complications of pregnancy and delivery can injure the fetal brain. The injury may be direct (e.g., by mechanical pressure) or indirect (e.g., by anoxia or various toxic substances).

Complications include eclampsia, uterine bleeding, placenta previa, prolapsed umbilical cord, damage by forceps, and many other factors. Low gestational age and low birth weight are also linked to many other pregnancy and delivery complications and to neuropsychiatric deficits. The multitude of potential complications and their interrelated nature hinder the development of a uniformly accepted rating scale for these events. Thus, research groups vary in their definitions of pregnancy and delivery complications and in the scoring of the severity of these complications. The standard instrument used in published studies is the Apgar score, which describes the neonate's condition in the first 5 minutes after birth. Adverse effects of prenatal exposure to alcohol were not appreciated until the description of fetal alcohol syndrome in the late 1960s; therefore, the early studies of pregnancy complications miss this important aspect.

The late effects of prenatal and perinatal complications may include behavioral deviance (Pasamanick and Knobloch 1960); extremely high rates of such complications among blacks (compared with whites) was an incidental finding. The possibility that criminal behavior—specifically, violent crime—may be related to prenatal and perinatal factors was addressed in a longitudinal study of a cohort of 1,976 males born at the University Hospital in Copenhagen, Denmark, between 1936 and 1938 (Litt 1972). Detailed hospital records describing the course of pregnancy, delivery, and the neonatal period were kept at that hospital. In the 1960s, a classification system for pregnancy and birth complications was developed and applied to these hospital records. The system was used as a rating scale, and the ratings were coded in 1970 onto magnetic tapes. Also in 1970, the Central Criminal Register of the Danish Ministry of Justice was searched to ascertain which of the 1,976 males had criminal records. Violent crime was not directly related to pregnancy or birth complications. However, the complications interacted with social class: violent crime was associated with pregnancy and birth complications in the middle social class but not in the low social class. Perhaps environmental factors favoring violence are relatively more powerful in the low class, whereas biological factors are more important in the middle class. The environmental factors in the low class might be generally described as a "subculture of violence" (Wolfgang and Ferracuti 1967). For a more specific analysis, it is useful to assess specific relevant aspects of the rearing environment such as physical abuse, neglect, and foster home placement. Collectively, these assessments have been used to determine whether a person suffered from psychosocial deprivation in childhood. As described in Chapter 4, researchers in California classified murderers in this way as "deprived" or "nondeprived," and it was the nondeprived subset that showed more brain pathology (Raine et al. 1998a). This finding was interpreted to mean that in this subgroup, the environmental circumstances likely to elicit deviance are minimized, and therefore the apparent effect of brain pathology on violence is relatively enhanced. This interpretation is consistent with the results of the Copenhagen study described above (Litt 1972).

These findings and their interpretation cannot be easily reconciled with the literature on compensatory environmental influences that appear to protect individuals who suffered perinatal injury against later dysfunction. Such protective compensatory influences are present more in advantaged than in disadvantaged families (Denno 1990, p. 10). Thus, the link between complications of pregnancy and birth and criminality would be expected to be stronger among disadvantaged (lower class) individuals than among middle-class individuals.

The Collaborative Perinatal Project, launched in 1959, generated the largest data set available for the study of pregnancy and perinatal factors in child mortality and development (Niswander and Gordon 1972). This project studied close to 60,000 pregnant women in 15 participating medical centers nationwide and provided for a follow-up of their offspring. One of the collaborating centers in the Collaborative Perinatal Project was the Pennsylvania Hospital, contributing information on nearly 10,000 pregnancies and deliveries between 1959 and 1965. This subsample was selected for a longitudinal study of violence and crime because of its location: the funding for the study was awarded to the Sellin Center for Studies in Criminology and Criminal Law, located in Philadelphia.

Pennsylvania Hospital was a public facility providing inexpensive care. The mothers were predominantly (88%) black and disproportionately young, and their socioeconomic status was slightly lower than that of the United States population as a whole. The proportion of white subjects was seen as inadequate for the study of delinquency, and the final sample studied was therefore limited to blacks. A subset of the offspring (n=987) was selected for a follow-up for criminality with a focus on violence (Denno 1990). The sample consisted of 487 males and 500 females. It is not clear how this final selection was made.

The results indicated that juvenile and adult crime is related to various neuropsychiatric dysfunctions, but not to pregnancy or delivery complications. On the basis of the results obtained in the Copenhagen birth cohort (Litt 1972), this lack of relationship would be expected in a sample with low average socioeconomic status (see above).

The Kauai Pregnancy Study focused on perinatal complications and quality of the childhood environment in a cohort of 866 children born on the island of Kauai, Hawaii, in 1955 and 1956. Perinatal complications had effects on physical status and mental and social development at age 2 years (E. Werner et al. 1967). At age 10 years, however, the effects of perinatal complications were almost completely overshadowed by environmental effects such as socioeconomic status, educational stimulation, and emotional support (E. Werner et al. 1968). Many outcome variables were assessed. One of them is of particular interest: a group of problems labeled "persistently overaggressive" included acting out, bullying, violent temper, and destructiveness. Persistent overaggressiveness was unrelated to perinatal stress; however, it was strongly associated with low socioeconomic status, low educational stimulation, and low emotional support.

The studies discussed above were not focused on any specific perinatal problem, and their equivocal results could be explained by this heterogeneity: it is unlikely that all the subtypes of pregnancy and perinatal complications are associated with identical behavioral consequences. This problem of heterogeneity was somewhat alleviated in a study that focused on very low birth weight (Breslau et al. 1988). In that study, teachers rated the behavior of 9-year-old children (n=65) who had very low birth weight (less than 1,500 g) and of 65 control (full-term) children individually matched for age, gender, race, and school. The long-term consequences of very low birth weight were profound in boys but minimal in girls. Among other behavioral problems, the boys were more likely than the control subjects to be aggressive and delinquent. These effects were not mediated by a difference in intelligence (which predictably favored the control subjects). More recently, structural magnetic resonance imaging was used to compare a sample of 8-year old preterm children with term control children comparable in age, sex, maternal education, and minority status (Peterson et al. 2000). Many regional cortical volumes were significantly different in the preterm children, and certain volume decreases were associated with lower full-scale, verbal, and performance IQ scores.

Parental psychopathology interacted with delivery complications in increasing rates of violent crime in another sample (Brennan et al. 1993). The subjects (all males) were selected either for a parental history of psychopathology (n=72) or as matched control subjects (n=36). Delivery complications were associated with an increased level of violent offending in subjects whose parents had a history of mental illness. No effect of delivery complications on violent offending was noted among control subjects.

The subjects in the study were selected from a birth cohort of 9,125 individuals born at a Copenhagen hospital between 1959 and 1961. An attempt to replicate this study in a larger sample drawn randomly from the same birth cohort yielded similar results, which, however, did not reach the level of statistical significance; this partial failure to replicate was attributed to a lower level of parental psychopathology in the random sample (Brennan et al. 1993).

The presence or absence of hyperactivity and attention deficit was determined for all subjects in both samples studied by Brennan et al. In the smaller sample, a pediatric neurologist examined the subjects when they were between 11 and 13 years old. A behavioral rating scale was used to determine whether hyperactivity or attention deficit was present. In the larger (random) sample, that determination was based on an interview with the mother; the interview, administered when the subjects were 18–22 years old, contained retrospective questions concerning the hyperactive and inattentive behavior of the subjects as young children.

Although the methods used for these estimations differed in the two samples, the results were virtually identical: delivery complications were associated with major increases in violent offending among the hyperactive subjects. These results are presented in Figure 5–3.

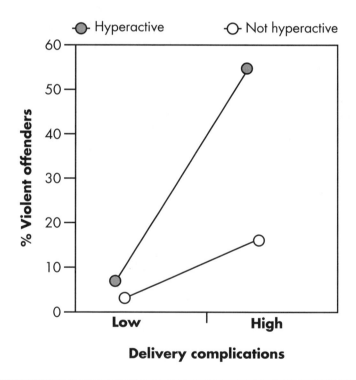

Figure 5–3. Delivery complications, hyperactivity, and violent criminal offenses among the sons of psychiatrically disturbed parents ($N=71$). The interaction is statistically significant ($\chi^2=12.5$, $P<0.001$).

Source. Reprinted from Brennan PA, Mednick BR, Mednick SA: "Parental Psychopathology, Congenital Factors, and Violence," in *Mental Disorder and Crime.* Edited by Hodgins S. Newbury Park, CA, Sage Publications, Inc., 1993, pp. 244–261. Used with permission.

An additional analysis of this Danish birth cohort focused on a subset of 4,269 males (Raine et al. 1994). These analyses were undertaken to establish whether early maternal rejection interacts with birth complications in predicting violent criminality in the offspring (Raine et al. 1994). Maternal rejection was defined as a factor based on a combination of three variables: unwanted pregnancy, attempt to abort fetus, or public institutional care of the infant for more than 4 months in the first year of life. Criminal status was determined when the subjects were age 17–19 years. The Danish National Crime Register was searched. The results showed that birth complications combined with early rejection was associated with an increase in violent offending. Neither birth complications alone nor rejection alone had this effect: the statistical interaction between these two factors was highly significant. Similar results were found in a more recent study of this birth cohort that extended the follow-up period for violent offending from 18 to 34 years (Raine et al. 1997a).

Taken together, the results of these Danish-American studies suggest that predisposition to violence may be phenotypically expressed (activated) by perinatal brain injury, which first elicits hyperactivity and later impulsive violent behavior. Another scenario involves prenatal or perinatal brain injury combined with environmental effects such as maternal rejection.

Given that early maternal rejection increases the risk for violent behavior in the offspring, would crime rates be reduced if unwanted pregnancies are terminated by abortion? This question was addressed by studying the impact of legalization of abortion on crime. As expected, crime rates began to decrease approximately 18 years after the legalization of abortion (Donohue and Levitt 2000). It appears that legalized abortion may account for as much as 50% of the recent reduction in crime rate in the United States. This is a highly controversial study whose scientific, legal, and ethical aspects are eliciting considerable discussion.

Prenatal Exposure to Toxic Substances and Nutritional Deficiency

Alcohol

All the studies of genetic, prenatal, and perinatal influences described above share an important weakness: they pay almost no attention to the maternal consumption of alcohol during pregnancy. This is understandable because they were all designed before alcohol's adverse effects on the fetus were fully appreciated. Fetal alcohol syndrome (K. L. Jones et al. 1973) includes the following characteristics: growth deficiency of prenatal origin, facial anomalies, microcephaly, delayed development, seizures, hyperactivity and attention deficits, intellectual deficits, and learning disabilities.

Partial expression of the syndrome is called *fetal alcohol effects.* In one of the samples studied (Streissguth et al. 1991), the average IQ in patients with fetal alcohol syndrome was approximately 66; in patients with fetal alcohol effects it was around 80. These values were obtained at age 8 years and did not change substantially at age 16 years. Approximately 50% of the adolescents and adults with fetal alcohol syndrome or effects were engaged in bullying; impulsiveness is frequent among these patients (Streissguth et al. 1991). They generally fail at school, even those with normal intelligence; attention deficit and hyperactivity interfere with their functioning in regular classes (Shaywitz et al. 1980). No follow-up of criminal behavior of such patients has been published to date.

The mechanisms of impulsive, aggressive, and hyperactive behavior elicited by fetal exposure to alcohol are not clear. Studying such mechanisms in humans is extremely difficult because the effects of prenatal exposure to alcohol cannot currently be separated from those caused by rearing by an alcoholic mother. Such a separation cannot be accomplished without appropriately designed adoption studies, which are not yet available. Under these conditions, animal studies in which one can cross-foster the prenatally exposed offspring to a nonexposed (control) mother are particularly important. These studies demonstrated increased levels of aggressive and locomotor activity and lowered brain levels of serotonin in the offspring of mice given alcohol during gestation (see Chapter 2).

Thus, the behavioral effects of prenatal exposure to alcohol in humans (including impulsiveness, bullying, and perhaps hyperactivity) might be caused by a disturbance of the serotoninergic system; this neurotransmitter and its role in aggression is discussed in detail elsewhere (see Chapter 3). Central serotoninergic function is deficient in alcohol abusers (Roy et al. 1990) and perhaps in hyperactive persons (Brase and Loh 1975). Hyperactivity is also involved in interactions among parental psychopathology, delivery complications, and violent offenses (Brennan et al. 1993).

Prenatal exposure of rodents to various psychotropic medications may also result in increased aggression (see Chapter 2).

Smoking

Maternal prenatal smoking was associated with behavior problems in children (Weitzman et al. 1992), and specifically with conduct disorder

(Wakschlag et al. 1997). The effect of this fetal exposure may persist in adulthood, as demonstrated by a Finnish study of 5,966 male members of a birth cohort, of whom 355 (6.0%) had committed a crime (Rantakallio et al. 1992). The incidence of delinquency by age 22 was 4.6% among the sons of the mothers who did not smoke during pregnancy and 10.3% among those of the smokers. The association of maternal smoking with delinquency persisted after controlling for a number of social and demographic variables.

The clearest demonstration of the effect of prenatal smoking on adult criminality was provided by a study of 4,169 males comprising a Danish birth cohort (Brennan et al. 1999) (Figure 5–4). Arrest histories of these males were checked when they were age 34 years. There were dose-response relationships between the number of cigarettes smoked in the third trimester of pregnancy and arrests for nonviolent and violent crimes, and these relationships remained significant after potential demographic, parental, and perinatal risk factors were controlled for.

The demonstration of the dose-response relationship and the control for demographic factors make it unlikely that the association between maternal smoking and offspring criminality is simply symptomatic of a certain lifestyle and norm-breaking behavior that adversely affect the rearing environment of the future criminals.

Nutritional Deficiency

In the winter of 1944–1945, the German army blockaded food supplies to large parts of the Netherlands. This was a deliberate retribution; the Germans intended to collectively punish the Dutch for assisting the Allied armies invading Europe. This shameful act of revenge against the civilian population resulted in varying degrees of nutritional deficiency affecting, among others, a large number of pregnant women. In the 1960s, Dutch men who were exposed as fetuses to this wartime famine (and their counterparts who were not exposed) were given psychiatric examinations as a routine part of their induction into the Dutch army. This sequence of events has provided a unique opportunity to study the effects of prenatal nutritional deficiency on deviant behavior in adulthood.

The military records for more than 100,000 Dutch men, including the psychiatric diagnoses, were obtained from the Dutch government, and the men were classified as to the degree of nutritional deficiency to which they were exposed during in the first, second, or third trimester of fetal development (Neugebauer et al. 1999). This classification was based on the place of residence of their pregnant mothers during the German

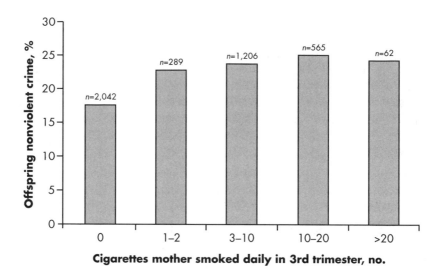

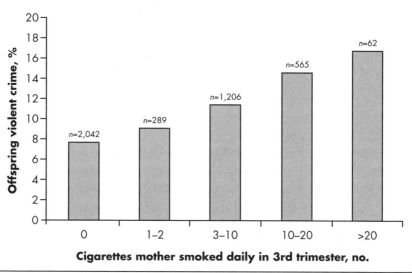

Figure 5–4. The relationships between maternal prenatal smoking and offspring nonviolent (*top*) and violent (*bottom*) criminal arrest. Both relationships are statistically significant.

Source. Reprinted from Brennan PA, Grekin ER, Mednick SA: "Maternal Smoking During Pregnancy and Adult Male Criminal Outcomes." *Archives of General Psychiatry* 56:215–219, 1999. Used with permission.

blockade. The results indicated that men exposed prenatally to severe maternal nutritional deficiency during the first 6 months of pregnancy had an increased risk for developing antisocial personality disorder, including aggressive behavior. The prevalence of antisocial personality disorder among those exposed to severe deficiency was 18.2/10,000; the prevalence was 11.2/10,000 among the unexposed. These numbers, although significantly different from each other, are remarkably low. The DSM-IV estimate of prevalence for (American) community males is 3% (approximately 25 times higher than in this Dutch sample). A 1948 Dutch version of the manual of the International Classification of Diseases was used for the diagnoses; perhaps differences in the diagnostic criteria contributed to the vast difference in prevalence.

In summary, pregnancy and perinatal factors have effects on violence. Emerging evidence suggests that these factors may interact with rearing environment in general in eliciting violent behavior. Many older studies virtually ignored maternal alcohol intake and smoking during pregnancy—a major design flaw. Animal studies have already demonstrated increased aggressiveness in rodents exposed to alcohol during pregnancy and suggested a possible mechanism of this effect. Prenatal nutritional deficiency may be an important factor on a global scale, particularly in developing countries where famine is not uncommon. Replication studies in other cultures with modern diagnostic criteria would be very interesting, but I think that such studies would be exceedingly difficult to do.

GENDER

Gender Difference in Violence: Samples Not Selected for Mental Illness

In the United States in 1998, the male to female ratio for arrest rates for murder, robbery, and aggravated assault was approximately 4.8:1 (Pastore and Maguire 2000, p. 350). Thus, the proportion of arrests of women for violent crime (excluding rape) is approximately 17% of the total arrests; the proportion is somewhat lower when rape is included. Certain caveats should be considered when interpreting arrest rates. These statistics count the number of arrests, not the number of persons arrested. Men commit crimes at higher rates than women; thus, the average man contributes more to arrest rates than the average woman. Therefore, the proportion of women participating in violent crime (relative to all participants) is somewhat higher than the proportion of arrests of women.

The ratio of men to women among persons arrested for homicide in Finland is 11.1:1 (Eronen 1995); the analogous ratio in the United States is 7.9:1 (Pastore and Maguire 2000, p. 350).

Women tend to kill in situations in which the victim (usually a male partner) started or threatened physical aggression (Jurik and Winn 1990). This self-protective character of homicide suggests that women are even less likely to initiate aggression than is suggested by the ratio of arrests.

The value of official statistics such as arrest or conviction rates as measures of criminal behavior has various limitations (see Chapter 1). Victimization surveys compensate for some of these limitations. It is therefore important that the victimization surveys have generally supported the predominance of men among perpetrators of violent crime (Aman et al. 1991, p. 113).

Criminal and noncriminal violent behavior was estimated by self-reports of adults living in the community (Swanson et al. 1990). Among persons without any psychiatric disorder, the 1-year prevalence of violent acts (such as hitting another person, spanking a child, fighting, and using weapons in a fight) was 2.74% in men and 1.11% in women. However, this gender difference was considerably reduced among community residents diagnosed with major affective disorders or schizophrenia, and it disappeared among those with alcohol or drug disorders (Swanson et al. 1990, p. 765).

A preponderance of men among perpetrators of illegal or violent behavior was observed in a community survey involving self-reports of arrests, fighting, and hurting someone badly (Link et al. 1992). A large community-based study in Israel examined the relationship between mental illness and violence (Stueve and Link 1998). Self-reports of fighting during a 5-year period were provided by an epidemiologic sample of 2,678 Jews in Israel who were interviewed when they were 24–33 years old. The interviews also yielded information on diagnoses and mental health treatment. The men reported more fighting than women, but this difference was reduced among recipients of mental health services.

In summary, arrest rates, victimization surveys, and self-reports confirm the preponderance of men among perpetrators of violence. The gender difference is particularly prominent for serious violent acts such as those resulting in an arrest. The difference is less pronounced for less serious (but much more common) violent acts described in self-reports. Psychiatric disorders reduce or eliminate the gender difference.

Gender Difference in Violence: Psychiatric Patients

The size of the gender gap with respect to violence in community residents with mental illness depends on the diagnosis (Swanson et al. 1990). It is not surprising, therefore, that the research on gender differences in violence in samples of psychiatric patients with varying diagnoses yielded confusing results. In addition to the gender gap variation imparted by the diagnoses, there are additional effects due to the various degrees of severity of mental illness and the related effect of the patient's environment (in or out of the hospital).

Patients' Violent Behavior in the Community

Violent behavior among identified psychiatric patients. Patients' violent behavior was assessed prospectively when they were outpatients, or the data on their community behavior were collected retrospectively shortly after they became hospitalized. The second method of patient selection is expected to yield a higher prevalence of violence because patients are frequently hospitalized as a result of violent behavior.

The first method of selection was used in a study of 2,905 outpatients (1,196 males and 1,709 females). Assaultiveness was detected in 4.26% of males and 1.40% of females (Tardiff and Koenigsberg 1985). (In this and some of the subsequent reports discussed in this section, I rearrange or abstract information from tables to facilitate comprehension.)

The second method of selection (i.e., after hospitalization) was used by the same principal author (Tardiff and Sweillam 1980) in the study of 9,364 patients (5,232 males and 4,132 females). Assaultive behavior before hospitalization was present in 11.4% of the males and 7.89% of the females. Remarkably similar results were obtained by another author (Craig 1982), who used a similar method to study 876 patients (514 males, 362 females) newly admitted to public psychiatric hospitals: assaultive behavior was seen as a problem by the admitting psychiatrist in 12.84% of the males and 7.98% of the females. Overrepresentation of males among patients who were assaultive during the 2-day period immediately preceding admission was reported in a sample of 1,687 patients (64.8% males); 341 of these patients (70.1% males) were assaultive (Rossi et al. 1986).

A very thorough review using multiple sources of information about violent behavior during the 4 months preceding hospitalization was conducted in 331 subjects (54% male) (Hiday et al. 1998). Several measures of violence were used, and males had a greater incidence of more serious violence involving weapons or injuries. There was no gender difference in a more inclusive measure of violence that involved threats and fights without weapons or injuries.

A similar interaction between gender and seriousness of violence was reported when arrest records were used to estimate the violent behavior of 172 psychiatric patients in the community: males were significantly more likely to be arrested for violent crimes than females, and the crimes for which they were arrested were more serious than those of female patients (Grossman et al. 1995). These patients were diagnosed with major mental disorders (schizophrenia, schizoaffective disorder, or mood disorder).

Population-based studies. A study of criminality in an unselected Swedish birth cohort (N=15,117) found that men with major mental disorders were approximately 4 times more likely to have been convicted of a violent offense than men with no mental disorder (odds ratio 4.2); the analogous odds ratio for women was 27.4 (Hodgins 1992). Similar gender differences in odds ratios were found for persons diagnosed with mental retardation or substance abuse. At the same time, men were in general more likely than women to have been convicted of violent offenses. The author noted that men with psychoses had less opportunity to commit crimes because they were hospitalized for long periods of time; the ratios were not adjusted for the time when the subjects were not able to offend for this reason.

Such adjustment was implemented in a longitudinal study of a cohort of all incident schizophrenia patients (N=538) between 1964 and 1984 in Camberwell (a London borough) and a nonschizophrenic control group (Wessely 1998). The odds ratio of conviction for a violent offense was 2.1 for men and 3.1 for women. Similar to the Swedish study (Hodgins 1992), the men were in general more likely to have been convicted of violent offenses than the women. There were numerous methodological differences between these two studies. Nevertheless, both studies demonstrated three things: First, men, mentally ill or healthy, are more likely to commit violent crimes than are women. Second, major mental illnesses (or schizophrenia) increase the risk for violent offending relatively more in women than in men. And third, major mental illnesses (or schizophrenia) increase the risk for violent offending in both sexes; this is discussed in Chapter 9.

Patients' Violent Behavior in the Hospital

The investigations of a gender gap with respect to violence in inpatients showed variable findings (Depp 1976; Haller and Deluty 1988; Karson and Bigelow 1987; Tardiff 1981). Taken together, these reports suggest that once the patients are in the hospital, the men are not more likely than the women to be assaultive. Women may actually have a higher rate of violent incidents, but men cause injuries that are more serious (Convit et al. 1990a). A countrywide study of risk for violence among long-stay psychiatric patients (N=2,946) showed that men were significantly more violent than women, but this difference lost statistical significance after controlling for age (Rabinowitz and Mark 1999).

Thus, male patients are more violent than female patients in the community, but this gender gap is absent in hospitalized psychiatric patients. This difference between hospitalized and nonhospitalized (community) samples could be due to a change in patients' behavior after hospitalization or to patients' selective admission because of violent behavior: if men and women are admitted because they have exceeded a threshold of tolerable violent behavior, and if that threshold is identical for both sexes, then this threshold will effectively equalize the violent behavior during the early part of hospital stay for both sexes. This threshold might actually be higher for women; one could speculate that violent behavior by women induces less fear than violence by men and therefore is easier to tolerate by caregivers and other people in the community.

The literature reviewed so far does not clarify these issues. To determine whether patients' behavior changes after hospitalization, one would have to follow up a patient sample before and after hospitalization. One group (Binder and McNiel 1990) interviewed patients on hospital admission about their violent behavior during a 2-week period preceding the admission and then followed them up during the first 3 days of hospitalization. There were 132 men and 121 women in this sample. During the 2-week prehospitalization period, 60.4% of the men and 39.6% of the women committed physical attacks. After hospitalization, the respective numbers were 40.9% for men and 59.1% for women. Thus, men were relatively more violent than women before hospitalization, but the opposite was true in the hospital.

Because all patients in this sample were admitted, this follow-up study supports the hypothesis of patients' changed behavior rather than the hypothesis of selective admission outlined above. It is possible that the deterioration of mental state, presumably a proximate cause of hospital admission, decreased the female patients' adherence to their expected nonviolent gender roles. That would explain the increase in their assaultiveness, but it would not explain the decreased assaultiveness of the admitted men. The authors did not report any data on patients' medication; it is possible that the men received higher doses of antipsychotics than the women (perhaps because the staff was more afraid of them); this difference in treatment could have explained the difference between men and women in the reported trend in assaultiveness after admission. The notion that the staff overestimates the risk of violence in men relative to women has been supported by a study of 226 newly admitted psychiatric inpatients (McNiel and Binder 1995).

In summary, male psychiatric patients in the community are more likely to be violent than their female counterparts. This gender gap appears to be smaller than that observed among nonpatients, and its size probably depends on patients' diagnoses. Although female patients in the community are less violent than their male counterparts, mental illness results in a relatively greater incremental risk for violence in women than in men.

The male overrepresentation among the violent patients disappears (or may even be reversed) once the patients are hospitalized. This phenomenon may be explained by differential gender-specific changes in postadmission behavior or by hospital policy stipulating violence as an important criterion for admission.

Origins of Gender Difference in Aggressiveness

The gender difference in aggressiveness develops in preschool years (Maccoby and Jacklin 1974), and it is fully expressed by puberty. The gender difference obviously has multiple causes, many of which are societal. Child-rearing practices in the United States and in most other societies promote expectations of more aggressive roles for males. Television, sports participation, peer groups, and many other societal influences shape the gender differences in aggressiveness (Eron and Huesmann 1989).

Biological effects on gender differences in human aggressiveness are suggested by several lines of evidence. In a majority of mammalian species, including nonhuman primates, males are more likely than females to fight under most conditions (see Chapter 2). These conditions include intermale aggression (which is largely a form of competition for access to females). The effects of testosterone levels on aggression in animals are discussed in Chapter 2, and their effects on aggression in humans are discussed in Chapter 3; these effects are complex and impinge on functions beyond reproduction. In most species, males also show more irritable aggression than females. This type of aggression is elicited by stress; thus, the male propensity for aggression cannot be fully explained by factors directly related to reproduction.

In general, adult males are larger than adult females in mammalian species (including humans), but there are many exceptions (Ralls 1976). Perhaps the animal's size (relative to conspecifics) is related to its aggressiveness, and if the females are larger than males, they would be more aggressive. This is true for some species (Skirrow and Rysan 1976). But interfemale aggression is generally less frequent than intermale aggression, and this difference is difficult to explain by the animal's size.

Certain forms of aggression are related to disturbances in serotoninergic transmission, as is demonstrated in many mammalia including humans. Experimental reductions in plasma leve. tophan—a serotonin precursor—increased certain aggressive behaviors in male (but not in female) vervet monkeys (see "Serotonin" in Chapter 2) (Chamberlain et al. 1987). Thus, males may be more vulnerable to the aggression-stimulating effects of reduced serotoninergic transmission. Furthermore, an association between irritable or impulsive aggressiveness and the tryptophan hydroxylase genotype was found in male (but not in female) patients with personality disorders (New et al. 1998). Similarly, an association between assaultiveness and the catechol-*O*-methyltransferase genotype was found in male (but not in female) patients with schizophrenia or schizoaffective disorder (Lachman et al. 1998) (see Chapter 3).

It was suggested that the dominant hemisphere is particularly vulnerable in males and that early lesions of that hemisphere account for the combination of aggressiveness and diminished verbal (as opposed to performance) IQ in violent males (Flor-Henry 1974). Electroencephalographic and neuropsychological literature suggests that recidivistic violence in adults is associated with dysfunctions of the dominant hemisphere (see Chapter 4). Most subjects in these studies were male; in general, gender interactions have not received appropriate research attention. However, when the gender effect was tested (Yeudall and Fromm-Auch 1979), lateralization of dysfunction to the dominant hemisphere was indeed more pronounced in the males.

Males are more likely than females to develop alcohol abuse and alcoholism. These conditions are sometimes associated with violence, and thus they further widen the gender gap in the propensity for aggression.

Biological and societal effects promoting male aggressiveness interact in ways that are not completely understood. The main reason for this lack of understanding is that these two classes of factors are rarely studied in the same subjects.

RACE

The relationships between race and violence are more complex than those regarding gender. The difference in the degree of complexity becomes clear as soon as one attempts to define *race*. The notion of gender is so obvious that no definition is needed. The notion of race is so obscure that no generally approved definition exists. Most available data are concerned with "whites" and "blacks." My discussion of race is for the most part limited to these two large groups.

Racial Differences in Violence: Samples Not Selected for Mental Illness

In the United States in 1998, the white-to-black ratio for arrest rates for violent crime was 1.4:1 (Pastore and Maguire 2000, p. 352), but the white-to-black ratio in the population was 6.1:1 (U.S. Census Bureau 2000). Thus, the arrest rates for blacks are much higher than those for whites relative to their proportions of the population. However, inferences concerning criminal behavior that are based on arrest rates have various limitations (see Chapter 1). One of these limitations is that the police officers (who are predominantly white in most police departments) may be arresting black suspects more readily than white ones. The police have some discretionary power in decisions concerning arrest; that power may be misused to discriminate against blacks and thus bias arrest rates.

The arrest data, however, are supported by victimization surveys, which are much less vulnerable to such bias (see Chapter 1 for survey methods). In 1999, the offender's race perceived by victims of all violent crimes was recorded. The white-to-black ratio among offenders was 2.7:1. The ratio specific for robbery was 0.91:1, and that for aggravated assault was 2.0:1 (Pastore and Maguire 2000, Table 3.26). Thus, relative to their proportion in the population, the blacks are overrepresented among the perpetrators of violent crimes. They are also overrepresented among the victims of violent crimes (Pastore and Maguire 2000, Table 3.0002).

A principal article (Swanson et al. 1990) describing self-reports of criminal and noncriminal violent behavior of adults living in the community is somewhat unclear regarding the effects of race. It states that "race was not related to violence when socioeconomic status was controlled" (p. 764). Another community sample study used self-reports of arrests, fighting, hurting someone badly, hitting others, and weapon use (Link et al. 1992). Blacks self-reported significantly more of the first three events than the other two groups (whites and Hispanics); however, socioeconomic status was not controlled.

In summary, the arrest rates, the victimization surveys, and self-reports confirm the relative preponderance of blacks over whites among perpetrators and victims of violent crime in the United States.

Racial Differences in Violence: Psychiatric Patients

Racial differences have not been systematically studied in psychiatric patients. If it is considered at all, race is usually introduced only as a confounding variable. The definitions of race are sometimes confusing; for example, a group introduced a variable called "race/ethnicity" that contained the mutually exclusive groups "white," "black," and "Spanish-speaking" (Rossi et al. 1986). (The "Spanish-speaking" group could obviously include white, black, American Indian, or any mixture of these). Other researchers created three mutually exclusive racial groups labeled "white and Asian," "black," and "Hispanic" (Tardiff and Koenigsberg 1985), or "white," "black," and "other"; the latter racial groups were subsequently reduced (in the same article) to "whites" and "nonwhites" (Tardiff and Sweillam 1980).

Patients' Violent Behavior in the Community

The reported effects of race on violent behavior by patients were variable. Race was shown to have no effect (Craig 1982); an equivocal increase in violence among black and Hispanic patients compared with that among whites and Asians (Tardiff and Koenigsberg 1985); increased assaultiveness in nonwhites that was reduced (but not completely eliminated) by stratification according to educational levels (Tardiff and Sweillam 1980); and a similar increase in assaultiveness that was not affected by an analogous stratification (Rossi et al. 1986). Patients from minority groups were more likely to be arrested for violent crimes than white patients (Grossman et al. 1995)

A sample of 304 adult men who were considered to be "potentially violent" were admitted as psychiatric inpatients and then followed up in the community for a year after their discharge (Klassen and O'Connor 1988a). Blacks were significantly more likely than whites to be readmitted for violence, and they were also (nonsignificantly) overrepresented among those arrested for violent crimes. However, a 6-month follow-up of the same sample yielded no significant effect of race on a composite variable that included arrests for violent crimes and readmissions "for an act that could have resulted in violent crime" (Klassen and O'Connor 1988b, p. 149). The effect of race was tested jointly with 66 other potential predictor variables; it is possible that an effect of race was accounted for by some of these other variables.

Patients' Violent Behavior in the Hospital

Patients' violent behavior in the hospital was studied in a large sample ($N=5,164$); no statistically significant difference between white and nonwhite patients with respect to assaultive behavior was detected (Tardiff 1992). No significant effect of race on in-hospital violence was detected in another study (Myers and Dunner 1984). Nevertheless, clinicians overestimate the risk of violence among nonwhite relative to white patients (McNiel and Binder 1995).

In summary, black patients in the community are perhaps more violent than white patients. This difference was not detected among inpatients. In general, research on race and violence among psychiatric patients has serious methodological problems.

Origins of Racial Differences in Aggressiveness

Many theories attempt to explain racial differences in aggressiveness; most of them address primarily the difference between blacks and whites in the United States. The theories were grouped into four broad categories (J.Q. Wilson and Herrnstein 1986, p. 466) according to the purported causative factors: constitutional differences between races, inadequacies of self-control (inability to delay gratification), a "subculture of violence," and economic deprivation.

The constitutional factors are "present at or soon after birth" (J.Q. Wilson and Herrnstein 1986, p. 466) and thus include genetic, prenatal, and perinatal influences. There is no evidence for genetic differences between blacks and whites in their propensity for violence. However, in the United States, most blacks probably receive inferior prenatal and perinatal care compared with most whites (C. McCord and Freeman 1990). This difference is reflected in higher rates of pregnancy and birth complications; studies relating these complications to violence and crime are discussed under "Pregnancy and Perinatal Factors" in this chapter.

Inadequacy of self-control or inadequate socialization is assumed to be related to child-rearing practices; single-parent families are particularly vulnerable. Single-parent families occur frequently in inner cities; this and other problems with families are discussed elsewhere (W.J. Wilson 1987). Inadequacies of self-control are probably related to aggressiveness, but I am not aware of empirical evidence demonstrating that blacks, in general, have less self-control than whites.

The subculture of violence theory (Wolfgang and Ferracuti 1967) states that criminals break the law because they reject the values of the larger society. It is possible that blacks are particularly likely to reject the values of the white-dominated society that has been oppressing them for hundreds of years.

The economic deprivation of blacks in the United States is well documented. Links between black poverty, unemployment, family dissolution, social dislocation, and crime were subjected to a penetrating analysis that focused on the history of social and economic discrimination that resulted in the current condition of the inner cities (W.J. Wilson 1987). This analysis emphasized the fact that the black middle and working classes moved out of the inner cities and were replaced by migrants who are not well equipped to compete in the shrinking job market. Thus, inner-city youths no longer have contact with successful mainstream role models; instead, they see drug dealers and other criminals. The social and economic pressures of the inner city have resulted in breakdowns of the family system, the schools, and other important institutions that in other communities teach young people discipline and respect for the law. These social dislocations in the inner cities thus increase crime rates even more than would be expected on the basis of current economic deprivation alone.

Current socioeconomic status, however, remains a powerful factor in explaining a large proportion of the black versus white difference in crime rates. A race effect on self-reported violent behavior was absent when socioeconomic status was controlled (Swanson et al. 1990). Intraracial domestic homicide rates in Atlanta were higher in the black than in the white households, but that difference disappeared when the researchers controlled for the effect of crowded households (Centerwall 1984, 1995). Crowding can be seen as a measure of (low) socioeconomic status.

Similar phenomena were observed in an analysis of childhood homicide in Ohio: "Blacks as a whole had higher rates than white children, but the difference tends to fade when socioeconomic status is taken into consideration, particularly for older children" (Muscat 1988, p. 822). Another investigation focused on the homicide victimization rate in New Orleans (Lowry et al. 1988). (Race-specific victimization rates are closely related to offending rates because most homicides are intraracial.) Blacks had higher victimization rates than whites. When the rates were presented as a function of the percentage of households below poverty level in the neighborhood, it was clear that the black versus white gap was larger in the poor neighborhoods than in the rich ones (Figure 5–5).

Although the interaction between neighborhood and race was apparently not formally tested, the data in Figure 5–5 suggest that the racial difference in homicide victimization is greatest among persons of low socioeconomic status, and it decreases as that status improves.

Nevertheless, even in the richest neighborhood studied, there was still an overrepresentation of blacks among homicide victims, suggesting that socioeconomic status could not completely account for the racial differences in homicide victimization. Similarly, black versus white differences in the rate of juvenile offending persisted after accounting for socioeconomic status (Wolfgang et al. 1972).

Blacks and whites, however, are difficult to match for socioeconomic status. One method of matching is to assign the same status to everybody

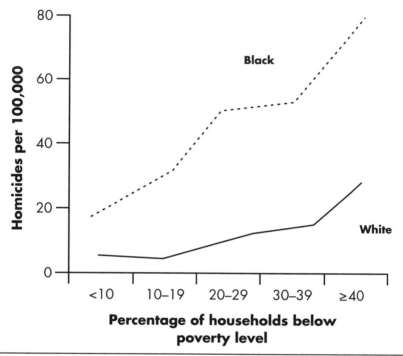

Figure 5–5. Mean annual homicide rate in New Orleans by race and poverty level of victim's neighborhood.

Source. Reprinted from Lowry PW, Hassig SE, Gunn RA, et al.: "Homicide Victims in New Orleans: Recent Trends." *American Journal of Epidemiology* 128:1130–1136, 1988. Used with permission.

who lives in the same census tract (Wolfgang et al. 1972); however, the incomes of blacks may be different than those of their white neighbors living in the same tract. Attempts to account for socioeconomic differences by stratification according to educational level (Rossi et al. 1986; Tardiff and Sweillam 1980) are not satisfactory; for example, high school graduates from inner-city schools are clearly different in socioeconomic status from those graduating in wealthy suburbs. More generally, stratification of a continuous variable (e.g., income) may result in overaggregation if the strata (or categories) are too broad (Leon 1993). For example, blacks may have a lower income than whites within the same stratum. Thus, the intended effect of stratification—adjustment for socioeconomic status—is defeated; moreover, this defeat is not appreciated by the researcher and his or her readers, who assume that the confounding effects of socioeconomic status were adequately controlled by the stratification. Therefore, a failure of the procedures used for matching blacks and whites on socioeconomic status may explain at least some of the racial differences in violent crime that remain after socioeconomic status has supposedly been accounted for.

Discrimination and economic deprivation have powerful effects on health. Links between illness or injury and violent behavior are incompletely understood. Besides the prenatal and perinatal complications discussed under "Pregnancy and Perinatal Factors" in this chapter, there are other (postnatal) health problems that have an impact on violent behavior.

Substance abuse is common in inner cities, and the violence associated with gang activity and drug marketing affects minority youths. The effects of alcohol and other abused substances on aggression are discussed in Chapter 8.

In addition to these obvious threats, there are other health risks that may be related to violence among underprivileged blacks. Lead intoxication, which in the past resulted mainly from the exposure of children to lead paint in substandard housing, may be associated with juvenile delinquency (see Chapter 4). Anemia showed a similar association with delinquency (Denno 1990). Lead interferes with several red cell enzyme systems, and thus lead exposure may lead to anemia. In any event, iron-deficiency anemia was (and probably still is) more prevalent among black children than among white children (Malina 1973, p. 59).

A landmark study on high mortality rates in Harlem (New York City) demonstrated the enormous health problems in inner cities (C. McCord and Freeman 1990). The causes of excessive mortality included homicide, drug dependency, and alcohol use—all directly or indirectly related to violence. Part of the excessive mortality was due to neonatal disorders. The study has attracted a lot of well-deserved attention; some of the commentators pointed out that similar health problems prevail in Philadelphia (Liebman et al. 1990) and probably in other American cities. Low availability of health care in inner cities, which is well documented (C. McCord and Freeman 1990), contributes to the poor health of the people living there.

In summary, the difference in violent behavior between blacks and whites in the United States can be largely explained by social forces. Biological mechanisms triggered by differences in the quality of health care probably contribute to the difference.

AGE

Arrest records and victimization surveys agree that the age distribution of perpetrators of violent crime peaks between ages 15 and 25 years (J. Q.

Wilson and Herrnstein 1986, p. 129). Self-reports of violent behavior by community residents yielded a similar result in one study (Swanson et al. 1990), but the results were equivocal in another study (Link et al. 1992).

Effects of age on violence in mentally ill offenders are somewhat different than those in the general population. The peak age of German violent offenders diagnosed with schizophrenia is somewhat higher (30–35 years) than that of violent offenders without a mental disorder (21–25 years) (Hafner and Boker 1982). Somewhat similar British data are presented in Figure 5–6.

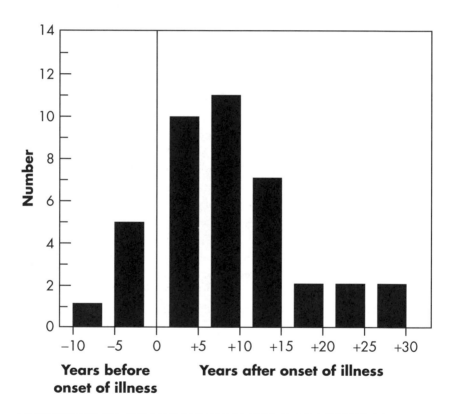

Figure 5–6. The relationship between age at onset of schizophrenia and the first infliction of injury against another person ($N=40$).

Source. Reprinted from Taylor PJ: "Schizophrenia and Crime: Distinctive Patterns in Association," in *Mental Disorder and Crime.* Edited by Hodgins S. Newbury Park, CA, Sage Publications, Inc., 1993, pp. 63–85. Used with permission.

As portrayed in Figure 5–6, the onset of aggression typically occurs during the first 5 or 10 years after the onset of illness (P.J. Taylor 1993, pp. 71–72). The average age at onset (time 0 in Figure 5–6) was 23 years (P.J. Taylor, personal communication, June 26, 1993). Thus, the average age at the first reported manifestation of aggression was 23–33 years, which is later than that in the general population. Figure 5–6 also shows that aggressive acts may precede the onset of illness. More detailed information on the incidence of aggressive acts before the illness onset, after the onset but before the first contact with psychiatric services, and after the first contact was provided in a study of first-episode psychosis (Milton et al. 2001) (see also Chapter 9). The younger age at onset of mental illness is associated with a worse outcome in terms of criminal behavior in the community (Wessely 1998) and persistent inpatient assaultiveness (Krakowski et al. 1988a).

Assaultive outpatients were younger than nonassaultive ones (Tardiff and Koenigsberg 1985), and younger mentally ill persons in the community were more likely to be arrested for violent crimes (Grossman et al. 1995). Among patients whose preadmission behavior in the community was examined after they were hospitalized, assaultive behavior was particularly common in males younger than 24 years (Tardiff and Sweillam 1980). However, another study using a similar strategy found no effect of age on preadmission assaultiveness (Rossi et al. 1986). In a study following up on psychiatric patients in the community for a year after their hospitalization, subjects ages 18–24 years had higher rates of arrest for violent crimes than older subjects (Klassen and O'Connor 1988a, p. 308). Similar results were reported for a 10.5-year follow-up of a cohort of patients discharged from a forensic hospital (Buchanan 1998): lower age at discharge was associated with higher conviction rates.

Similar age effects were documented among inpatients (Tardiff 1984; Tardiff and Sweillam 1982). Assaultiveness among inpatients was greatly reduced after age 30 years, but there was a slight increase in assaultiveness among women after age 65 years (Tardiff 1984).

It is regrettable that more is not known about interactions between age, violence, and the other factors just mentioned. It is quite possible that the age effects on violence vary with patients' diagnoses (similarly to the gender effect). Such interaction might explain the occasional inconsistencies of the age effect (Rossi et al. 1986).

The reviewed studies of the effect of age on violence were all cross-sectional. Information on fluctuations of violent acts over time within individuals was obtained in longitudinal studies. There is evidence suggesting continuity of aggressive behavior within individuals between childhood and age 30 years: people who are aggressive at one age are likely to be aggressive at another age. These issues are discussed in Chapter 6.

On the other hand, the reader should recall that the total number of crimes committed in a time period depends on the number of persons committing crimes and on the frequency of offending (see Chapter 1). Thus, the evidence for the peak age of perpetrators reviewed above could mean that the proportion of persons committing violent crimes increases in that peak age range or that violent criminals in that age range are particularly active (committing more crimes per year). Both of these mechanisms may be operating; the cross-sectional studies discussed above cannot address this issue. Longitudinal studies focusing on criminal careers suggest that the increased activity of criminals in this age range plays a role in the increased age-specific crime rates (Farrington 1986; Wessely and Taylor 1991).

Longitudinal information is available on psychopathic individuals. An age-related decrease in criminality (described by Hare as "burnout") has been clearly demonstrated for nonviolent crimes; surprisingly, the decrease for violent crimes appears much less dramatic and seems to occur as late as age 40 years (Hare et al. 1988).

Origins of Age Differences in Aggressiveness

Explanations of three events are needed: the onset of aggressive behavior, the decline and cessation of the behavior, and the reemergence of the behavior in elderly demented patients. At this point, I deal only with the first two events.

The onset of aggressive behavior at puberty is common among many mammalian species; it is preceded by increasingly serious play fighting. The activational effect of testosterone is discussed in Chapter 2. Maturational changes include physical growth and increased strength and agility; these features make real fighting (including potential damage to the fighters) much more feasible.

Additional effects operate in humans. Teenagers receive less supervision than younger children, peer pressures are stronger, and cravings for sex, money, and adventure are stronger than they are before puberty. Furthermore, some teenagers start using illicit drugs and alcohol.

If the patients whose mental illness starts early tend to be more violent than those with a later onset, this phenomenon may contribute to the frequently reported link between young age and violence. The relation between an early onset of mental illness and violence is intriguing. Perhaps these early-onset cases are related to an early neurodevelopmental effect causing both persistent aggression and mental illness.

The decline of aggressive behavior with age may be explained by the individuals' experience with the consequences of violent offending, increased responsibility to one's family and community, less intense cravings, decreased impulsiveness, or decreased physical strength and agility. "It is not hard to find or invent explanations by the dozen" (J.Q. Wilson and Herrnstein 1986, p. 144). The problem is that empirical support for these explanations has been lacking. What is needed is a better understanding of factors that switch aggression on at a certain age and then switch it off later. Such factors could be useful in the design of prevention and remediation efforts.

In summary, violent behavior peaks between ages 15 and 25 years among community residents and between ages 25 and 35 years among schizophrenic patients. Future research should focus on interactions between age and these other factors.

The age-related decline of violent behavior may be somewhat slower among psychopathic individuals. A slight increase in violent behavior among inpatients occurs after age 65 years.

Many explanations were offered for the age differences in aggressiveness. These explanations do not have firm empirical bases. If we understood the mechanisms increasing aggression in the teens and decreasing it in the late twenties, we would be in a better position to control violence.

SUMMARY AND CONCLUSIONS

Congenital effects on violence result from additive or interactive influences of genetic, prenatal, and perinatal factors.

Twin and adoption studies provided strong evidence for congenital and at least partly genetic effects on crime, aggressiveness, impulsiveness, and irritability. The propensity toward violent behavior results from interactions between genetic, prenatal, and perinatal factors. The effect of these factors is then modified by the rearing environment.

Studies of the effects of prenatal and perinatal factors on violence have yielded equivocal results. These factors are probably heterogeneous in their long-term effects on future violent behavior. The study that narrowed its focus to very low birth weight yielded clear effects, demonstrating increased levels of aggression and delinquency in boys at age 9 years.

The studies were designed before the effects of fetal exposure to maternal use of alcohol and cigarette smoking were fully appreciated, and the effects of these toxins were missed. This omission reduced the value of studies of prenatal and perinatal factors, as well as of adoption studies.

Men are more physically aggressive than women. This difference evolves in preschool years and is fully developed by puberty. Arrest rates, victimization surveys, and self-reports confirm this gender difference. The gender gap in violence is less expressed among psychiatric outpatients and disappears altogether among inpatients.

The gender gap has societal and biological origins. Males are more aggressive than females in most mammalian species. Testosterone is involved in maintaining this gender difference. In humans, males are more susceptible to alcohol abuse than females; alcohol elicits aggression under many conditions.

In the United States, race breakdowns of arrest rates and victimization surveys indicate that blacks perpetrate more violent crime than whites (relative to their proportions in the population). Blacks are also more frequently victimized than whites. This race difference appears to be less expressed among psychiatric patients in the community, and—similar to the gender effect—it disappears among inpatients.

The black-white difference in violent behavior can be largely explained by economic and social deprivation experienced by blacks. Increased risks for various disorders (e.g., substance abuse) and injuries, as well as the inferior health care available to poor blacks, probably contribute to the difference in violent behavior. These biological mechanisms are driven at least in part by social forces.

Among all the biological and social factors discussed, age has the most robust association with violent behavior. Arrest records, victimization surveys, and self-reports agree that most violent acts are perpetrated between ages 15 and 25 years. The peak age for violent behavior is 25–35 years in schizophrenic patients.

Interactions among age, violence, and other factors (such as gender, race, and diagnosis) have not been adequately studied. We need more data about the mechanisms subserving the age-related changes in violence.

6 | Developmental Antecedents of Violent Behavior

Neuropsychiatric disease, brain injury, or adverse environmental changes may cause a sudden emergence of violent behavior in adults who had been placid and untroubled all their lives. More frequently, however, violent behavior develops over a long period. Its antecedents can be congenital (see Chapter 5). Environmental influences that interact with the child's congenital endowment include family, school, peers, and community. The child's response to these influences affects those environments; the dynamic interplay developing over time between the individual and the environment is captured by the transactional model discussed in this book's introduction.

In this chapter, I first review evidence illuminating the continuity of aggressive and other deviant behavior from childhood to adulthood. This evidence, obtained largely in longitudinal prospective studies, contains information on developmental antecedents of violent (and criminal) behavior. The antecedents may be defined as one-dimensional behavioral measures (e.g., a teacher's ratings of aggressivity) or as more complex descriptions of a child's behavior (e.g., those included in a psychiatric diagnosis). Children diagnosed with attention-deficit/hyperactivity disorder (ADHD) may be at risk for violent and antisocial behavior as adults; this problem has been studied, and I review that work. General medical conditions are other antecedents of adult aggressive or criminal behavior.

Many studies of developmental antecedents were designed before the importance of child abuse and neglect for adult violent behavior was fully appreciated; therefore, these important developmental antecedents were largely ignored. Literature on child abuse is also reviewed.

Much of the aggressive behavior in children and adults has been learned. Some research indicates that it is the inhibition of aggression that has to be learned if a child is to develop into a responsible, law-abiding adult. A learning theory is described.

DEVELOPMENT AND CONTINUITY OF VIOLENT AND ANTISOCIAL BEHAVIOR

Strong evidence for the continuity of antisocial behavior has been obtained in longitudinal studies of several cohorts (Robins 1978). These studies demonstrated close relationships between juvenile and adult delinquency. Juveniles who start their criminal careers earlier are more likely to develop into recidivistic offenders than are those who start later. The probability of committing an offense increases with the number of previous offenses; for example, in a male cohort in which the probability of the first violent offense was 0.26, the probability of the sixth violent offense was 0.57 (Wolfgang 1983, p. 15). Thus, past behavior is a good predictor of future behavior.

Several classic longitudinal prospective studies (Glueck and Glueck 1950; Robins 1974) described the development of multiple aspects of deviancy; I now discuss other projects that dealt more specifically with violent behavior. In the Cambridge-Somerville Youth Study (J. McCord 1983, 1988), 227 boys selected between the ages of 5 and 9 years were followed up through their late 40s. Counselors visited the boys' families twice a month between 1939 and 1945 and provided descriptions of family environment, including the behaviors of the subjects and their parents. Child aggressiveness was rated. The counselors' reports also noted parents' aggressiveness (which included verbal and physical aggression), their affect, types of discipline exercised over the child, supervision of the child's activities outside of school, conflict between parents, and deviancy of the role model presented by each parent.

Criminal records of these subjects were obtained between 1976 and 1978, when they were in their 40s. The subject's aggressiveness as a child, history of inconsistent discipline or corporal punishment, absence of supervision, absence of parental affection, and parental aggressiveness were related to the development of registered criminality, including violent crime.

Another well-known project has a confusingly similar title: the Cambridge Study in Delinquent Development. This was a prospective longitudinal study of 411 boys who were first contacted in 1961–1962. At that time, they were 8 years old and living in a working-class area of London, England (Farrington 1989). They were selected because they attended schools in the vicinity of the researchers' office. Eight interviews of the subjects were completed between ages 8 and 24 years. Additional information was obtained from parents during home visits, from teachers, and from official records of criminal convictions.

The study provided evidence for the continuity of aggressive behavior. The best predictors of violent behavior fell into six categories of theoretical constructs: economic deprivation, family criminality, poor child rearing, school failure, hyperactivity-impulsivity-attention deficit (see "Attention-Deficit/Hyperactivity Disorder" below), and antisocial child behavior. Many variables defined each of these constructs. Even though Farrington provided extensive tables, it is difficult to evaluate the individual contributions of these constructs (or their component variables) to the variance of the four dependent variables (adolescent aggression, teenage violence, adult violence, and convictions for violence). Four multiple regression analyses were performed, and multiple r values ranged from 0.37 for the convictions to 0.49 for teenage violence (Farrington 1989, Table 4). Thus, the proportion of explained variance ranged from 14% to 24%.

A review of 16 studies indicated considerable stability (longitudinal consistency) of aggression in males over decades, although the size of a stability coefficient decreased linearly as the time between the measurements increased (Olweus 1979). Interindividual differences in aggressiveness manifested themselves by age 3 years. Subsequent work confirmed and extended the conclusions of this review.

Aggressiveness was assessed in an American (semirural) sample population of more than 600 subjects, their parents, and their children (Huesmann et al. 1984). Subjects who were more aggressive than others at age 8 years were also more aggressive at age 30 years. Early aggressiveness also predicted criminal convictions by age 30 years. In addition to the within-subject stability of aggression, these authors studied that stability across three generations. The stability across generations was not of a different order than the stability within the subjects' life span. Thus, the grandparents' aggressiveness was transmitted to their grandchildren. This study used path analysis (the method is discussed in Chapter 5).

In a Swedish prospective study (Stattin and Magnusson 1989), 517 boys were followed up from late childhood through age 26 years. Those rated as more aggressive by their teachers at age 10–13 years committed more violent crimes as adults than those who were rated as less aggressive. The proportions of variance in violence explained by the predictors were similar to those reported from Britain (Farrington 1989). These studies were not concerned with psychiatric patients. Continuity of aggressive behavior in psychotic patients over short time spans has been studied (Krakowski et al. 1988b; Volavka and Krakowski 1989), but we do not know enough about the long-term changes.

An important longitudinal prospective study is in progress in Mauritius (an island in the Indian Ocean). All children born in 1969 in two towns (N=1,795) were recruited into the study when they were age 3 years (in 1972 or 1973). A recent report from this study indicated that fearlessness, stimulation-seeking, and large body size at age 3 predisposes to aggressive behavior at age 11 (Raine et al. 1998b). Inspired by this report, a group of Finnish researchers analyzed the appropriate data from their longitudinal prospective study of the 1966 Northern Finland Birth Cohort. They found a similar (albeit weak) relationship between large body size in childhood and *adult* violent crime (Rasanen et al. 1999). The relationship may have interacted with gender in the Finnish sample (it was apparently more expressed in males), but not in the Mauritius sample.

Some of the empirical data reviewed above were used to set up complex theoretical models of the development of deviant behavior. One of these models posits four stages leading to delinquency and antisocial behavior (Patterson et al. 1992, p. 10).

In the first stage, parental effectiveness breaks down in repeated disciplinary confrontations. The child learns that aversive behaviors such as whining, crying, yelling, or hitting will turn off parental demands for compliance with various requests (e.g., a request to help with domestic chores). These exchanges between the child and other family members are termed coercive. These coercive confrontations gradually increase in frequency and in amplitude (the likelihood of hitting increases). Children who learn that physical aggression in family interactions brings desired results will resort to it with increasing frequency (Patterson et al. 1992, p. 53). The child eventually coerces the family to reduce supervision; this gives the child an opportunity to associate with similarly deviant peers in the street.

The second stage is linked to the child starting school. The abrasive, coercive style these children learned at home leads to failure in the development of social relationships with their peers. Furthermore, they soon fail academically because they avoid homework (and work at school) using the coercive techniques learned in their preschool years at home. These children are rejected by their parents, their teachers, and their schoolmates.

The third stage consists of the child's response to these multiple rejections. The only peers who will not reject him are those who are similar to him. Association with similarly deviant peers leads to truancy, substance abuse, and juvenile delinquency. The juvenile delinquent develops into an antisocial adult (stage four).

Thus, defects in social skills acquired before the child starts school may lead to peer rejection at school and to later antisocial outcomes. It is possible that growing up with siblings gives a preschool child a better opportunity to learn social skills than growing up alone. If this is true, one might expect that growing up as an only child would increase the risk for antisocial behavior in adulthood. This hypothesis was tested in male subjects in the northern Finland birth cohort (N=5,587). The risk for violent (but not nonviolent) crimes later in life was increased among the only children (Kemppainen et al. 2001). The relationship between being the only child and later violence appeared to interact with various other risk factors (e.g., perinatal) described elsewhere (see Chapter 5).

Summarizing some of the evidence reviewed in this book, I developed a mini-theory of the intergenerational transmission of violent behavior (Figure 6–1).

According to this mini-theory, the offspring learns aggressive behavior from the abuser as a target or as a witness of abuse (or both). Violent parents may also neglect their offspring, which may lead to later aggression, perhaps via inadequate supervision (Patterson et al. 1992). The abuse may result in head injuries; ample literature on the relationship between head injuries and violence exists (see Chapter 4). Alcohol may acutely increase the likelihood of the abuser's violent behavior (see Chapter 8); furthermore, hyperactivity, impulsiveness, bullying and fighting, and other antisocial behaviors may be late consequences of fetal exposure to toxins via maternal use of alcohol (Streissguth et al. 1991) or smoking cigarettes (Brennan et al. 1999) during pregnancy, or to maternal malnutrition during pregnancy (Neugebauer et al. 1999). Early maternal rejection may interact with obstetric complications to increase the risk for violent crime in the offspring (see Chapter 5) (Raine et al. 1997a). Finally, recent evidence indicates that genetic influences interacting with rearing environment affect the propensity for violent behavior (see Chapter 5).

In summary, there is robust evidence for the continuity of violent and antisocial behavior from childhood to adulthood and from one generation to another. Inappropriate parenting practices play a large role in the development of children's deviant behavior: inconsistent discipline, physical punishment, and inadequate supervision are some of the important adverse influences. Fetal exposure to toxins, parental alcohol abuse, head injuries, and other biological effects are also involved.

ATTENTION-DEFICIT/HYPERACTIVITY DISORDER

Attention-deficit/hyperactivity disorder is one of the most common behavior disorders in children, particularly boys. The children are over-

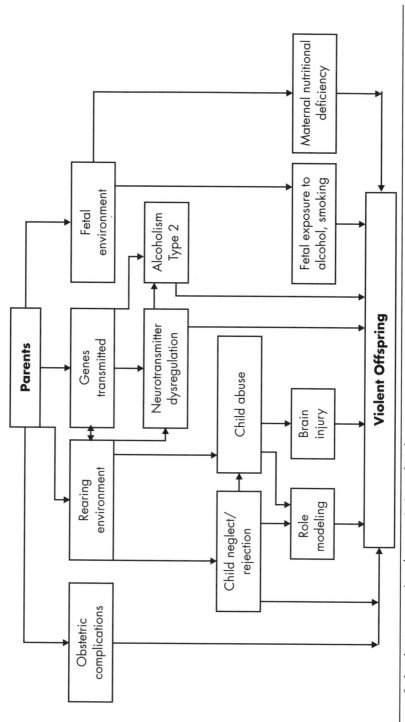

Figure 6–1. Intergenerational transmission of violence.

active, easy to distract, impulsive, and aggressive. These problems and the associated learning disability lead frequently to academic failure at school; that failure may be a link in the chain of events that eventually leads to delinquency. (See the preceding section; also Patterson et al. 1992.) What happens to these children when they grow up has been a concern for several decades, and several prospective studies have addressed this question.

An early study examined 83 children (75 boys and 8 girls) between ages 12 and 16 years who were diagnosed with the "hyperactive syndrome" 2–5 years earlier (W. Mendelson et al. 1971). At follow-up, 51% of the children were involved in fighting, 34% threatened to kill their parents, 59% had some contact with the police, and 17% were involved with the police three or more times. No control group was used; thus, it cannot be determined whether these behaviors deviated from those commonly observed among teenagers in the community in which these subjects lived. Nevertheless, the authors felt that this degree of involvement in antisocial behavior was unusually high. In a similar but less elaborate study, half the boys who had been hyperactive in grade school experienced major conflicts with authority by age 14 years (Ackerman et al. 1977).

Somewhat more optimistic results were reported by a Canadian group in a 10-year prospective follow-up study of young adults (average age, 21 years) who had been diagnosed as hyperactive in childhood (Hechtman et al. 1984). This study used a comparison (nonhyperactive) group. All information reported in this study (including the offenses and court referrals) was obtained by interviewing the subjects. No official criminal records were available.

Aggression was more pronounced in the hyperactive group before age 15 years, but it ceased around that age. Court referrals tended to be more frequent in the hyperactive group, but the difference from control subjects did not reach the level of statistical significance. A similar lack of difference was observed in tests comparing the seriousness of offenses (including violent offenses) between the groups. However, at the follow-up, the sample was reduced to 73% of its original size because of refusals or inability to trace subjects. Unfortunately, there was also a trend ($P<0.06$) for the dropouts to have higher initial scores on aggressiveness. Thus, the relatively optimistic outcome reported by these researchers may have been influenced by a biased attrition of the final sample.

Many of the methodological shortcomings of the work just discussed (Hechtman et al. 1984) were avoided in another prospective study that relied on official arrest records; this information was obtained for 100% of the subjects (Satterfield et al. 1982). Two groups of boys (average age,

17 years) were studied: one group (*n*=110) had been diagnosed in childhood with attention-deficit disorder (ADD), and the second group (*n*=88) consisted of psychiatrically healthy control subjects. The ADD group had a significantly higher arrest rate for serious offenses than the control subjects, and the difference was not attributable to socioeconomic status.

Another prospective follow-up study examined 103 males (ages 16–23 years) who had been diagnosed with attention-deficit/hyperactivity disorder (ADHD) between ages 6 and 12 years and 100 psychiatrically healthy control subjects (Mannuzza et al. 1989). The official arrest records indicated that significantly more probands than control subjects had been arrested (39% versus 20%), convicted (28% versus 11%), and incarcerated (9% versus 1%). Arrests for aggressive offenses defined as robbery, assault, property destruction, and weapon use were significantly more frequent among probands than among control subjects (18% versus 7%). These differences between probands and control subjects were mediated by the development of an antisocial personality in early adulthood. There was a subgroup of ADHD children (approximately 25%) who developed antisocial personality disorder, and this subgroup was at a particularly high risk for arrests.

Hyperactivity may interact with parental psychopathology and perinatal complications in the development of violent crime (Brennan et al. 1993); this work is reviewed in the section on congenital factors (see "Pregnancy and Perinatal Factors" in Chapter 5).

In summary, despite the methodological differences among studies (which include changing diagnostic criteria for hyperactivity syndrome), there is a clear preponderance of evidence that male children with ADHD are at risk for later involvement in noncriminal and criminal violence, as well as in other types of criminal activity. The mechanism is unclear. Perhaps the children become delinquent because of a failure to develop proper social bonds; their persistent academic failure could be involved here. Perhaps hyperactivity, unimportant by itself, is a marker of prenatal or perinatal brain damage that predisposes to aggressive or antisocial behavior, perhaps interacting with a genetic or environmental influence of parental psychopathology.

The behavior of a hyperactive child can frustrate the parents; that frustration may lead to a punitive style of child rearing. There is some evidence for this punitive style (Weiss and Hechtman 1986, p. 173). Details are not known, although it is possible that hyperactive children are more frequently abused than others. Effects of child abuse are discussed in the next section.

CHILD ABUSE AND NEGLECT

"Violence Breeds Violence—Perhaps?" is the title of an early essay (Curtis 1963) considering the possibility that today's abused children will grow up to be tomorrow's murderers (a "cycle of violence"). A lot of work has been done in this area since that article was published, but much of the uncertainty suggested by the article's title remains to be resolved.

Child abuse and neglect are ascertained retrospectively by self-reports of juveniles or adults, by official court records, or by interviewing and observing children and family members in their home environment or elsewhere. The subjects selected for the study of child abuse are most frequently criminal offenders or psychiatric patients; "normal" subjects or community samples are studied less frequently. One can classify the studies of child abuse and neglect according to the method of ascertainment and the type of subjects studied.

Retrospective self-reports of abuse by juveniles or adults are used in studies that share certain design features. Most of these studies identified violent subjects who were asked about their childhood. The subjects were either offenders (Climent et al. 1973; Corder et al. 1976; C.H. King 1975; Lewis et al. 1985, 1988, 1989; Sendi and Blomgren 1975) or psychiatric patients (Else et al. 1993; Felthous 1980; A. Rosenbaum and Hoge 1989; Yesavage 1983a); the dividing line between offenders and patients was not always clear. These studies generally yielded the expected result: the subjects said that they had been abused.

Exceptionally, self-reports of child abuse were obtained in patients who were *not* selected for violence (or any other specific behavioral problem). In such patients, reports of childhood physical and sexual abuse were associated with adult dissociative experiences (Goff et al. 1991). However, adult reconstruction of childhood events is unreliable and difficult to corroborate in patients with multiple personality disorder (Frankel 1993) and probably in other patients as well. The reliability of these reconstructions is particularly doubtful in offenders who might expect that a history of child abuse could reduce their culpability.

Furthermore, the studies lack control groups; the frequency at which nonviolent, otherwise comparable patients or offenders report child abuse is not known. When control groups were used, they were too small for meaningful comparisons (Lewis et al. 1985; Sendi and Blomgren 1975).

"Normal" subjects (persons not selected among offenders or patients) were interviewed about childhood experiences. College students revealed that corporal punishment of children was a widely used method of behavior management; it was reported by 95% of the sample ($n=170$).

This high percentage, however, was due to the inclusion of relatively benign forms of corporal punishments such as light slaps. High levels of corporal punishment were associated with reports of aggression, lack of friends, and delinquency (Bryan and Freed 1982).

A set of "normal" Danish males ($N=201$) were interviewed at age 18–21 years in the context of a study of alcoholism (Pollock et al. 1990). Some reported physical beatings in childhood, and these self-reports were associated with current aggressive behavior.

The reports on normal subjects suggest an association between child abuse and adult aggressive behavior. However, the retrospective nature of these reports makes it difficult to determine whether the currently observed aggressive behavior developed before or after the physical abuse in childhood. If a causal relationship between these two phenomena exists, retrospective-report studies do not permit us to determine the direction of the relationship (i.e., identify cause and effect). Contemporaneous interviews of children were used in several longitudinal prospective studies. The data provided in interviews of family members—including the children themselves—are presumably less distorted by inaccuracies inherent in the retrospective self-reports of childhood experiences by adults.

In the Cambridge-Somerville Youth Study (see "Development and Continuity of Violent and Antisocial Behavior" above), men reared by aggressive parents became aggressive adults (J. McCord 1983). Those reared by parents who were generally nonaggressive but severely disciplined their children became self-centered adults.

In another prospective study (Huesmann et al. 1984), parental aggressiveness was measured by the severity of punishment of the subjects (who were 8 years old when this information was collected). Information on the aggressiveness of the subjects' children (age 6–12 years) was obtained when the subjects were 30 years old. Remarkably, the punishment meted out by the subjects' parents to the subjects was correlated not only with the subjects' aggression at age 8 years, but also with the subjects' children's aggression. Even more remarkably, the correlation coefficients between generations 1 and 2 and generations 1 and 3 were equal (Huesmann et al. 1984, p. 1131). These data suggest that aggression can be transmitted across at least three generations.

The studies mentioned up to this point show a wide variation in the way they defined and ascertained the independent variables (abusive or aggressive behaviors toward children) and the dependent variables (the aggressive behaviors exhibited by the children after they grew up). This variability makes it difficult to compare, generalize, and replicate the results of these studies.

One way to reduce this variability is to rely on official records of child abuse and of violent crime. These records may underreport child abuse, but once a record exists, it is probably better substantiated and less ambiguous than much of the data obtained by interviews. Therefore, a well-known study accessed all court records of substantiated sexual and physical child abuse and neglect in a metropolitan area in the Midwest that were processed during the years 1967 through 1971 (Widom 1989b). The children ($n=908$) were less than 11 years old at the time of victimization. Widom established a matched control group of children who had no official record of being abused or neglected ($n=667$).

At the time when the subjects' average age was 25.7 years, juvenile and adult official records (local, state, and federal) were searched to trace their criminal histories. Arrests for violent offenses occurred in 15.8% of the physically abused subjects compared with 7.9% of the control subjects. Subjects who were physically abused or neglected as children had a significantly higher likelihood of an arrest for violent crime than the control subjects. This result was obtained when sex, age, and race were accounted for. However, each of these three factors appeared to have a considerably greater effect on the likelihood of arrest for violent crime than did the history of child abuse or neglect (Federal Bureau of Investigation 1987, p. 164, Table 3). Additional details can be found elsewhere (Widom 1989a).

Most abused children did not grow up to be violent adults, and most adults arrested for violent crimes had not been victims of child abuse. Nevertheless, Widom's results provide important support for the existence of the cycle of violence. The childhood experiences she reports were clearly antecedent to the arrests for violent crime; the clarity about this sequence of events was missing in most previous research. Of course, the behavior that eventually led to the adult arrest might have developed gradually in childhood and perhaps elicited the abuse. This speculation is based on the extensive literature on the continuity of aggressive behavior reviewed above.

As pointed out in a "friendly amendment" by two geneticists (DiLalla and Gottesman 1991), Widom did not consider the possibility that the abusing parents might have been criminal and that the propensity for violent crime was transmitted genetically. In addition to the possibility of direct genetic transmission resulting in a set of congenital properties, there may be a genetic component even in later influences that are traditionally considered environmental; these masked genetic components influencing child development have been estimated quantitatively by using data from several adoption studies (Plomin et al. 1985). Surprisingly, neither the critique (DiLalla and Gottesman 1991) nor Widom's response (Widom 1991) explicitly considers the possibility that genetic (and, more generally, biological) factors may interact with the rearing environment (see Figure 6–1).

In summary, strong evidence for the intergenerational transmission of violence exists. The mechanisms of this transmission are not quite clear. "Researchers in the areas of violence and criminality need to keep an open mind and eye on both the social and biological literature" (Widom 1991, p. 131) and plan their work accordingly: future research projects should include both social and biological variables. Unless both types of variables are investigated in the same subjects, it will not be possible to understand the mechanisms of intergenerational transmission of violence.

LEARNING LAW ABIDANCE

Repeated fights or assaults constitute one of the diagnostic criteria for antisocial personality disorder (see Chapter 7). Persons with this disorder (or *psychopathy*, to use the classic term) lack remorse and shame, show general poverty of affect, fail to learn by experience, and do not conform to laws or other social norms. It is possible that low emotionality leads to a failure to learn law abidance; violence may then be a final manifestation of that failure.

Important components of moral sense, such as sociability and empathy, are detectable very early in life and may be innate (J.Q. Wilson 1993). However, much socialized, law-abiding behavior has to be learned. It is not clear how this learning takes place, and which anatomical structures in the nervous system are recruited for this purpose at what developmental time period. Orbital prefrontal cortex lesions occurring before 16 months of age preceded defective social and moral reasoning in two adult patients, suggesting that the learning of moral rules had been impaired by these lesions (see Chapter 4) (Anderson et al. 1999). Thus, this area may play a role in the early development of moral sense.

Arousal and fear are thought to play a role in this learning process. Therefore, these two emotional states are worth studying in this context. Observable, overt reflections of these emotional states can be detected and measured in heart rate, skin conductance, and electrical brain activity. Each measure can be taken under resting or stimulated conditions. Heart rate is a relatively simple measure requiring no special explanation. Electrical brain activity and its acquisition and analyses are discussed in Chapter 4. Skin conductance requires some explanation.

Skin Conductance Technique and Measures

To measure skin conductance, electrodes are attached to two fingers of the same hand. These two electrodes form a bipolar lead. A small current from an external source is passed across the electrodes through the skin, and resistance (the reciprocal of conductance) to its passage is measured. Conductance is measured and recorded continuously. In the display, the vertical axis is calibrated in units of conductance; conventionally, the increase in conductance is indicated by an upward deflection. These deflections are called skin conductance responses (SCRs). An SCR may occur as a response to a stimulus or "spontaneously" (i.e., without a stimulus controlled by the experimenter). The latter type is called nonspecific SCR (NS-SCR). In addition to the SCRs, one can measure the basic skin conductance level (SCL). A schematic representation of the SCR is presented in Figure 6–2.

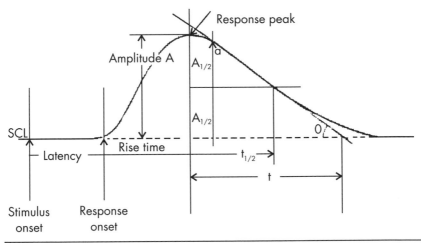

Figure 6–2. Schematic representation of the skin conductance response. Before the stimulus onset *(left side of figure)*, one can see the skin conductance level (SCL). t=recovery time; $t_{1/2}$=half-recovery time; $A_{1/2}$=half-amplitude.

Source. Reprinted from Venables PH: "The Recovery Limb of the Skin Conductance Response in 'High-Risk' Research," in *Genetics, Environment and Psychopathology* (North-Holland Research Series on Early Detection and Prevention of Behaviour Disorders, Vol. 1). Edited by Mednick SA, Schulsinger F, Higgins J, et al. Amsterdam, Netherlands, North-Holland, 1974, pp. 117–133. Used with permission.

Figure 6–2 shows the magnitude of the response (amplitude) and its three temporal aspects: latency (time between stimulus onset and response onset), rise time (time between response onset and peak), and recovery (time between peak and a defined decrease of amplitude). The recovery time can be difficult to measure because the response may not recover completely for a long time and because it may not be easy to determine exactly when the full recovery (return to baseline) occurred. The half-recovery time is a more practical measure to use. The half-recovery rate can be calculated by dividing the half-amplitude by the half-recovery time. Details can be found in the original publication (Venables 1974, pp. 117–121). The half-recovery rate was used as a measure of speed of recovery in most of Mednick's work described below.

Learning and Arousal

Pavlovian conditioning is one method for the gradual socialization of children. Antisocial actions are punished, and because they are repeatedly associated with punishment, eventually even contemplation of such actions is accompanied by conditioned fear and perhaps guilt. Thus, conscience can be seen as a conditioned reflex (H.J. Eysenck 1964, p. 110; H.J. Eysenck and Gudjonsson 1989, p. 111).

Pavlovian literature indicates that low arousal inhibits conditioning. Therefore, if the learning of socialized behavior (and law abidance) is accomplished via conditioning, one would expect children with habitually low levels of arousal to have more difficulty learning socialized behavior and to be more likely to break laws when they grow up.

There is empirical support for a connection between low arousal and (nonviolent) criminality. Persuasive evidence for this link came from a longitudinal prospective study that started with 101 English schoolboys. When the subjects were 15 years old, arousal was estimated by the following measures: power in six electroencephalographic frequency bands, NS-SCR and SCL (see the previous "Skin Conductance Technique and Measures" section for explanations), and heart rate (Raine et al. 1990b). In addition, autonomic orienting responses were obtained by using skin conductance and heart rate (Raine et al. 1990a).

Criminal status was assessed when the subjects were approximately 24 years old. Official records indicated that 17 of the 101 subjects were found guilty and sentenced; the offenses were mostly burglary and theft. These 17 subjects were designated "criminals," and the remaining 84 subjects were designated "noncriminals." These two groups were compared on the skin, heart, and electroencephalographic measures collected when they were approximately 15 years old. As predicted, the future criminals had fewer NS-SCRs, lower SCL, lower heart rates, and more electroencephalographic power in lower frequency bands than the noncriminals. Each of these differences indicated a lower level of arousal among the future criminals (Raine et al. 1990b). The orienting responses were smaller in the future criminals, indicating a deficit in autonomic orienting (Raine et al. 1990a). The measures of arousal used by the authors are partly genetically determined, and the measures were taken before the start of most subjects' criminal careers. For these reasons, the authors speculated that the low arousal may be a biological manifestation of a genetic predisposition to criminality.

Unfortunately, the sample was too small to separately present the results for violent and nonviolent crime. Furthermore, the absence of criminal activity among the "noncriminals" at age 24 years is uncertain (because not all criminals are sentenced). In addition, some of the "noncriminals" at age 24 may have become "criminals" later. Nevertheless, these papers (Raine et al. 1990a, 1990b) and the literature they cite suggest that low arousal may be an antecedent of nonviolent crime.

In summary, inhibition of antisocial behavior is learned, conditioned reflexes are involved in that process, conditioning in general is hindered by low arousal level, and low arousal level precedes the development of some forms of criminality. It is not yet clear whether violent crime is associated with low arousal.

Learning, Anxiety, and Fear

Experimental support for the role of conditioned anxiety in the learning of prosocial behavior first emerged in studies of psychopathic individuals. One of the earliest studies compared prisoners meeting diagnostic criteria for psychopathy (Cleckley 1976) with other prisoners and with nonprisoner control subjects (Lykken 1957). Compared with control subjects, the psychopathic individuals were less able to develop conditioned anxiety (as measured by SCR) to auditory stimuli previously associated with painful electric shocks. The psychopathic individuals were also relatively incapable of avoidance learning. Criminal or other behaviors of the subjects outside of the experimental situation are not mentioned; it is not known whether they were violent. This pioneering paper influenced subsequent research and is still widely quoted.

So far I have discussed three variables derived from skin conductance measurement: NS-SCR, SCR, and SCL. I now turn to skin conductance recovery. Slow recovery was associated with antisocial behavior (although not necessarily with aggression) in studies summarized elsewhere (Mednick and Volavka 1980, pp. 119–122).

Mednick's mini-theory based on the data I have discussed so far explains the development of inhibition of antisocial aggression (Mednick and Volavka 1980, pp. 116–119). The theory posits the following sequence of events:

1. Child contemplates aggressive action.
2. Because of previous punishment, he or she experiences fear.
3. Fear inhibits the aggressive action.
4. Fear dissipates. Fast dissipation is a natural reinforcer of the inhibitory response. The faster the reduction of fear, the more effective the reinforcement.

The speed of the fear reduction is partially controlled by the autonomic nervous system; it can be estimated by the speed of the skin conductance recovery. If the speed of the conductance recovery (and the concomitant fear reduction) is too slow, the reinforcement for inhibiting the aggressive action will be inadequate and the child will not learn to inhibit aggression.

It should be noted that the first three steps follow the lines suggested by H.J. Eysenck (1964); the core of the hypothesis is in step 4. Additional discussion of Mednick's mini-theory can be found elsewhere (Mednick et al. 1982).

SUMMARY AND CONCLUSIONS

Harbingers of violent behavior are present in early childhood, well before the school years. The development of a future violent person is affected by inappropriate parenting practices, including inadequate supervision and inconsistent, punitive discipline. ADHD increases the risk for later violent behavior (including violent crime) and nonviolent crime. Child abuse has similar effects. Interergenerational transmission of violence is effected by interactions between genetic, prenatal, and perinatal factors that modify the child's response to the rearing environment. A mini-theory that seeks to integrate these mechanisms is presented.

Specific physiologic traits may predispose to the development of antisocial (including aggressive) behavior by interfering with the child's ability to learn the inhibition of such behaviors. One such trait is a low level of arousal as demonstrated by central and peripheral measures. Another trait may be a slow recovery of skin conductance responses; Mednick's mini-theory explaining the effect of this trait on learning to inhibit aggression is reviewed.

7 | Personality Disorders and Impulse Control

The diagnostic separation of personality disorders from impulse control disorders was introduced with DSM-III in 1980 (American Psychiatric Association 1980). The previous version of the manual, DSM-II (American Psychiatric Association 1968), included the diagnostic category "explosive personality disorder" among personality disorders. This diagnostic category was replaced in DSM-III by "intermittent explosive disorder," which was removed from the group of personality disorders and placed in the new group of impulse control disorders.

Impulsive behavior is included among the diagnostic criteria for antisocial and borderline personality disorders (American Psychiatric Association 1994). Problems of impulse control are seen not only in the impulse control disorders and personality disorders but also in eating disorders, substance abuse disorders, and some other diagnostic groups. An overarching category was therefore proposed: a "multi-impulsive personality disorder" (Lacey and Evans 1986). Even if not formally accepted, such a category could stimulate useful research into neurobiological features shared by persons classified in these categories. In any event, personality disorders and impulse control disorders are both discussed in this chapter.

PERSONALITY DISORDERS

Maturational or developmental factors are generally recognized to play a role in the causation of personality disorders, and the DSM-IV diagnostic criteria for antisocial personality disorder (ASP) formally incorporate childhood and adolescent behaviors (American Psychiatric Association 1994). The DSM-IV criteria stipulate that the diagnosis of ASP cannot be made in patients younger than 18 years, but this age limit is arbitrary.

Many incarcerated offenders meet the other criteria for the diagnosis of ASP before age 18 years (Eppright et al. 1993).

In general, personality and its disorders can be described in terms of a multidimensional space or in terms of categories. The dimensional approach respects the graded nature of personality traits, whereas the categorical approach follows the traditional medical model based on diagnoses. In violence research, the diagnostic approach is less useful than the dimensional one. Certain personality dimensions (such as impulsiveness) cut across diagnostic categories and have better-defined neurobiological underpinnings than do diagnoses. As a result, research on links between personality dimensions and violence is inherently more interesting than research on (categorical) personality disorders and violence. Furthermore, some personality disorder diagnoses include aggressive and criminal behavior among the diagnostic criteria. This makes the relationship between violence and personality disorders tautological. The tautology can be mitigated by removing from the lists of diagnostic criteria those items that directly reflect violence or crime; I return to this issue in a subsequent discussion of ASP. Despite these disadvantages, personality disorder diagnoses have been widely used, and much literature is set within the diagnostic framework. Diagnoses of personality disorders will inevitably continue to be used in forensic and general psychiatric practice.

The most influential model of personality was developed by Eysenck, who proposed three principal orthogonal dimensions: extraversion-introversion, neuroticism, and psychoticism. The model was used to explain aspects of criminal behavior (H.J. Eysenck 1964; H.J. Eysenck and Gudjonsson 1989). Another dimensional approach was taken by Zuckerman (1979), who sought to explain disinhibited behavior by "sensation seeking."

Dimensional and categorical aspects of personality were reconciled in a model with three dimensions to describe traditional personality disorder diagnostic categories (Cloninger 1987). The dimensions were "novelty seeking" (pursuit of excitement and avoidance of monotony, similar to Zuckerman's sensation seeking), "harm avoidance" (inhibition of behavior to avoid punishment), and "reward dependence" (marked responsiveness to reward or to relief of punishment). The principal neuromodulators proposed for these dimensions were, respectively, dopamine, serotonin, and norepinephrine. In this theoretical model, high novelty seeking was associated with impulsive behavior. Aggressive behavior was associated with high novelty seeking and low harm avoidance. ASP was defined as a combination of high novelty seeking, low harm avoidance, and low reward dependence. It is surprising that this elegant, intellectually appealing model has apparently not yet stimulated much research in the area of violence.

Antisocial Personality Disorder and Psychopathy

Among the subtypes of personality disorder, ASP has the closest links to violence and is partly defined by acts of violence. In DSM-IV-TR (American Psychiatric Association 2000), diagnostic criterion C calls for evidence of conduct disorder with onset before age 15 years. Seven of the 15 behaviors defining conduct disorder involve physical aggression against people or animals: bullying, fighting, using weapons, physical cruelty to people, physical cruelty to animals, robbing, and forcing someone into sexual activity. Robust evidence for the continuity of violent behavior (see Chapter 6) indicates that some of the enumerated violent behaviors continue into adulthood.

The validity of the definitions of ASP in DSM-III and DSM-III-R (American Psychiatric Association 1987), which are closely related to the current DSM-IV-TR definition, is supported by neurobiological studies (e.g., Virkkunen et al. 1994). Nevertheless, these definitions of ASP have some disadvantages for violence research. Because only 7 of the 15 behaviors defining conduct disorder in DSM-IV-TR involve physical aggression, and because only 3 of the 15 criteria need to be met for the diagnosis of conduct disorder, criterion C for ASP can be met without a history of violence, or it can be met exclusively (or partly) with items reflecting violence. Criterion A can be met with or without violence. Thus, without the individual criteria leading to the diagnosis (which are rarely published), the ASP diagnosis per se does not allow an inference about violence.

Thus, the answer to the question "Does ASP predict violent behavior?" depends on the items constituting the diagnosis in individual cases. Because the mix of items varies among subjects and studies, results concerning violent behavior based on a diagnosis of ASP are difficult to replicate.

Furthermore, the list of ASP diagnostic criteria contains many behaviors that are against the law. The criteria needed for the ASP diagnosis can be met without any history of illegal behavior, or they can be met exclusively (or partly) by items reflecting illegal behavior. The diagnosis of ASP per se does not allow any inference about illegal behavior. However, it can be assumed that offenders who meet the ASP criteria do so primarily for the same reasons that brought them to the attention of the criminal justice system. Thus, the utility of the ASP diagnosis is reduced in studies of prisoners and similar populations: a diagnostic procedure is not needed to determine that these subjects broke laws.

Another more general problem regarding ASP is that the diagnostic criteria are repeatedly revised. This problem applies to any diagnostic system and is not specific to ASP or the DSM. The problem with ASP is not only that the criteria for the disorder are revised; even the name of the disorder changes. *Psychopathy* and *psychopathic personality* were replaced by *sociopathic personality disturbance*, subsuming *antisocial reaction* as well as *addiction* (American Psychiatric Association 1952, p. 38). The term *ASP* emerged in DSM-II.

These changes in terminology were related to a profound transformation of the underlying concepts. These transformations have a particularly important impact on longitudinal prospective studies that span several revisions of the diagnostic criteria.

Comorbidity of ASP with other disorders may affect the likelihood of violent behavior. ASP diagnosis was associated with violent crime among jail detainees (Abram 1989); the number of arrests for violent crime was further increased among detainees who had substance abuse disorders co-occurring with ASP (Abram 1989, p. 140). Most jail detainees with major mental disorders (schizophrenia or mood disorders) also met criteria for ASP or substance abuse disorders (Abram and Teplin 1991). In a sample that was representative of male penitentiary inmates in Canada, 63% of schizophrenic inmates also met diagnostic criteria for ASP (Cote and Hodgins 1990). Co-occurrence of schizophrenia and ASP may cause clinical problems in individual cases; failure to recognize schizophrenia in ASP patients may deprive them of appropriate antipsychotic treatment (Travin and Protter 1982). A subtype of alcoholism, which is transmitted genetically from fathers to sons and starts early in life, is associated with many of the behaviors common in ASP. Frequent fights, particularly after drinking, are characteristic (see Chapter 8) (Cloninger et al. 1981).

Some of the biological concomitants of ASP are reviewed in sections on CSF 5-HIAA, glucose tolerance, and monoamine oxidase (see Chapter 3), frontal lobes (see Chapter 4), adoption studies (see Chapter 5), and learning law abidance (see Chapter 6).

Psychopathy was a loosely used term until Cleckley (1976) endowed it with specific content, conceptual framework, and classic clinical descriptions. *The Mask of Sanity* (Cleckley 1976) influenced several generations of clinicians and researchers, including Hare (1986), who has continued to use the term *psychopathy* although it was discarded by the American Psychiatric Association decades ago. Discarded terms, of course, are no longer revised by an official committee; this can be seen as an advantage by researchers who may dislike repeated redefinitions of the disorders they study.

Hare developed several versions of a psychopathy checklist based on Cleckley's work. One of them is called the Psychopathy Checklist–Revised (PCL-R). This checklist has 20 items; a brief description and references to appropriate manuals is elsewhere (Hart et al. 1994; Kaye and Shea 2000, pp. 729–732). Unlike the current ASP criteria, which focus largely on criminal behavior, the checklist emphasizes personality traits and psychological processes. These traits and processes may be more difficult to define and ascertain than discrete criminal behaviors such as an arrest for driving while intoxicated. Therefore, one would expect the checklist to have a relatively low reliability. Surprisingly, the indices of checklist reliability (α coefficients and intrarater and interrater reliability) were very high (Schroeder et al. 1983). Psychopathy is a narrower concept than ASP: most psychopaths meet the diagnostic criteria for ASP, but most individuals with ASP are not psychopaths.

Several studies demonstrated that psychopathy was associated with violent crime (Hare and McPherson 1984). The checklist was typically used to classify offenders into two or three categories (psychopaths and nonpsychopaths; or psychopaths, mixed, and nonpsychopaths).

Psychopaths as defined by the checklist showed a higher mean number of criminal charges (including charges of violent crime) per year out of prison compared with nonpsychopaths. Convictions for violent crimes were more frequent among the psychopaths (85%) than the nonpsychopaths (54%). A very similar proportional difference was observed between the groups for violent behavior in prison (Hare and McPherson 1984).

Hare and his associates developed a shorter version of the psychopathy checklist, the Psychopathy Checklist: Screening Version (PCL:SV) (Table 7–1), which was tested in populations with various major psychiatric disorders (Hart et al. 1994).

Table 7–1.   Items in the Psychopathy Checklist: Screening Version (PCL:SV)

Factor 1: "interpersonal/affective"	Factor 2: "social deviance"
1. Superficial	7. Impulsive
2. Grandiose	8. Poor behavior controls
3. Manipulative	9. Lacks goals
4. Lacks remorse	10. Irresponsible
5. Lacks empathy	11. Adolescent antisocial behavior
6. Doesn't accept responsibility	12. Adult antisocial behavior

Source.   Adapted from Hart SD, Cox DN, Hare RD. *The Hare Psychopathy Checklist: Screening Version.* Toronto, Ontario, Canada, Multi-Health Systems; 1995.

The items are scored according to specific criteria on the basis of interview and collateral case history information. Each item is scored on a 3-point scale: 0=doesn't apply, 1=applies to an extent, 2=applies. Standard cutoffs for the PCL:SV total score classify individuals scoring 12 or less as nonpsychopathic. Those who score 18 or higher are classified as psychopathic. Scores of 13 through 17 indicate possible psychopathy. Analyses of the PCL:SV have yielded two factors. Factor 1 reflects personal and affective characteristics; Factor 2 reflects a socially deviant, unstable lifestyle. Hare argues that the ASP criteria should be revised to include more personality traits (such as those comprising Factor 1 of the PCL:SV) in future editions of the DSM (Hare 1996). I think that he is right.

Comorbidity of psychopathy with major mental disorders is an issue that has clinical, legal, and policy implications. Schizophrenia is associated with an increased risk for violence (see Chapters 9 and 10), and not all violent acts by schizophrenic patients can be clearly linked to psychotic symptoms. Individuals with schizophrenia may commit violent acts that are premeditated and similar in their apparent motivation to those committed by persons without mental illness (Rice 1997; Volavka et al. 1995). Thus, comorbidity with psychopathy may explain some of the violent behavior in schizophrenia patients.

Comorbidity of psychopathy with schizophrenia in general forensic patient populations is less than 4% (Hart and Hare 1989; Rice and Harris 1995). However, the comorbidity rate was 17% in a small sample of mentally ill patients selected for extreme dangerousness or violence (Rasmussen and Levander 1996). It is possible that the persistent, repetitive violent behavior in schizophrenic or schizoaffective patients is linked to underlying comorbid psychopathy. This hypothesis was tested in a study that compared the PCL:SV in 26 persistently violent patients with 25 matched nonviolent patients (Nolan et al. 1999b). There were statistically significant differences on the following items: "Lacks remorse," "Lacks empathy," "Doesn't accept responsibility," "Impulsive," "Poor behavioral controls," "Irresponsible," "Adolescent antisocial behavior," and "Adult antisocial behavior" (Nolan et al. 1999b, Table 3). Using the standard cutoff values, 5 violent patients (19%) were classified as psychopathic, 13 (50%) as possibly psychopathic, and 8 (31%) as nonpsychopathic. All of the nonviolent patients were classified as nonpsychopathic. Consistent with these results, psychopathy was strongly associated with violent recidivism in the community by discharged psychiatric patients when assessed by PCL:SV (Douglas et al. 1999) or PCL-R (Tengstrom et al. 2000).

The relation between antisocial behavior and schizophrenia is complex, and its underpinning is unclear. The term *pseudopsychopathic schizo-*

phrenia was used in the 1950s to describe cases that started as conduct disorder–type behavioral problems preceding the development of psychosis (Bender 1959). It is possible that the patients diagnosed with schizophrenia who exhibit psychopathic traits have a previously unclassified subtype of schizophrenia (Nolan et al. 1999a). It appears that early damage to certain brain structures (e.g., prefrontal cortex) (Anderson et al. 1999) (see Chapter 4) interferes with the normal development of moral sense. At least some cases of schizophrenia have a neurodevelopmental basis; it seems reasonable to speculate that the same neurodevelopmental problem may predispose to a phenotype that eventually meets the criteria for both "psychopathy" and "schizophrenia."

Borderline and Other Personality Disorders

Borderline personality disorder is defined in part by impulsiveness, recurrent anger with lack of control reflected by physical fights, and suicidal threats or behavior (American Psychiatric Association 1994). Borderline (or antisocial) personality traits were found among men who physically abuse women (Else et al. 1993).

Behavioral patterns of patients diagnosed with borderline personality disorder are linked to a central serotonin disturbance. Some important studies of the biological aspects of personality disorders are concerned with central serotoninergic function; this work is discussed in Chapter 3. Briefly, dysfunction of the central serotoninergic system was associated with impulsive aggressive behavior in male patients with personality disorders but not in patients with mood disorders.

Among 17 patients meeting diagnostic criteria for various personality disorders, 8 with borderline personality disorder showed a particularly pronounced dysfunction of the central serotoninergic system, and they may have largely accounted for the reported relationship between aggressive behavior and serotoninergic dysfunction (Coccaro et al. 1989).

In summary, ASP is partly defined by violent and criminal behaviors, making it difficult to avoid a tautological error when using ASP as a concept in research on violence and crime. With this caveat, it should be noted that the likelihood of violent behavior may be increased when ASP co-occurs with other disorders such as psychoses or substance abuse. *Psychopathy,* a term discarded by the American Psychiatric Association, was redefined in a way that is less dependent on criminal and violent behavior than ASP is. Prisoners defined as psychopaths were more likely than other prisoners to have committed violent crimes. Borderline personality disorder is partly defined by impulsive and aggressive behaviors; such behaviors have been related to a disturbance of the central serotoninergic system.

IMPULSE CONTROL

Impulse control is a concept of pivotal importance for the neurobiology of violence. It links criminologists' explanations of criminal propensity due to inadequate "self-control" (Gottfredson and Hirschi 1990, pp. 87–94) or impaired "impulse control" (J. Q. Wilson and Herrnstein 1986, pp. 435–437) to the data on the role of serotonin in impulsive violence (Virkkunen and Linnoila 1993) and to the animal research on the capacity to wait (to delay response) (Soubrie and Bizot 1990). The concept of impulse control might become a cornerstone of a future Grand Unified Theory of Aggression. Unfortunately, impulse (or impulse control) is not uniformly defined despite a large effort (Barratt and Patton 1983; Schalling 1993).

Meanings of the Word *Impulse*

In English literature, the word *impulse* has two slightly different meanings: "a sudden spontaneous inclination or incitement to some usually unpremeditated action" or "a propensity or natural tendency usually other than rational" (Webster 1991, p. 607). In general psychiatry, the term *impulsive* usually applies to swift action without forethought or conscious judgment, whereas in psychoanalysis *impulsive* and *instinctive* are generally used interchangeably (Hinsie and Campbell 1960, p. 378). A modern psychiatric glossary defines *impulse* as "a psychic striving, usually refers to an instinctual urge"(E. M. Stone 1988).

Thus, impulse is a psychic striving that 1) comes on suddenly, 2) is instinctual and urgent, and 3) leads to swift (impulsive) action that is taken without forethought.

Hence, we consider impulsive individuals (who have inadequate impulse control) and impulsive acts.

Impulsive Individuals

Inadequate impulse control may be a relatively permanent personality attribute (impulsiveness as a trait). Similar to the definitions of personality discussed above, the definition of impulsiveness may be seen as dimensional or categorical.

Dimensional Definition

A well-known dimensional system (Barratt 1985b) describes three aspects of disinhibitory psychopathology that partly define syndromes or diagnostic categories. These aspects or subtraits were labeled motor, cognitive, and "nonplanning" impulsiveness. *Motor impulsiveness* (physical activity without forethought) is a core symptom of attention-deficit/hyperactivity disorder (see Chapter 6); furthermore, it is negatively related to a measure of central serotoninergic activity in patients with personality disorders (Coccaro et al. 1989) (see also Chapter 3). *Cognitive impulsiveness* involves rapid and careless decision making.

Nonplanning impulsiveness implies lack of concern for the future. This subtrait is conceptually very close to "time discounting" (J.Q. Wilson and Herrnstein 1986, p. 50). People pay most attention to the events surrounding them here and now, whereas the importance of the events looming in a distant future beyond a "time horizon" is discounted. Individuals vary in the extent to which they discount time. The more an individual discounts time, the more he or she acts on the spur of the moment without regard for negative consequences in the future (e.g., incarceration). Because the rewards of violent behavior usually precede its penalties, time discounting can be seen as a mechanism underlying nonplanning impulsive violence.

The existence of the three subtraits was supported by a factor analysis of the Barratt Impulsiveness Scale (BIS), and various laboratory tests suggest that the subtraits may differ in their psychophysiologic bases (Barratt 1985b). The BIS (Barratt 1985a; Hollander et al. 2000, pp. 691–693) has been used by biological researchers studying the role of serotonin in aggression (C.S. Brown et al. 1989; Coccaro et al. 1989) (see also Chapter 3). Most of the subjects in these studies did not have major mental disorders. The BIS was originally developed by using populations without mental disorders (such as students). Subsequently, Barratt developed a version of the BIS for use in persons with major mental disorders (Steadman et al. 1994).

Other researchers (Schalling et al. 1988) used other scales developed to measure impulsiveness (S.B.G. Eysenck and Eysenck 1978) in psychiatrically healthy volunteers; high impulsiveness was related to low levels of platelet monoamine oxidase (see Chapter 3). In a similar study, impulsiveness in psychiatrically healthy volunteers was negatively related to plasma cortisol level; the interpretation of this finding is not clear (R.J. King et al. 1990). Impulsiveness measured by a scale (S.B.G. Eysenck and Eysenck 1977) was related to the amount of alpha activity in the resting electroencephalogram (EEG) in psychiatrically healthy volunteers

(O'Gorman and Lloyd 1987). These findings might link impulsiveness to arousal, but alpha activity levels may be affected by many influences besides arousal.

Categorical Definition

DSM-IV-TR has a special section on impulse control disorders not elsewhere classified. The class contains several categories, two of which are relevant for this topic: intermittent explosive disorder and pyromania. Intermittent explosive disorder has the following (abbreviated) diagnostic criteria (American Psychiatric Association 2000):

A. The occurrence of episodes of failure to resist aggressive impulses that result in serious assaultive acts or destruction of property.
B. The degree of aggressiveness during the episodes is grossly out of proportion to any precipitating psychosocial stressors.
C. The aggressive episodes are not better accounted for by antisocial or borderline personality disorders, psychosis, or attention-deficit/hyperactivity disorder, and they are not due to the direct effects of a substance or a general medical condition (e.g., a personality change due to head injury).

Many patients diagnosed in the 1960s and 1970s with "episodic dyscontrol syndrome" (Monroe 1970) or with "explosive personality" (DSM-II) would now be diagnosed with intermittent explosive disorder. Patients diagnosed with episodic dyscontrol syndrome showed numerous signs of neuropsychiatric dysfunction (Bach-y-Rita and Veno 1974; Bach-y-Rita et al. 1971; Monroe 1978). Such signs are probably also detectable by careful examination in many patients diagnosed as having intermittent explosive disorder today. The signs may not be obvious to clinicians (who therefore use this residual diagnostic category). It is not clear how many patients would retain the diagnosis of intermittent explosive disorder if careful examination was done for the presence of the disorders enumerated in criterion C above (which must be ruled out before this diagnosis can be made).

Offenders diagnosed (by DSM-III criteria) with explosive personality disorder were among the impulsive violent criminals reported to have low cerebrospinal fluid 5-hydroxyindoleacetic acid (CSF 5-HIAA) levels (Linnoila et al. 1983) (see also Chapter 3). Serotoninergic dysfunction could be a neurobiological basis of explosive personality disorder. All subjects with explosive personality disorder, however, also had a diagnosis of borderline personality disorder, and their violent behavior occurred frequently under the influence of alcohol. It is uncertain how many of these subjects would meet the DSM-IV-TR diagnostic criterion C for intermittent explosive disorder.

Pyromania

The abbreviated diagnostic criteria from DSM-IV-TR for pyromania are as follows:

A. Deliberate, purposeful, and repeated fire setting.
B. Tension before the act.
C. Fascination with fire.
D. Pleasure or relief when setting fires or witnessing their aftermath.
E. The fires are not set for money, politics, to conceal another crime, to express anger, or in response to psychotic symptoms.
F. The fire setting is not better accounted for by ASP, conduct disorder, or a manic episode.

DSM-IV-TR states that "individuals with pyromania may make considerable advance preparation for starting a fire" (p. 669). These preparations of course imply premeditation, which is inconsistent with the lack of forethought, an essential element in the definition of *impulse* (see "Meanings of the Word *Impulse*" above).

A relationship between a childhood history of fire setting and adult violent crime (murder, assault, robbery, and rape) was reported among prisoners examined at a psychiatric forensic unit (Hellman and Blackman 1966). Fire setting alone—as well as a combination of fire setting, enuresis, and cruelty to animals—was reported more frequently among prisoners charged with violent crimes than among other prisoners.

Twenty adult arsonists "who apparently did not set fire for economic gains" were compared with 20 habitually violent offenders and 10 psychiatrically healthy control subjects (Virkkunen et al. 1987). The arsonists had lower CSF levels of two monoamine metabolites, 5-HIAA and 3-methoxy-4-hydroxyphenylglycol (MHPG) (see Chapter 3), than the other groups and had low glucose nadirs in the oral glucose tolerance test. Nineteen of the 20 arsonists were diagnosed (DSM-III) with borderline personality disorder and 17 with alcohol abuse. Eighteen set fires under the influence of alcohol, raising questions about the relationships between serotonin dysfunction, dysthymia, self-medication with alcohol, and hypoglycemia (see Chapter 3). It is not clear whether the arsonists' primary impulse was to drink alcohol or to set fires. Impulsive features are shared by impulse control disorders, substance abuse disorders, eating disorders, and personality disorders (Lacey and Evans 1986). The neurobiology of impulse control disorders (Stein et al. 1993) may also be shared by other disorders that are currently not regarded as impulse related (see "Impulsive-Compulsive Dimension" below).

To summarize, low 5-HIAA levels suggest that fire setters (who may or may not meet the diagnostic criteria for pyromania) have a disturbance of the serotoninergic system; that disturbance may be implicated in a common neurobiological basis of impulse control disorders. The role of alcohol abuse in the neurobiology of fire setting remains to be clarified, and it would be useful to replicate these results with arsonists who do not abuse alcohol and who set fires while sober.

Impulsive Acts

Acts are included in the definitions of impulse and impulse control disorders. The discussion so far has focused on impulsive individuals. In criminology, the focus is shifted from individuals to their acts (crimes). Violent acts are of greater concern to society—and they are easier to describe—than the mental condition of the individuals committing them. Furthermore, access to police records that contain descriptions of the acts is easier to obtain than access to incarcerated individuals and their collaboration with interviewers. As in the study of individuals, dimensional and categorical approaches are used to define impulsive acts.

Dimensional Definition

A 10-item rating scale to measure "self-control attributes" or "impulsivity" of crimes was constructed (Heilbrun 1979; Heilbrun et al. 1976). The scale uses information gleaned from criminal records; no direct contact with offenders is involved. Students used the scale to evaluate 251 individual criminal records; 11 crimes were ranked according to their average impulsivity (Table 7–2). The most impulsive (least premeditated) crime was manslaughter; the least impulsive crime was arson (the investigators probably did not exclude cases of arson for monetary gain). Table 7–2 shows that violent crimes tend to be rated as more impulsive (less premeditated) than the other crimes.

Categorical Definition

In an early study (Hill and Pond 1952), homicides were defined as "clearly motivated" or "apparently motiveless" (see Table 4–2 in Chapter 4). The motiveless killings were unpremeditated; today, they would probably be classified as impulsive. The electroencephalographic records of

Table 7–2. Impulsivity of crimes

Crime	Impulsivity rating
Manslaughter	2.31
Murder	2.52
Assault	2.56
Rape	2.83
Auto theft	3.08
Robbery	3.15
Drug violation	3.25
Larceny	3.31
Burglary	3.33
Forgery	3.38
Arson	3.42

Note. Ratings of impulsivity for 11 crimes were obtained by averaging rating scale scores of 251 individual criminal case records. Scores ranged from 1 (most impulsive) to 10 (least impulsive).
Source. Adapted from Heilbrun 1979.

impulsive homicide offenders were more frequently abnormal than were those of other offenders.

Violent crimes were deemed impulsive "when the victim was unknown to the offender, no provocation was evident, and the motivation of potential monetary gain was ruled out" (Virkkunen et al. 1989a, p. 604). The other violent crimes were deemed nonimpulsive. Very similar (but not identical) definitions were used in the other work by this group (Linnoila et al. 1983; Virkkunen et al. 1989b). For each subject in these studies, the index offense—somewhat biblically called "the original crime" (Virkkunen et al. 1989a, p. 604)—was thus classified as impulsive or nonimpulsive. The subjects were then individually classified as impulsive or nonimpulsive on this basis. Their hypothesized neurobiological *traits* (CSF monoamine levels) were thus inferred from a police description of a single act of violence that occurred several months or years before the CSF samples were obtained. It is surprising that the hypothesis was supported; the subjects' CSF monoamine metabolite levels were indeed distributed according to the classification of a single violent act. These results suggest that a single crime may inform us about certain neurobiological (and perhaps other) traits of the offender and, conversely, that these traits determined by a single examination may affect the characteristics of crimes committed over a long period by that offender (see also Virkkunen et al. 1989b).

Impulsive-Compulsive Dimension

Hollander and his colleagues have formulated an integrated theory linking a number of disorders that share an inability to delay repetitive deviant behaviors (Hollander and Rosen 2000). Compulsivity can be seen as a drive to reduce anxiety, and impulsivity as a drive to obtain pleasure or gratification. The impulsive-compulsive dimension may be viewed as a continuum of disorders, with obsessive-compulsive disorder at one end and ASP at the other end of the spectrum. The obsessive-compulsive part of the spectrum is characterized by the patients' overestimation of potential harm, whereas the impulsive part is associated with an underestimation of harm. Obsessive-compulsive disorder, body dysmorphic disorder, anorexia nervosa, and hypochondriasis are among the disorders in the obsessive part of the spectrum. ASP, borderline personality disorder, sexual compulsions, pyromania, and self-injurious behaviors are among the disorders in the impulsive part of the spectrum; disorders in this part of the spectrum are characterized by aggression or loss of control. The advantage of this scheme is that it provides a common theoretical framework for the investigation of underlying neurobiology and psychopharmacologic interventions (Hollander 1999).

In summary, impulse and its control are pivotal issues in theories of aggression, but neither concept is uniformly defined. Investigation of impulse control focuses either on impulsive individuals or on impulsive acts. Impulsiveness in individuals may be defined by dimensional or categorical characteristics. The dimensional approach is represented by the work of Barratt, who defined three subtraits: motor, cognitive, and nonplanning impulsiveness. The categorical (nosologic) approach is represented by several DSM-IV-TR diagnostic categories, two of which are discussed: intermittent explosive disorder and pyromania. Similarly to impulsive individuals, impulsive acts may also be defined by dimensional or categorical characteristics. The concept of impulsive-compulsive dimension provides a framework for future research.

Impulsive features of individuals and their acts have been associated with dysfunctions of the serotoninergic system, glucose metabolism, and electrical brain activity. Relationships between these types of dysfunctions should be explored in future studies (see Chapter 12).

8 | Violence and Psychoactive Substance Abuse

ALCOHOL

The notion that drinking leads to fighting has been a part of folk wisdom for centuries. However, the relationships between alcohol and aggression turn out to be surprisingly complex. The mechanism of action of alcohol on aggression has not been elucidated.

In most species, the dose-response relationship is nonlinear; in short-term experiments, low doses of alcohol elicit or facilitate aggression, whereas high doses reduce it. This relationship is dependent on many factors, such as the experimental method used to induce aggression, the animal's species, its previous exposure to aggression, and probably its current levels of testosterone (Miczek 1987) (see also Chapter 2).

Human studies first addressed the relationship between alcohol and violent crime. By necessity, these studies (which generally used offenders as subjects) were naturalistic and correlational. More recently, psychological experiments using psychiatrically healthy volunteers who ingested alcohol under controlled conditions were conducted in an effort to explain causal relationships between alcohol and aggression. Other studies explored relationships between alcohol abuse, drug abuse, and neuropsychiatric illness. Current interest in biochemical mechanisms underlying aggression has inspired studies of neurotransmitters—particularly serotonin—in aggressive alcohol abusers.

Short-Term Effects of Alcohol and Violent Crime: Naturalistic Observations

A classic study (Shupe 1954) established that 87% of 882 persons arrested shortly after committing a crime (violent or nonviolent) had measurable urine alcohol levels. A reanalysis (Murdoch et al. 1990) of Shupe's data demonstrated that higher alcohol levels occurred more frequently among the perpetrators arrested for violent compared with nonviolent crimes. The notion that violent crimes are more frequently committed after drinking than nonviolent ones has been supported by other studies based on police records (Cordilia 1985) or on forensic assessments (Langevin et al. 1982b). An exhaustive study of homicide offenders in northern Sweden (Lindqvist 1986) found that 66% of the offenders were intoxicated at the time of the killing. The evidence linking violent crime to short-term effects of alcohol appears impressive, but it has certain limitations.

The subjects of these studies (Cordilia 1985; Langevin et al. 1982b; Shupe 1954) shared an important feature: they were all apprehended. However, most offenses committed do not result in an arrest. It should therefore be determined whether the offenses (and the offenders) analyzed in these studies constitute representative samples. These samples are biased in at least two ways. First, alcohol intoxication probably decreases the perpetrators' ability to evade arrest. Second, nonviolent offenses are less likely to result in an arrest than violent ones (Maguire et al. 1993, p. 451). For these reasons, the intoxicated violent offenders were probably overrepresented in the studies discussed above (Cordilia 1985; Langevin et al. 1982b; Shupe 1954). Therefore, these and similar studies do not necessarily imply that getting drunk leads to violent crime or that violent criminals drink too much.

To understand the relationship between drinking and crime, it is necessary to know the overall drinking patterns in the community from which the criminal population is derived. For example, the finding that 60% of homicide offenders had been drinking before the crime (Wolfgang 1958, p. 166) does not reveal much about the relationship between alcohol and homicide unless it is known how many nonoffenders had also been drinking. This issue was addressed in a case-control study of risk factors for injury to women from domestic violence (Kyriacou et al. 1999). The study sites were eight emergency departments. The subjects were 256 women who had acute injuries resulting from a physical assault by a male partner. The 659 control subjects were women treated for other conditions in the same emergency departments. All women were interviewed to obtain the characteristics of their partners. There were substantial differences between the partners of the injured women and the partners of control women. For example, alcohol abuse was reported in 67.7% of the partners of the intentionally injured women, but only in 26.3% of the control subjects' partners. Furthermore, 51.6% of the injured women reported that their partners had been drinking just before the assault. The risk of inflicting injury was associated with the following characteristics of the partners: alcohol abuse (adjusted relative risk, 3.6; 95% confidence interval, 2.2–5.9); drug use (adjusted relative risk, 3.5; 95% confidence interval, 2.0–6.4); intermittent employment (adjusted relative risk, 3.1; 95% confidence interval, 1.1–8.8); recent unemployment (adjusted relative risk, 2.7; 95% confidence interval, 1.2–6.5); having less than a high school graduate's education (adjusted relative risk, 2.5; 95% confidence interval, 1.4–4.4); and being a former husband, estranged husband, or former boyfriend (adjusted relative risk, 3.5; 95% confidence interval, 1.5–8.3).

To understand the relationship between drinking and violence at the level of individual incidents, one should study not only violent events (with or without alcohol involvement) but also drinking events (with or without violence). These issues were addressed in a large anthropological study of alcohol use and aggression (Pernanen 1991). That study used three types of data: interviews with a representative sample of community residents, police reports, and systematic observations in bars in the community. The study confirmed that alcohol is indeed implicated in criminal violence and that it is also "abundantly present in the day-to-day violent confrontation" (Pernanen 1991, p. 193).

The inquiry on the impact of alcohol on crime cannot be limited to the assailant's drinking. The victim's behavior frequently precipitates violence by the assailant. In his classic book, Wolfgang (1958) coined and defined the concept of the "victim-precipitated homicide." Approximately one-quarter of the homicides in his sample were precipitated by the victims. Ingestion of alcohol by the victim was identified as one of the precipitating factors (Wolfgang 1958, p. 256). The important role of the male (but not the female) victim's drinking in precipitating violence has been confirmed by the anthropological study mentioned above (Pernanen 1991). The probability of aggression between two people is "greatest when both are intoxicated, intermediate when one person is intoxicated, and least probable when both are sober" (Murdoch et al. 1990). In the study of intentionally injured women in the emergency rooms (Kyriacou et al. 1999), 22.7% of these victims reported that they themselves abused alcohol; this contrasted with the 7.1% reported by the control subjects. It is unclear how many of the victims drank alcohol just before they were assaulted.

Intoxication may lead to victimization in several ways. It is possible that alcohol reduces fear so that the future victim continues to participate in a dangerous activity (Pihl and Peterson 1993) such as a quarrel. It is interesting that alcohol-free mice, rats, and squirrel monkeys increase their aggressive behavior when confronted by an alcohol-treated opponent (Miczek 1987, p. 239). Perhaps the intoxication reduces the organism's ability to perceive threats, to evaluate risks, or to respond appropriately to a threatening situation.

Overall, the extensive literature reviewed elsewhere (Murdoch et al. 1990) indicated that the assailants were under the influence of alcohol in more than 50% of assaults and homicides and that this percentage was lower for nonviolent criminal offenses. Furthermore, alcohol ingestion by the victims was a factor that precipitated assault and homicide. An association between the short-term effects of alcohol and violence was thus overwhelmingly supported by correlational studies. However, such studies do not directly address the causal relationships and mechanisms underlying that association. Studies of alcohol effects under controlled laboratory conditions are better suited to this purpose.

Short-Term Effects of Alcohol and Human Aggression: Experimental Studies

Theoretical explanations of the effects of alcohol on aggression can be classified into several groups (Bushman and Cooper 1990). For the purposes of this discussion, the scheme can be simplified by positing only two types of effects: pharmacological ("direct") and psychological effects, which include factors such as expectancy, motives, and predisposition.

These effects were tested by experimental studies that generally shared certain design features such as the type of subjects, beverage administration, and measures of aggression. The subjects were usually healthy men free from obvious mental disorders who had used alcohol (social drinkers) but denied alcohol dependence. Small to moderate doses of alcohol were used, mostly ranging between 0.1 and 1.0 g/kg. Such doses yielded peak blood alcohol levels (BALs) well below 100 mg/dL (0.5 mg/kg yielded approximately 35 mg/dL) (Pollock et al. 1983). The researchers using the placebo design told all subjects that they would be receiving alcohol, but in reality, some subjects received only a nonalcoholic beverage. This design failed to control for the expectancy of alcohol, because all subjects expected to get it. In the balanced placebo design, half the subjects were told that they would be getting alcohol, and the other half were told to expect a nonalcoholic beverage. Half the subjects within each of these groups received alcohol, and the other half did not. This arrangement yielded a condition opposite to placebo ("antiplacebo"), in which the subjects did not expect alcohol, but in fact did receive it. The general outline of this design is shown in Table 8–1.

Table 8–1. Balanced placebo design for beverage administration

	Subjects told they would receive	
Subjects received	Alcoholic beverage	Nonalcoholic beverage
Alcoholic beverage	Alcohol	Antiplacebo
Nonalcoholic beverage	Placebo	Control

The principal purpose of the balanced placebo design was to separate the direct effects of alcohol from the effect of subjects' expectancy: the comparison of antiplacebo and control groups provided a measure of direct alcohol effects uncontaminated by expectancy. Conversely, the comparison of placebo and control groups provided a measure of expectancy (uncontaminated by the direct effects of alcohol).

Most measures of aggression were obtained by using variations of the Buss-Taylor paradigm (Bushman and Cooper 1990; Pihl and Peterson 1993; S.P. Taylor et al. 1976). This paradigm used one real and one fictitious ("confederate") subject. The real subject was instructed to exchange electric shocks with the confederate for reasons that varied among experiments. The subject controlled the intensity and duration of these shocks intended for the confederate; both intensity and duration (which jointly defined aggression) were used as the principal dependent variables in most experiments of this type.

A meta-analysis of 30 studies (Bushman and Cooper 1990) yielded effect sizes for four contrasts: alcohol versus control, alcohol versus placebo, antiplacebo versus control, and placebo versus control. The results of the meta-analysis are summarized in Table 8–2.

The effect sizes significantly greater than zero were yielded by the contrasts of alcohol versus placebo and alcohol versus control; the other two contrasts were not significant. These results indicated that alcohol does elicit aggression. However, the effect on aggression was not direct because the antiplacebo versus control contrast was not significant (see above). Furthermore, purely psychological effects such as expectancy did not alone account for the alcohol effect on aggression, as evidenced by the nonsignificant contrast of placebo versus control. Thus, these experiments collectively suggested that pharmacological (direct) and psychological aspects of alcohol consumption exert a joint effect on aggression. The alcohol versus control condition (which had a significant effect) appeared to be the closest one to real life: if the bartender is honest, every customer knows what kind of beverage he or she is getting.

Another meta-analysis of alcohol experimental studies investigated the role of several sociopsychological mechanisms involved in the modu-

Table 8–2.   Effects of alcohol on human aggression: results of meta-analysis

Effect tested	Contrast (see Table 8–1)	Effect size
"Direct" effect of alcohol alone	Antiplacebo versus control	n.s.
Expectancy alone	Placebo versus control	n.s.
"Direct" effect plus expectancy compared with expectancy alone	Alcohol versus placebo	$P<0.05$
"Direct" effect plus expectancy compared with baseline	Alcohol versus control	$P<0.05$

Note.   n.s.=not significant.
Source.   Adapted from Bushman and Cooper 1990.

lation of aggression in humans (Ito et al. 1996). The difference in aggression between sober and intoxicated subjects decreased as intensity of provocation, level of frustration, and self-focused attention increased.

Short-Term Effects of Alcohol in Neuropsychiatrically Impaired Individuals

The elegant experiments described in the preceding section typically used "normal" male college students as subjects. Such men sometimes commit violent crimes, but most real-life violence is not perpetrated by college students. Typical violent offenders differ from college-student subjects in many respects. Their educational achievement is generally lower, and therefore they may have limited resources and outlets to express hostility verbally (rather than physically). Unlike college students, many violent offenders grew up in what was termed *a subculture of violence* (Wolfgang and Ferracuti 1967); this background made them prone to violence because of the established pattern of such behavior in their community. Thus, violent offenders may be more likely than college students to expect increases in aggressiveness after drinking. Furthermore, violent offenders may differ from college students in other areas of functioning besides the aggressive behavior; such differences may facilitate that behavior. For example, violent offenders frequently meet the criteria for psychopathy (Milich and Kramer 1984) or antisocial personality disorder (American Psychiatric Association 1994).

Above and beyond personality disorders, many violent offenders show signs of neuropsychiatric impairment resulting from various types of brain damage (e.g., head injuries). Brain damage is an important intervening variable between drinking and violence because it changes the organism's response to alcohol (Finger and Stein 1982). The relationship between the dose of alcohol and the person's response may be changed quantitatively and qualitatively. *Alcohol intolerance* may be described as a largely *quantitative* change: the sequence of intoxicated behaviors proceeds as usual from initial excitement to sleep, but the dose of alcohol required to elicit the effect is reduced. This intolerance can be expressed quantitatively as a shift of the dose-response curve to the left.

Furthermore, certain *qualitative* features of the alcohol effect may be altered. Compared with control subjects, violent offenders reported more frequently that alcohol ingestion made them feel paranoid and inferior (Langevin et al. 1987). These offenders also tended to show more neuropsychiatric impairment on a test battery than the control subjects. Such feelings may conceivably account for some instances of violence under the influence of alcohol.

Qualitatively deviant alcohol effects were also reported in persons whose brain function was impaired due to a combination of factors that may act in an additive or interactive fashion. Thus, schizophrenic individuals who also abuse drugs may be particularly likely to become assaultive under the influence of alcohol (Yesavage and Zarcone 1983).

These results (Langevin et al. 1987; Yesavage and Zarcone 1983) were based on self-reports of alcohol effects; alcohol doses were not controlled. Perhaps the violent individuals drank more than others, and the differing effects on mood and assaultiveness were due to a higher dose of alcohol. Nevertheless, it appears that neuropsychiatric impairments predispose to a qualitatively different, maladaptive response to alcohol. The nature of such impairments and the disorders responsible for them remain unclear. It is certain, however, that alcohol is sometimes associated with aggressive behavior that is incongruous with the personality of the drinker, inappropriate to the situation, and apparently independent of the dose of alcohol ingested.

Pathological intoxication (also known as "idiosyncratic intoxication") may represent an extreme example of this effect. This category is controversial. Although it had been listed in previous DSM editions, DSM-IV (American Psychiatric Association 1994) omits it because of lack of supporting evidence that it is distinct from regular alcohol intoxication. However, pathological intoxication is discussed in a body of American and European literature, and use of this concept in forensic psychiatry (perhaps with a different label) is likely to continue on both sides of the Atlantic despite its exclusion from DSM-IV. Therefore, I briefly review this concept.

In a person with pathological intoxication, assaultive or other maladaptive behavior that is atypical when he or she is not drinking occurs shortly after ingestion of a small amount of alcohol. Amnesia for such behaviors is frequently reported. The definitions of the "small amount" varied slightly as the criteria developed. Early criteria stipulated a "minimal alcohol intake" (DSM-I and DSM-II [American Psychiatric Association 1952, 1968]); this was changed to an "amount of alcohol insufficient to induce intoxication in most people" (DSM-III and DSM-III-R [American Psychiatric Association 1980, 1987]). This change was probably intended to deflect the obvious question: What is "minimal intake"? Unfortunately, the change has not helped. The questions have just become more difficult to answer: Who are "most people"? What is their age, gender, and race? What is their history of alcohol use? All these factors have powerful and well-known effects on tolerance to alcohol, rendering the loose concept of "most people" rather useless in this context. Some European textbooks state that small amounts of alcohol are "frequently" sufficient to elicit pathological intoxication (Dufek 1975; Huber 1987; Tolle 1988). Predisposing factors for idiosyncratic intoxication include brain damage due mostly to trauma or encephalitis; other factors include unusual fatigue or debilitating physical illness.

Behavioral manifestations of pathological intoxication start and stop rather suddenly, the behavior is incongruous with the patient's personality and with the situation, and amnesia is frequent. These clinical features make it similar to temporal lobe epilepsy. Indeed, a syndrome indistinguishable from idiosyncratic intoxication apparently may be elicited by alcohol in epileptic patients, particularly in patients with temporal lobe epilepsy (complex partial seizures).

In general, alcohol use increases the likelihood of seizures in epileptic patients. It is well known that seizures may be elicited as a part of the alcohol withdrawal syndrome. However, alcohol may increase the risk of seizures in epileptic patients more directly, without any withdrawal (S.K. Ng et al. 1988). Short of clinical seizures, the epileptogenic effect of alcohol may be manifested by electroencephalographic "activation"—in other words, induction of electroencephalographic abnormalities not apparent before the administration of alcohol or enhancement of preexisting electroencephalographic abnormalities.

For all these reasons, epileptic persons are advised not to drink, but some do anyway. Although there is no evidence that epilepsy in general leads to violent behavior (see Chapter 4), it appears that violent behavior with amnesia may be elicited in epileptic persons by relatively small doses of alcohol. Such behavior has never been demonstrated in epileptic persons after experimental alcohol administration under controlled conditions; however, electroencephalographic activation by approximately 60–90 mL of alcohol by mouth was demonstrated in a series of patients with posttraumatic epilepsy who had a history of violent episodes after ingestion of alcohol (Marinacci and Von Hagen 1972). It is important to note that the patients did not show any aggressive behavior during these electroencephalographic activation tests. Attempts at electroencephalographic activation by means of intravenous alcohol in 10 patients with a clinical history of pathological intoxication (some of whom had epilepsy) failed (Bach-y-Rita et al. 1970).

However, another author elicited behavioral changes similar to those described by others in persons with pathological intoxication (Maletzky 1976). Subjects were selected for this study because of their history of violent or psychotic behavior while under the influence of alcohol; presumably they were not epileptic. They were given relatively large amounts of alcohol (100–300 mL iv), and 11 of the 22 subjects developed "inappropriate rage." The BALs in two of the subjects (measured around the time of their violent reaction) were, respectively, 117 mg/dL and 210 mg/dL. (To put these results into context, note that drivers with BALs of 100 mg/dL and above are legally considered intoxicated in most jurisdictions.) The electroencephalographic effects of alcohol observed in this study were diagnostically nonspecific and were not related to violent behavior. Most of the subjects in this study were alcohol abusers; some were alcohol dependent. Maletzky argued that the diagnostic criterion stipulating that pathological intoxication is elicited by a small amount of alcohol makes little sense in patients who have an increased tolerance due to antecedent chronic use or abuse of alcohol.

Pathological intoxication is an important forensic concept because it offers "perhaps the only genuine exculpating condition linked to acute drug use" (Mitchell 1990). The defense may claim that the defendant's action was caused not by simple drunkenness but by an unusual reaction to alcohol that was due to an underlying brain disease. Numerous objections have been raised against this argument, but a critical analysis of these objections suggested that pathological intoxication provides "a potentially significant defense in many serious cases" (Tiffany and Tiffany 1990, pp. 49–50).

Thus, idiosyncratic reactions to alcohol remain controversial from the standpoint of psychiatry, neurology, clinical pharmacology, electroencephalography, and the law. Everybody is confused. Pathological (or idiosyncratic) intoxication is a concept that has eluded a clear and generally accepted definition. Its very existence has been doubted (Small 1987; Tiffany and Tiffany 1990). Despite all the confusion, it is clear that links among epilepsy, alcohol, amnesia, and violence do exist. However, one should keep in mind that alcoholic blackouts are frequent and that they occur in persons without any evidence of seizure disorder.

In summary, it appears that interactions among various types of underlying neuropsychiatric impairments and the short-term effects of alcohol account for a proportion of alcohol-associated violence. Such an interaction has been proposed (Langevin et al. 1987) but not tested. This presents an interesting opportunity for future research.

Alcohol Abuse, Alcohol Dependence, and Violent Crime

Until now, I have only discussed the short-term effects of alcohol, disregarding the pattern of its use. Some of the violent crimes committed under the influence of alcohol (see above) were probably committed by offenders who would have met the diagnostic criteria for alcohol abuse or dependence (American Psychiatric Association 1994). However, the data needed to diagnose those offenders are not available. The prevalence of alcohol abuse among newly incarcerated offenders was estimated at 20% (Petrich 1976) or 15% (Schuckit et al. 1977), but the relationship of these diagnoses to violent crime is not clarified by these data. Alcohol abuse or dependence may be more prevalent among violent criminals, particularly among violent recidivists. Among 129 male homicide offenders in Finland, 59 (46%) were diagnosed with alcohol dependence (with or without personality disorder) (Tiihonen et al. 1993). Among 36 homicide recidivists (persons who committed two or more homicides) in Finland, 24 (67%) were diagnosed with "alcoholism" combined in most cases with a personality disorder (Eronen et al. 1996a).

The rates of drinking by the offender during or immediately before the commission of a violent crime are generally above 50%. In relation to violent crimes, there may be a distinction between short-term effects of alcohol and a diagnosis of alcohol abuse or dependence (Abram 1989; Collins and Schlenger 1988). This distinction received support from a major longitudinal prospective study of a New Zealand birth cohort (Arseneault et al. 2000). In that study, alcohol dependence marginally increased the odds ratio for violent crime (OR=1.9, confidence interval 1.0–3.5), but that increase was largely explained by actual alcohol use shortly before offending. This distinction implies that persons who are dependent on alcohol are not at an increased risk for offending as long as they are sober. Of course, such persons are by definition at a very high risk for not staying sober.

Most authors reporting links between alcohol use and violent crime have not controlled for co-occurring disorders. Therefore, it is possible that such links are mediated by a third variable such as antisocial personality disorder (see Chapter 7). Data supporting this possibility have been published (Abram 1989). Alternatively, a subtype of alcohol abuse may be inherited jointly with antisocial personality disorder. Cloninger and his group demonstrated the existence of two types of alcohol abuse (Cloninger et al. 1981). Type 2 abusers frequently fight (and get arrested) under the influence of alcohol. This type of alcohol abuse is transmitted from fathers to sons, and it develops early in life. Patients with type 2 alcohol abuse show many features characteristic of antisocial personality disorder. Furthermore, there is evidence suggesting that type 2 alcohol abusers also have abnormalities of serotoninergic transmission reflected by low cerebrospinal fluid levels of 5-hydroxyindoleacetic acid (Virkkunen and Linnoila 1990). Such abnormalities are known to be linked to impulsive aggressive behavior (see Chapter 3).

In general, offenders frequently have multiple disorders (e.g., alcohol and drug abuse, personality disorders, neurological syndromes). Clinicians know that these disorders interact with each other, but the interactions have not yet received sufficient attention in research.

DRUG ABUSE AND DEPENDENCE

In North America, it would be difficult to find anyone unaware of links between drug abuse and crime. These links, illustrated by the daily portions of gore provided by newspapers, have been popularized by politicians who know that voters are extremely concerned about crime. It is probably fair to speculate that much of the recent funding for neuroscience research into drug abuse has been allocated at least in part to address this concern about crime. The available scientific data support the links between violent crime and certain illicit drugs.

Crime and Acute Effects of Drugs

In 1999, illicit drugs were detected in urine samples of 49%–77% of the arrested males in 34 United States cities (Pastore and Maguire 2000, p. 380). Cocaine and marijuana were the drugs most frequently detected. Cocaine was detected in the urine of arrested males at rates ranging from 22% in Omaha, Nebraska, to 49% in Miami, Florida (Pastore and Maguire 2000, p. 380). The detection rates for marijuana were generally comparable. Some of these positive-testing persons were arrested for possession or sale of drugs, having committed no other crime. In the

United States, however, drug violations account for fewer than 11% of offenses charged (Pastore and Maguire 2000, p. 338).

Taken together, these data suggest that illicit drug use may increase the likelihood of committing crimes above and beyond drug violations. However, these correlational observations do not prove a causal relationship between drugs and crime. Similarly to the analogous data on alcohol in arrested persons, such information is difficult to interpret without urine samples from persons in the same community who were not arrested. Such control samples are needed because short-term drug effects may increase the likelihood of arrest of those who commit crimes, and because comparable persons in the same community who do not commit crimes (other than drug possession) may be using drugs at rates that are similar to those of the arrested persons. The need for control samples is illustrated by self-reports of recent (within last 30 days) drug use among young adults in the United States in 1999: marijuana was used by 15.6% and cocaine by 1.9% of the respondents (Pastore and Maguire 2000, p. 242).

Crime and Drug Abuse

Evidence for linkage between drug abuse and crime varies depending on the drug. The most persuasive data on linkage exist for opioids. This availability of evidence is not primarily due to specific pharmacologic effects of opioids on aggression; rather, it is due to the long history and relatively high prevalence of opioid abuse in the United States and the history of funding for research in this area. One of the major achievements of the methadone treatment programs in the 1970s was a dramatic reduction in the arrest rates of their clients. The arrest charges were not specified in the major follow-up reports (Dole and Joseph 1978; Gearing and Schweitzer 1974). However, the decline of arrest rates was so great that perhaps one can assume fewer arrests for violent crime in patients currently receiving methadone treatment (in addition to the obvious reduction in arrests for drug possession). The arrest rate returned to the original (pretreatment) high levels in patients who dropped out of the methadone programs (Gearing and Schweitzer 1974).

Hanlon et al. (1990) interviewed 132 opioid addicts about their drug use and criminal activity. The interviews covered, on average, a period of 15 years. During that time, the subjects experienced periods of "addiction" and "nonaddiction." A period of opioid addiction was defined as a "period of one month or more while at large in the community during which the subject illicitly used opiates 4 or more days a week." This definition, albeit idiosyncratic, yielded data on long-term fluctuations of opioid intake; such fluctuations are generally related to changes in the severity of substance use disorders.

Self-reported criminal activity was higher during the addiction periods than during the nonaddiction periods. Furthermore, there was a long-term trend for the criminal activity (including violent crime) to decrease after a peak occurring during the first period of addiction.

These results emphasized the importance of close temporal relationships between the level of drug use and crime: most crime was committed during periods when the offender was using maximal amounts of drugs. This finding may explain why a diagnosis of drug-use disorder (lifetime or current) did not account for significant proportions of variance of criminal activity (Abram and Teplin 1990): the diagnosis misses important information on temporal fluctuations of the amount of drugs used. Similar data emphasizing the importance of the temporal relationship of drinking to crime (rather than the diagnosis of alcohol abuse or dependence) were mentioned in the preceding section on alcohol.

The data discussed so far suggest a relationship between drug abuse and crime, including violent crime. I now turn to the nature of that relationship. Drug-related violence may be broadly classified into three types: psychopharmacologic, economic-compulsive, and systemic (Goldstein 1985).

Psychopharmacologic mechanisms elicit violence directly; they involve intoxication or drug withdrawal. Economic-compulsive violent crime is committed by drug-dependent individuals to obtain money to purchase drugs. Some of these individuals are driven to criminal violence by withdrawal symptoms; these cases blur the difference between the psychopharmacologic and the economic-compulsive types of violent behavior. Systemic violence is intrinsic to involvement with illicit drugs. Typical examples include territorial fights among dealers, elimination of informers, and punishment for selling adulterated drugs or for unpaid debts. Systemic violence may be committed under the influence of drugs, which again somewhat blurs the distinction between psychopharmacologic and other types of violence.

Each of these three types of drug-related violence affects the drug users and distributors (as aggressors or victims) as well as innocent people not involved with drugs who are victimized intentionally (e.g., in a robbery) or unintentionally (e.g., hit by stray bullets in gun battles). The relative importance of the three types of drug-related violence was explored by interviewing a group of persons receiving methadone maintenance treatment and a group of untreated control subjects (Spunt et al. 1990a). The interviews were concerned with violent events occurring over a sample period of 8 weeks. Slightly more than 50% of all violent events reported by these subjects were drug related. Within this drug-related subset, psychopharmacologic and systemic violence occurred with similar frequencies, whereas economic-compulsive violence (mostly related to cocaine) was less frequent. The statistics in this report are presented in a somewhat confusing way. However, the authors give interesting quotes from the interviews. The quotes illustrate the perceived reasons for violent events and reveal the participants' attitudes. An event that had a systemic dimension was described by a participant:

> Went to cop some herb for this girl late Saturday night. She gave me $5. She's saying "I gave you $20." I copped, but she says, "Where's the change?" Her boyfriend say, "We'll kill you, give me the change!" After 15 minutes of her yelling and his giving me bullshit, I snapped. I swung and missed, 2nd shot I hit his nose, I think I broke it. I go down to get him on the ground. He got me in the eye.... There was no hustle, I got her a good nickel of smoke. She was running bullshit by me. (Spunt et al. 1990a, p. 92)

A subsequent report by this group (Spunt et al. 1990b) indicated that the proportions of psychopharmacologic, economic-compulsive, and systemic drug-related violent events depended on the race and gender of the participants. The involvement of white males tended to be classified as psychopharmacologic, whereas the black males were relatively more involved in the systemic subtype of violence. The psychopharmacologic subtype predominated among females irrespective of their racial or ethnic identification.

Psychopharmacologic Features of Drugs of Abuse

Psychopharmacologic features that relate to violence or aggression are described below.

Psychostimulants

The psychostimulants most frequently involved in violence are cocaine and amphetamine. Effects of stimulants on aggression in animals have been extensively studied (see Chapter 2). These effects are variable, depending on the animal species, the dose of the drug (low doses may elicit aggression, but high doses may have an opposite effect), and the animal's social position in a group (dominant or subordinate individuals in primate groups).

Cocaine. Cocaine is used as either the hydrochloride salt or the freebase. Freebase can be prepared from the hydrochloride salt by individual users. Since the mid-1980s, preprocessed freebase ("crack") has become available on the streets of United States cities. Most users take the hydrochloride powder intranasally, or they dissolve it in water and inject it intravenously. Crack is volatile at temperatures above 90°C, which makes it more suitable for smoking.

Immediately after the intravenous administration or inhalation of smoked cocaine, the user experiences an extremely pleasurable feeling (a "rush") that lasts a few minutes. This rush is followed by feelings of anxiety, depression (a "crash"), and intense craving for more cocaine. The effects of intranasal administration are less intense and delayed (due to slower absorption). Intranasal or intravenous administration of single doses of cocaine to healthy subjects under experimental conditions did not result in any obvious hostility or aggression (Resnick et al. 1977). However, no specific experimental assessment of aggressiveness (similar to that done in the alcohol studies described under "Short-Term Effects of Alcohol and Human Aggression: Experimental Studies" above) has been performed in studies of the short-term effects of cocaine.

The craving during a crash may lead to immediate additional administration of cocaine, and the cycle is repeated until the drug supply is exhausted or the user becomes too incapacitated to continue. This type of binge use results in high cumulative doses that may elicit an intoxication or a delirium. Most of the violent behavior elicited by the pharmacologic effects of cocaine apparently occurs during these states. Other symptoms of intoxication or delirium include auditory, visual, and tactile hallucinations; paranoid and other delusions; irritability; confusion; and psychomotor agitation (sometimes extreme).

Violent behavior in patients presenting with cocaine intoxication was observed in hospital emergency rooms (Brody 1990; Brower et al. 1988; Honer et al. 1987; Manschreck et al. 1988). Violence was more pronounced in patients reporting higher levels of cocaine use in the preceding month (Brower et al. 1988), in patients presenting with psychotic symptoms (Manschreck et al. 1988), and perhaps in patients who smoked crack or used cocaine intravenously compared with intranasal users (Brower et al. 1986). This relationship between route of administration and violence may be mediated by the cocaine dose: intranasal users may be taking lower doses, and the cocaine dose they take is less efficiently absorbed. Cocaine plasma level curves after intravenous administration and smoking are very similar (Johanson and Fischman 1989, p. 7).

Symptoms of intoxication or delirium typically disappear within 2 days after the last dose of cocaine. However, a delusional syndrome may linger for a week or more after the last dose. This syndrome is characterized by persecutory delusions, which may elicit violence against misperceived "enemies." The emergency room reports (Brody 1990; Brower et al. 1988; Honer et al. 1987) do not contain sufficient clinical details to separate the delusional syndrome from the more acute manifestations (intoxication and delirium).

Drug-related violent events were classified as psychopharmacologic, economic-compulsive, or systemic (see "Crime and Drug Abuse" above). Specific data for cocaine indicate that violent events associated with this drug were primarily economic-compulsive among white males, systemic among black males, and psychopharmacologic among females of all ethnic and racial groups studied (Spunt et al. 1990b).

Violence may be elicited by cocaine alone. However, in addition to cocaine, many patients seen in emergency rooms are using other substances, including alcohol. These substances may contribute to the violent behaviors observed. Furthermore, violent behavior is one of the reasons why these patients were brought to the emergency rooms. This selection bias precludes use of these data to estimate the frequency of violent behavior elicited by cocaine in the general population. A similar selection bias applies to self-selected problem users of cocaine who provide self-reports of violent behavior (Washton and Tatarsky 1984).

It is clear (and fortunate) that violent behavior is exhibited by fewer than 50% of the patients presenting at emergency rooms with cocaine intoxication or other cocaine-related problems (Brody 1990; Brower et al. 1988; Honer et al. 1987). What makes these patients prone to violence? What protects the majority of cocaine-using patients against developing violent behavior? The effects of co-occurring personality disorders on cocaine-elicited violence remain largely unexplored.

Amphetamine. Amphetamine may cause intoxication, delirium, or a delusional disorder; these conditions are clinically indistinguishable from those produced by cocaine. Paranoid delusions may result in assault (Angrist and Gershon 1969; Ellinwood 1971) or homicide (Ellinwood 1971). The mechanism of the effects of amphetamine on aggression is unclear, but observations in subjects withdrawn from opioids suggest that opioid peptides may play a modulatory role in these effects of amphetamine (Miczek and Tidey 1989).

Phencyclidine

Phencyclidine (PCP) may be smoked or taken orally, intranasally, or intravenously. Intoxication is manifested by belligerence, assaultiveness, ataxia, dysarthria, muscle rigidity, seizures, and hyperacusis. Delirium caused by PCP may last longer than that caused by cocaine (because of a slower clearance of PCP); otherwise, it is clinically similar. PCP delusional disorder is similar to that elicited by cocaine. Early descriptions of PCP-related violence relied largely on self-reports (Fauman and Fauman 1979, 1980), which were not quite clear about the time elapsed between the last PCP dose and the violent act. Furthermore, some of the subjects reported using other drugs and alcohol in addition to PCP. Inpatients detoxifying from PCP were not especially assaultive (Khajawall et al. 1982). However, a history of PCP abuse given by male schizophrenic inpatients predicted their assaultiveness in the hospital (Convit et al. 1988c; Yesavage and Zarcone 1983). This finding might have been caused by co-occurring (but undiagnosed) personality disorders in the PCP users. Alternatively, schizophrenic patients may be especially vulnerable to some long-term effects of PCP that perhaps facilitate violence. On the whole, however, the links between PCP use and violence appear to be more tenuous and less important than the early reports implied (Fauman and Fauman 1980).

Cannabis

Cannabis preparations (marijuana and hashish) have been associated with violence in folk tales for centuries. The origin of the English term *assassin* can perhaps be traced, via the Arabic *hashashin,* to hashish; this etymology suggested to some that cannabis use was linked to violence (Abel 1977). The folklore was illustrated by the bug-eyed creeps high on marijuana committing unspeakable atrocities in the United States antidrug propaganda movie *Reefer Madness.*

However, evidence linking cannabis to violence has been scarce. In animals, cannabis extracts and its principal active component, Δ^9-tetrahydrocannabinol (THC), reduced aggressive behavior and increased flight and submission under most conditions (Miczek 1987, p. 257). THC tended to suppress aggression in healthy human volunteers in the experimental paradigm described above for testing alcohol effects (S.P. Taylor et al. 1976); see previous "Short-Term Effects of Alcohol and Human Aggression: Experimental Studies" section). A survey of adolescent delinquents indicated that cannabis was used for its calming effect and that it decreased assaultiveness (Tinklenberg et al. 1976). We have conducted numerous experiments studying the short-term and long-term effects of cannabis in American (Volavka et al. 1971a) and Greek (Fink 1977) users without noticing any hostility or violence; the administration of marijuana or hashish seemed to make the subjects more friendly. There is some anecdotal evidence that cannabis preparations may elicit violence in persons with various preexisting mental disorders (Abel

1977). In general, however, modern evidence suggests that cannabis preparations may be associated with violence only under exceptional conditions in predisposed persons.

Although marijuana has no clear pharmacologic effects that would result in increased risk for aggression, dependence on marijuana was associated with a clear increase of risk for violent crime in a large birth cohort (Arseneault et al. 2000). This is explained by systemic violence that is intrinsic to involvement with illicit drugs (see "Crime and Drug Abuse" above).

Opioids

Opioids generally suppress aggressive behavior in animals (Miczek 1987, p. 246). This suppression is nonspecific; other behaviors are suppressed as well by the overall sedative effect. However, when withdrawal from opioids occurs while other animals are present, aggressive or defensive behavior is displayed by rodents and rhesus monkeys (Miczek 1987, pp. 251–252).

In pain-free humans, short-term effects of morphine include mental clouding, sedation (but sometimes excitation), and euphoria (but sometimes dysphoria). The effects of heroin (diacetylmorphine) are similar to those of morphine. Heroin penetrates the blood-brain barrier faster than morphine; accordingly, its central effects have an earlier onset. Heroin is quickly metabolized to morphine. In persons dependent on opioids, the euphoria that follows an intravenous administration of heroin has two phases. The first phase (the "rush") is an intense orgasmic experience that usually lasts for several minutes after the injection. The second phase, lasting several hours, is experienced as a peaceful, pleasant, and sleepy period (the "nod"). In our studies, ex-abusers given moderate doses of heroin under experimental conditions (Volavka et al. 1974) became friendly and "mellow" rather than displaying any aggressive reaction.

In general, clinical observations suggest that opioids have short-term pacifying effects. Methadone was used to treat rage in a schizophrenic patient (Berken et al. 1978). Potential merits of opioids as an antiaggressive treatment were considered (Verebey et al. 1978), but ethical and practical considerations have precluded any systematic tests of opioid treatment for aggression.

Withdrawal from opioids increases aggressive behavior in animals under various experimental conditions (see "Dopamine" in Chapter 2). The evidence for this effect in humans is based on clinical observations rather than on controlled experiments. Dysphoria, irritability, and increased hostility were reported in humans (Tinklenberg and Stillman 1970). There are anecdotal reports of violent behavior elicited by withdrawal from opioids: for example, prostitutes in opioid withdrawal attacked and robbed their clients rather than just tricking them out of their money using more common nonviolent means (Goldstein 1985).

Benzodiazepines

Flunitrazepam is widely prescribed as a rapidly acting hypnotic in Europe and other parts of the world. It has not been approved for medical use in the United States; it is unlikely that this situation will change. Its pharmacologic effects are not qualitatively different from other benzodiazepines; nevertheless, it seems to be the preferred benzodiazepine among substance abusers (Woods and Winger 1997). Use of flunitrazepam, particularly in combination with alcohol, was associated with serious violent crimes among male juvenile offenders in Sweden (Daderman and Lidberg 1999).

Furthermore, illicit flunitrazepam has acquired a reputation as a "date-rape" drug in the United States (Anglin et al. 1997). It can be served to the prospective victim without her knowledge because it easily dissolves in water and is tasteless. Drowsiness and confusion caused by flunitrazepam, particularly in combination with alcohol, reduce the victim's ability to resist; anterograde amnesia reduces the ability to complain afterward. Other benzodiazepines, used to treat agitation and aggression, may occasionally produce a paradoxical increase of violent behavior; this is discussed in Chapter 11.

Anabolic Steroids

Anabolic steroids have been illegally misused by athletes and bodybuilders to enhance muscle growth, strength, and performance. Increased irritability and aggressiveness were recognized as unintended side effects of this practice in a series of published case reports (Anonymous 1993; Choi et al. 1989; Conacher and Workman 1989; Corrigan 1996; Dalby 1992; Moss and Panzak 1992; Pope and Katz 1988, 1990; Schulte et al. 1993). The reports typically describe young male athletes who had not demonstrated any aggressive behavior or other psychopathology until they started medicating themselves with various steroids, sometimes at high doses, to improve their performance or their size. After several weeks or months of self-medication, the men became irritable and combative, committing violent crimes that included homicide, assault, and robbery. Their irritability and violent outbursts disappeared within several months after they stopped using steroids. Mania, depression, and irritability was described in a study of 88 athletes who abused steroids (Pope and Katz 1994). However, risk of violent criminal behavior attributable to steroid abuse does not appear to be very large; interviews of 133 consecutive male convicts have detected only two steroid-induced crimes (Pope et al. 1996)

CO-OCCURRING DISORDERS

To simplify the presentation, the relationships between violence and substances of abuse have been discussed separately for each substance. In reality, however, polysubstance abuse is very common. Substances may be taken simultaneously, even in the same injection (such as the "speedball" combination of cocaine and heroin). Alcohol is frequently combined with drugs of abuse during the same occasion, or it may be used on separate occasions. Polysubstance use may result from a deliberate decision on the part of the user or from a drug supplier's decision to mix several substances together. These mixtures are then sold to users on the streets under various names that do not necessarily imply their true composition: no Food and Drug Administration regulations on product labeling protect these consumers. The user does not necessarily know that he or she is using more than one drug. The combinations of substances result in multiple interactions, and very little is known about the effects of these interactions on aggression in animals or on violence in humans.

Co-occurrence of substance abuse and other mental disorders is very frequent; the contribution of such co-occurring disorders to violent behavior is discussed in Chapter 9. Co-occurrence of substance abuse and antisocial personality disorder is particularly important in assessing the contribution of alcohol and drugs to violent behavior. As discussed above (see "Alcohol Abuse, Alcohol Dependence, and Violent Crime") and in Chapter 7, alcohol abuse or dependence may be related to crime—including violent crime—primarily via antisocial personality disorder (Abram 1989). Substance abuse and other psychiatric disorders were studied in relation to violent behavior in the community within the framework of the Epidemiologic Catchment Area survey (Swanson 1994; Swanson and Holzer 1991; Swanson et al. 1990). Substance abuse was associated with an increased level of self-reported violence, as was schizophrenia. Only Axis I diagnoses (DSM-III) were reported in this study; personality disorders remained unexplored.

In a follow-up study of discharged schizophrenic patients in Sweden, it was noted that violent crime was linked to co-occurring substance abuse (Lindqvist and Allebeck 1990). Similar results were obtained in a prospective study of a cohort of 331 severely mentally ill patients in North Carolina (Swartz et al. 1998a, 1998b) and in an unselected birth cohort (N=11,017) in northern Finland (Rasanen et al. 1998) (see also Chapter 9). Violent behavior among sober, hospitalized schizophrenic patients was related to a self-reported history of assaultive or "loud" behavior under the influence of alcohol or drugs (Yesavage and Zarcone 1983). The effects of alcohol in neuropsychiatrically impaired patients are described above (see previous "Short-Term Effects of Alcohol in Neuropsychiatrically Impaired Individuals" section).

In summary, studies of prisoners, hospital patients, and community samples suggest that the effects of alcohol and drugs on violence are co-determined by the mental disorders of the user. The evidence for interaction among substance abuse, violence, and antisocial personality appears convincing. Similar interaction data for schizophrenia and other disorders are emerging. Such interactions among co-occurring disorders and violence must be addressed in future research, prevention, and treatment efforts.

SUMMARY AND CONCLUSIONS

Alcohol and drugs have variable effects on violent behavior. The direction and size of these effects depend on the dose, the user's personality and his or her experience with the substance, and the social setting (including the availability and behavior of potential victims). The effects of alcohol and drugs on aggression are extremely complex, and it appears that many mechanisms are involved. To design appropriate studies of these mechanisms, one should consider the following factors related to the assailant, the victim, and the pharmacology of the substance:

1. The assailant's personality.
2. The assailant's underlying brain disorder, if any.
3. The assailant's expectancy about the effect of the substance.
4. The assailant's previous experience with the substance. Is the assailant tolerant to the substance? Is he or she dependent on the substance?
5. The victim's activity (including possible alcohol or drug intake) and other factors in the setting.
6. The dose of the substance and its bioavailability (blood and brain levels).

7. The effects of short-term and long-term administration. These may differ dramatically.

8. The effects of the parent compound compared with those of the metabolites. These effects may be different.

9. What receptors are affected. More is being learned about receptor function, and drugs that are more receptor specific are becoming available. However, aggression is mediated by many types of receptors; furthermore, the drug-receptor interactions depend on many of the factors enumerated above (e.g., dose).

9

Violent Behavior of Persons With Mental Disorders Outside of Hospitals

In the degree of public fear it inspires, violent behavior of mentally ill persons in the community overshadows other aspects of violence discussed in this book. The fear is highlighted by the few particularly heinous crimes that receive media attention. Several people with serious mental illness have pushed strangers onto the New York City subway tracks to their deaths (Dugger 1995; Winerip 1999), sometimes repeatedly (Perez-Pena 1993). Each offender had a history of major mental illness, was probably psychotic at the time of the crime, and was not receiving treatment. The question that troubles the general public is this: Are the mentally ill dangerous? The question can be rephrased: What is the relationship between major mental disorders and violence?

Mental health professionals are usually more interested in another question: Can we predict which persons with a mental disorder will become violent? The reason for the interest in prediction is obvious: mental health professionals must continually make practical decisions based implicitly or explicitly on the assessment and management of risk of patients' violent behavior. Each problem (the relationship between mental disorders and violence, and risk assessment) has generated a very large amount of research. This chapter thus consists of two parts: prevalence studies and risk assessment.

The major mental disorders discussed in this chapter include schizophrenia, diverse psychotic disorders not elsewhere classified, severe mood disorders, and various other Axis I disorders (excluding substance abuse, which is reviewed elsewhere). I group together this varied congregation of disorders because many reports on violence and mental illness are diagnostically nebulous when describing the offenders. Diagnostic uncertainty is somewhat more common in reports on patients' behavior in the community than it is for those in hospitals. Violent behaviors of patients in the community and in the hospital differ in many respects and are discussed separately.

PREVALENCE STUDIES

Prevalence studies aim to determine either the prevalence of violent behavior among persons with mental disorders or the prevalence of mental disorders among those who commit violent acts. Until recently, almost all research of the first type was limited to patients discharged from mental hospitals, whereas research of the second type was largely limited to violent criminal offenders. With the development of psychiatric epidemiology, it was soon realized that these samples were subject to various biases, and representative community samples were introduced. Adopting the approach used elsewhere (Monahan 1992, p. 514), we can classify the literature using the following criteria:

1. Violent behavior among persons with major mental disorders
    a) Among identified psychiatric patients
    b) Among representative community samples
2. Major mental disorders among persons exhibiting violent behavior
    a) Among identified violent criminal offenders
    b) Among representative community samples

Violent Behavior Among Persons With Major Mental Disorders

Violent Behavior Among Identified Psychiatric
Patients Estimated From Arrest Rates

I first review the evidence for increased arrest rates and then interpret that evidence. Subjects in the arrest-rate studies were identified as psychiatric patients if they had been discharged from an inpatient psychiatric facility or were registered outpatients. Arrest rates for violent crimes among patients were compared with the arrest rates for the same offenses among control subjects (usually the general public). Arrest rates for homicide and assault were higher in eight samples of discharged patients than they were in control subjects (Rabkin 1979, p. 6, Table 2). More recent studies of this problem showed similar results.

Arrest rates among clients of the Los Angeles County Department of Mental Health (i.e., patients) were compared with those of the adult population of the same county (Schuerman and Solomon 1984). Unlike many other studies that used arrest rates in the general public for comparisons, the county adult population data were adjusted to remove the patients. The ratio of the arrest rate for violent crime among patients to that for violent crime among the general adult population was 1.7:1 (computed from Table 4.1 of Schuerman and Solomon 1984, p. 91). As the authors pointed out, the arrest rate among patients was underestimated because of missing data. Nevertheless, this study is important because of the large size of the populations at risk (65,599 patients and 4,919,000 members of the general population).

Increased arrest rates for violent crime were observed among young adult psychiatric patients (Holcomb and Ahr 1988) and among psychotic individuals who had threatened the president or some other prominent political figure (the "White House Cases"), were hospitalized, and then were discharged (Shore et al. 1990). Similar results were suggested by a survey of patients' families (McFarland et al. 1989). High rates of arrest for violent crime were detected in a follow-up study of males discharged from a community mental health center, but these patients were selected because they were at risk for violent behavior (Klassen and O'Connor 1988b). Unselected patients discharged from another community mental health center in the same state had arrest rates comparable to those of the general population and lower than the arrest rates reported in many other studies of mental patients (Harry and Steadman 1988). The authors suggested that patients treated at community mental health centers differ from those treated at state facilities in terms of their criminal involvement. Another explanation of the relatively low arrest rate is the location of the center "in a small Missouri city"; small cities generally have lower arrest rates than large ones. Two other groups reported a lack of relationship between arrests and mental illness, but their samples of subjects with major mental disorders were too small to draw a useful conclusion: $N=52$ (Lafave et al. 1993) and $N=58$ (Teplin et al. 1993).

Taken together, the articles reviewed by Rabkin and the more recent results yield an approximate median ratio of patient to public arrest (for all offenses) of 3:1 (Link et al. 1992, p. 276). A median ratio specific for violent crimes could not be computed because the level of detail in the description of the offenses varies among studies; an inspection of individual studies giving this information suggests that the ratio for violent crime is at least as large as that for other offenses (e.g., Schuerman and Solomon 1984). It appears that the arrest rates of discharged mental patients have been increasing since the 1950s.

Homelessness may be associated with increased risk of arrest for violent crime in mentally ill persons. In New York City, the prevalence of homelessness among mentally ill persons is approximately 2%; however, 50% of the mentally ill offenders admitted to a major forensic facility serving the city's population are homeless (Martell 1991). The homeless mentally ill offenders were more likely to be charged with violent crimes than were the domiciled offenders (Table 9–1). Murder and assault were the most frequent violent offenses among the homeless mentally ill persons admitted to this forensic hospital. Schizophrenia was the most frequent diagnosis among these offenders (no substantial diagnostic differences between the homeless and the domiciled were seen).

The importance of homelessness as a risk factor for violent behavior in mentally ill persons was supported by a study of persons who pushed victims onto subway tracks in New York City (Martell and Dietz 1992). Of 36 perpetrators who acted alone, 25 were referred for psychiatric evaluation, and data on 20 of these evaluees were available. Nineteen were psychotic at the time of the crime, and 13 were homeless. These data support the overrepresentation of homeless persons among the mentally ill violent offenders in New York City. Furthermore, the case histories of these individuals described the delusions and hallucinations that led them to push innocent strangers to their deaths; for example, three men falsely believed that they rescued others by pushing perceived villains onto the tracks (Martell and Dietz 1992, p. 474).

Several interpretations of these data were considered (Martell 1991; Martell and Dietz 1992). The stresses of homelessness (such as difficulties in finding the necessities of food and shelter) overwhelm the already impaired coping mechanisms of mentally ill persons, eliciting or facilitating violent behavior. Another interpretation is based on a criminalization of homelessness and mental illness. The criminalization hypothesis (which is explained in more detail below) states that mentally ill persons are arrested for trivial behaviors that usually do not lead to arrest in persons who do not obviously have mental disorders. However, these people are charged with very serious offenses.

Table 9–1. Violent crime by domicile status

	Homeless		
Violent crime	No	Yes	Total
No	14 (20.3%)	5 (7.4%)	19 (13.9%)
Yes	55 (79.7%)	63 (92.6%)	118 (86.1%)
Total	69 (50.4%)	68 (49.6%)	137 (100.0%)

Source. Reprinted from Martell DA: "Homeless Mentally Disordered Offenders and Violent Crimes: Preliminary Research Findings." *Law and Human Behavior* 15:333–347, 1991. Used with permission.

I think that a principal reason for the overrepresentation of homeless persons among mentally ill violent offenders is that homeless mentally ill persons are even less likely to receive antipsychotic treatment than the domiciled ones. Homeless psychotic persons usually neither actively seek psychiatric treatment nor have relatives or friends to persuade them to go (or take them) to a psychiatric facility. The alarming data (Martell 1991; Martell and Dietz 1992) should compel the design and implementation of a system for delivering mental health services to homeless people on their terms (probably on their turf), rather than hoping they will spontaneously use the existing overburdened facilities. At the same time, it must be realized that the data do not mean that most homeless people are dangerous or that most violent crimes are committed by homeless people. Such misconceptions will aggravate the plight of homeless people and further complicate the problems of care for those who are both homeless and mentally ill.

In summary, identified patients with major mental disorders have increased arrest rates, including arrests for violent crime. However, serious flaws make the interpretation of these results difficult.

The interpretation of the arrest rate evidence is complicated by a number of problems. The main flaw is that patients discharged from public psychiatric hospitals are not representative of the general public. Many patients are admitted to such hospitals because they are violent in the community (Craig 1982; Rossi et al. 1985, 1986; Tardiff and Sweillam 1980). The best predictor of future violence is past violence (see Chapter 6). If patients are selected for admission because of violence, it is not surprising that the violence sometimes continues in the hospital and then after discharge. Furthermore, the poor and minorities are overrepresented among patients in public hospitals, and—at least in the New York metropolitan area—the majority of patients are male. These demographic factors are associated with violent crime. Unless these factors are accounted for, they (rather than mental illness) may be the basis for the observed increases in the arrest rates among discharged patients.

Another serious problem of these studies is inherent in the complexity of the processes leading to arrest (see Chapter 1). In general, only a small proportion of violent (or criminal) behavior is followed by an arrest. Furthermore, specific biases may affect arrests of suspects with mental disorders. Briefly, the offender's ability to avoid capture, the officers' perception of the offender, and the officers' experience, training, and bias determine whether an arrest or an alternative disposition will occur. From the officers' standpoint, arresting mental patients may be faster and surer than attempting to initiate emergency hospitalization; such attempts have a reduced rate of success because the standards for involuntary commitment have generally become more stringent.

Without adequate housing and treatment, patients experience exacerbations of their symptoms with concomitant disorderly, fear-inducing, or violent behavior in the streets. These behaviors may not be crimes, and even if they are, the offenses are frequently quite trivial. In the absence of adequate mental health resources, patients may be arrested just because they exhibit strange behavior in public, and they may be jailed with or even without criminal charges (Torrey et al. 1992). The term *criminalization of mental illness* was coined to describe this diversion of patients from the mental health system to the criminal justice system (Abramson 1972). Thus, the high arrest rate among discharged patients may reflect the presence of mental illness rather than underlying violent behavior (Teplin 1984). However, police sometimes rehospitalize rather than arrest assaultive ex-mental patients; thus, "police statistics concerning the criminal activity of ex-mental patients may radically underestimate the most serious behavior of ex-mental patients while overestimating the less serious behavior" (Steadman and Keveles 1972, p. 309).

Increasing numbers of people prone to violence and crime are served by public psychiatric facilities. This psychiatrization of criminal behavior (Monahan 1973) has resulted in an influx of persons with prior criminal records into patient populations. Many persons of this type are admitted to psychiatric facilities because of violence. It has been argued that the high arrest rates among discharged patients may reflect psychiatrization of their (previous) criminal violence rather than any relationship between mental illness and violence or crime.

The influx of patients with a prior criminal record, described as "changing clientele" (Steadman et al. 1978a), may be associated with changing characteristics of schizophrenic patients admitted to state hospitals. Between 1970 and 1986, the proportion of males among these patients increased from 50.7% to 70.6%, and the proportion of patients paying no fee increased from 34.8% to 58.2% (J.W. Thompson et al. 1993). In general, males with low incomes are overrepresented among violent criminals. A comparison of two inpatient admission cohorts (1968 and 1978) demonstrated that the number of patients with a history of a prior arrest for violent crime increased from 13.3% to 20.8% (Cirincione et al. 1992). Hospital downsizing has probably resulted in relatively higher numbers of aggressive patients; thus in a hospital in Maryland, the census decrease was consistently and uniformly associated with an increase in staff injuries over a period of 10 years (Snyder 1994).

Further evidence for the overlapping functions of the criminal justice and mental health systems was provided by data indicating that arrests and hospital admissions are correlated with each other: the more frequently persons are defined as criminal (arrested), the more frequently they are defined as mentally ill (admitted) (Klassen and O'Connor 1988a). Taken together, the data on criminalization of mental illness, psychiatrization of criminal behavior, and mutual penetration of the systems suggest the existence of unpredictable, arbitrary procedures that determine whether a person is arrested, hospitalized, or released. This renders the meaning of arrest (or admission) as an outcome variable quite ambiguous and obscures the interpretation of arrest studies.

Arrest studies were summarized and interpreted in a frequently quoted review that has had a profound influence on thinking about mental disorders and crime (Monahan and Steadman 1983). The authors studied the trends in arrest rates for discharged mental patients and concluded that these rates were increasing and that the increase could be accounted for by an increased number of patients with a prior criminal record being admitted to public psychiatric facilities (Steadman et al. 1978a). The increased arrest rate of discharged mental patients (compared with that of the general population) was explained by factors such as the patients' lower age, lower social class, and greater frequency of prior arrests. Once statistical adjustments were made to account for these factors, the arrest rates among discharged patients and the general population equalized. Discharged patients without a prior arrest had approximately the same or lower likelihood of arrest as the general population, which was also observed by another reviewer (Rabkin 1979).

However, comparison with the general population is not without problems. As pointed out by others (Link et al. 1992, p. 277), the general population consists of persons with various numbers of arrests. For example, comparing the arrest rate of patients with "no prior arrest" with the arrest rate of the general population is inappropriate, unless persons with prior arrests have been removed from the general population sample. This removal is not easy. The arrest rates of discharged mental patients can be compared with those of criminal offenders released from jails and prisons (Steadman et al. 1978b). One of the advantages of this comparison group is that its arrest rate history can be obtained with relative ease. Predictably, ex-offenders had much higher arrest rates than ex-patients after the prior arrests were controlled for (Steadman et al. 1978b).

Let us consider the statistical adjustments for social class and prior arrests. One of the authors of the original review (Monahan and Steadman 1983) observed that these adjustments were problematic (Monahan 1992, p. 514). I agree. Because mental illness is too vague a concept to discuss in this context, let us focus on schizophrenia—a principal cause of hospitalization in public psychiatric facilities. First, consider the relationship between social class and schizophrenia. There is general agreement that the highest prevalence of schizophrenia is in the lowest social classes, and many investigators believe that this overrepresentation is caused by a downward social drift of the patients (Babigian 1985, p. 649). By accounting for the effects of social class, a relationship between mental illness and arrests is obscured. However, the effect of social class on the future (postdischarge) arrest rate was relatively minor compared with that of the prior arrest rate.

Prior arrest rate is associated with postdischarge arrest rate among mental patients. The proportion of patients with prior arrest records has been increasing among those who are newly hospitalized, and the increase in the postdischarge arrest rate is attributable to an increase in the proportion of patients with prior records. But why has the proportion of newly admitted patients with prior arrests increased?

Steadman's concept of changing clientele (Steadman et al. 1978a) could mean either that different individuals are admitted or that the individuals are the same but their behavior is changing. Steadman meant a difference in individuals: "The issue is not so much that there are more mentally ill people at risk for criminal activity in the community; more accurately, the problem seems to be that there are more criminals in mental hospitals in the first place" (Steadman et al. 1978b, p. 1220). I think that this hypothesis implies that mental illness (e.g., schizophrenia) is unrelated to future arrests; the risk of future arrest is due to prior arrests, which are due to illegal behavior unrelated to mental illness.

Alternatively, it is possible that prior arrests are related to mental illness. I now discuss how that could be and why prior arrests may be increasing for clinical and social reasons.

In examining the prior arrest problem, the first question is: prior to what? Typically, investigators mean "prior to current hospitalization." But what does that mean in the course of a mental illness such as schizophrenia? Public psychiatric facilities do not generally admit first-break schizophrenic patients. At the two state hospitals in the New York metropolitan area that house our research units, newly admitted schizophrenic or schizoaffective patients had an average of six to eight previous hospitalizations, and the first symptoms occurred 7–10 years before the current admission (Volavka et al. 1992a, p. 356). This issue is important because the onset of schizophrenia and the onset of aggressive behavior may be related (see Chapter 5, Figure 5–6, and P.J. Taylor 1993). No violence or arrest information was obtained in our set of patients (Volavka et al. 1992a), but judging from the data of P.J. Taylor (1993), most of them had passed through the period of maximal risk for the onset of violence (which may have occasioned one or more "prior arrests") by the time we first saw them. Accounting for prior arrests (which may have been a result of schizophrenia) would thus obscure a relationship between schizophrenia and violence or arrest after discharge.

But how would Taylor's findings account for the increase in the number of prior arrests in the United States since the 1960s? The initial push for deinstitutionalization and subsequent continuing pressure to discharge patients from public hospitals have had two relevant effects.

First, patients' violent behavior no longer occurs in the hospital, where violence would usually not lead to arrest, but in the community, where arrest is a more likely response. Thus, if mental illness results in violent events independent of the environment but linked to the course of illness, discharging patients to the community would result in an increased likelihood of their arrest, depending on the course of illness.

Second, the likelihood of violent behavior and arrest in discharged patients may be increased by various risk factors whose effects are magnified by the inadequacy of outpatient psychiatric care and a lack of housing. The most obvious of these risk factors is patients' noncompliance with antipsychotic treatment. Discontinuation of maintenance antipsychotic medication greatly increases the likelihood of a relapse (Schooler 1991), with an exacerbation of hostility and irritability (Zander et al. 1981), antisocial behavior (Johnson et al. 1983), and violent behavior (Swartz et al. 1998b). Another obvious risk factor is alcohol and drug abuse. Comorbidity of substance abuse and schizophrenia has probably been rising (Cuffel 1992); this issue is discussed later in more detail.

Discontinuation of treatment may be caused by inadequacies of psychiatric care or by the patients' unwillingness (or inability) to take advantage of the opportunity offered by such outpatient psychiatric care that is available. Outpatient commitment to court-ordered treatment is a method that addresses this complicated issue. It is possible that if it is maintained for longer periods of time (more than 6 months) and is combined with intensive outpatient treatment, it may improve treatment compliance, reduce substance abuse, and decrease violent behavior (Swanson et al. 2000; Swartz et al. 2001). However, outpatient commitment may not be effective in all circumstances (Steadman et al. 2001).

The problems with arrest-rate studies were recognized by researchers who launched projects to correct them. Some uncertainties surrounding the process leading to arrest were resolved by direct observations of encounters between police and citizens (Teplin 1985). This study showed that mentally ill persons did not differ substantially from other citizens in their pattern of crime, and the author thus thought that her data "help dispel the myth that the mentally ill constitute a dangerous group prone to violent crime" (p. 593). However, only 20 police-citizen encounters were concerned with violent personal crimes; 3 of the suspects (10%) were among 30 citizens with mental disorders, and 17 of the suspects (3.6%) were among 476 citizens without mental disorders involved in encounters with police (Teplin 1985, p. 597, Table 2). These percentages, taken at face value, would support rather than dispel the "myth" of dangerousness. However, the number of observed encounters involving violent personal crimes was too small for definitive conclusions.

In summary, in earlier studies, many problems complicate the interpretation of arrest data in identified mental patients. These patients were usually included in studies after their hospital discharge, thus biasing the selection. Furthermore, the processes leading to arrest are complex and are likely to result in additional biases. There has been an increase in the arrest rates of mental patients. Possible explanations of this increase include criminalization of mental illness, psychiatrization of criminal behavior, discharges of large numbers of mental patients without a commensurate increase in community resources to care for them, and possibly increased rates of comorbidity of major mental disorders with substance abuse.

Violent Behavior Among Identified Psychiatric Patients Established Independently of Arrest

In this section, I discuss violent behavior in the community by identified psychiatric patients. The identification of a person as a psychiatric patient was provided by hospital or outpatient facility records. Most studies report on behavior during several days or weeks preceding hospital admission, with the admission records as the principal source of data. Other studies capture the patients' violent behavior over longer periods of their stay in the community. Both types of studies are retrospective.

Preadmission violence studies generally confirm that violent behavior is a frequent antecedent of admission to a psychiatric hospital. Physically violent acts against persons or objects occurred "recently" in 18% of newly admitted psychiatric patients ($N=321$). These researchers (Lagos et al. 1977) excluded patients diagnosed with personality disorder or a toxic condition due to alcohol and drugs; therefore, most of the violence reported was attributable to major mental disorders. The largest study of this type was based on 9,365 patients admitted to public psychiatric hospitals in Long Island, New York. Assaultiveness on admission was recorded in 923 (9.9%) patients (computed from Table 3 of Tardiff and Sweillam 1980, p. 165). In another study, psychiatrists recorded assaultiveness as "present" in 11% of 876 patients newly admitted to a psychiatric hospital (computed from Table 1 of Craig 1982, p. 1263). An analogous study reported that 20% of 1,687 patients were assaultive within 2 days before admission (Rossi et al. 1986). A total of 53 of 238 newly admitted patients (22%) engaged in physical attacks during the 2 weeks preceding hospitalization (McNiel et al. 1988).

Data from a World Health Organization (WHO) prospective study of the outcome of schizophrenia (Jablensky et al. 1992; Sartorius et al. 1986) were subjected to post hoc analyses focusing on the rate of physical assaults against other persons in a sample of 1,017 patients in 10 countries (Volavka et al. 1997). These patients were ascertained when they had their first-in-lifetime contact with a helping agency as a result of their psychotic symptoms. Among the 1,017 patients, 20.6% had a history of assault, which was more frequent in the developing (31.5%) than in the developed countries (10.5%) .

Aggressive incidents in first-episode psychosis were studied in a cohort of 166 consecutive psychotic patients making first contact with psychiatric services in a British town (Milton et al. 2001). Using multiple sources of information, the authors reconstructed the histories of aggressive incidents occurring before the onset of illness (Period A) and after the onset but before contact with services (Period B), and they reassessed the subjects' aggressive incidents during the first 3 years after the contact (Period C). In Period A, 9.6% of the subjects exhibited aggressive behavior; in Period B, 17.0%, and in Period C, 21.1%. Aggression in these incidents was rather widely defined; when only serious incidents were counted (any injury to victim, sexual assault, weapon use, or threat), the proportions of seriously aggressive patients for Periods A, B, and C were, respectively, 6.0%, 4.8%, and 4.8%. Overall, 9.6% of the subjects demonstrated at least one act of serious aggression, and 23.5% demonstrated lesser acts of aggression. The rate of serious aggression is similar to the 10.5% rate of physical assaults reported for the developed countries in the WHO study (Volavka et al. 1997).

These studies differ in the definitions of violence and in the methods of its ascertainment. Some studies (e.g., Craig 1982) apparently used data routinely collected by workers who received no special training or supervision by researchers; other studies applied a research rating scale to medical records (Lagos et al. 1977; McNiel et al. 1988; Rossi et al. 1986). The studies using raw data reported a rate of preadmission violence of approximately 10%; the others reported a rate of approximately 20%. Perhaps the methods used by the latter studies were more sensitive. In any event, the rates grossly overestimate the prevalence of violent behavior among psychiatric patients residing in the community; it should be remembered that these patients were selected for admission at least in part because of acts of violence. Violence probably peaks shortly before admission. Furthermore, because dangerousness to others or oneself is known to be a key condition for admission to public psychiatric facilities, it is conceivable that assaultiveness may be overreported by relatives or other persons interested in the patient's admission. However, patients who commit violent acts against members of their families are less likely to be admitted than those who assault strangers (Gondolf et al. 1991).

Violence not linked to admission was investigated in a prevalence study of 2,916 outpatients at clinics of two private hospitals; 3% of these outpatients exhibited recent assaultive behavior in the community toward other persons (Tardiff and Koenigsberg 1985). This study is unique in its choice of private facilities as research sites and in its focus on outpatients.

A small sample ($n=148$) of discharged mental patients was compared with a sample ($n=245$) of the general population and with ex-offenders ($n=141$) living in the community (Steadman and Felson 1984). The subjects were interviewed regarding their violent behaviors in the past year; these self-reports indicated that the patients' involvement in violent incidents was greater than that of the general population but smaller than that of the ex-offenders.

In a landmark project (MacArthur Violence Risk Assessment Study), mental patients ($N=1136$) who were followed up for a year after their discharge from the hospital were compared with community residents ($N=519$) (Steadman et al. 1998). The patients were recruited in hospitals in Pittsburgh, Pennsylvania; Kansas City, Missouri; and Worcester, Massachusetts. The community sample was recruited in Pittsburgh in the neighborhoods in which the patients resided after discharge. The patients and collateral informants were interviewed five times after discharge (every 10 weeks); the subjects in the community sample and informants were interviewed once. The information collected from patients and community subjects pertained to violent behavior and symptoms of substance abuse during the previous 10 weeks.

There was no significant difference between the prevalence of violence by patients without symptoms of substance abuse and that of the nonpatient community residents who were also without symptoms of substance abuse. Substance abuse was associated with increased rates of violence in both groups, more so among the patients. Patients had increased rates of substance abuse in comparison with nonpatients. Patient violence decreased during the 1-year follow-up period.

As the authors acknowledge, the sample attrition may have been biased; it has been suggested that more persistently violent patients would drop out first, and this would have explained the decline in the rate of violence that was observed (Czobor and Volavka 1999). This explanation would be consistent with the fact that the patients who were lost to follow-up were more likely to be diagnosed with alcoholism than those who completed the study (Steadman et al. 1998, Table 1). Furthermore, the rate of violent behavior among the nonpatient community residents was surprisingly high even in the subset of persons without substance abuse; this might have contributed to the lack of difference in the rates between the discharged patients and other community residents. Nevertheless, the community behavioral patterns may be representative of the environments into which patients are discharged from public urban psychiatric facilities in the United States.

Violence Among Persons With Mental Disorders in Community Samples

Two main problems complicate the studies of identified mental patients discussed above. First, the patients are usually identified through records of public hospitals. This method tends to select patients who are likely to be violent. Second, the main outcome measure—the arrest rate—is compromised by uncertainties surrounding the procedures leading to arrest.

These problems are avoided in the studies of persons with mental disorders who were detected in representative community samples. The first such study (Swanson 1994; Swanson et al. 1990) was done in the Epidemiologic Catchment Area (ECA) program (Regier et al. 1984). The ECA surveyed adult household residents. The Diagnostic Interview Schedule (Robins et al. 1981) was used to assess the community prevalence of mental disorders. The Diagnostic Interview Schedule recorded violent behavior (hitting someone, fighting after drinking alcohol, using a weapon in a fight). Demographic, diagnostic, and institutional-contact predictors of violent behavior in the community were analyzed by logistic regression (Swanson 1994, p. 127, Table 9). That analysis demonstrated that substance abuse was very strongly associated with violence. Major mental illness (schizophrenia spectrum and affective disorders) was also associated with violence, and that association remained significant after the effects of substance abuse, demographic variables, and institutional contacts (previous arrests and hospitalizations) were accounted for statistically. The analysis also demonstrated strong effects of demographic variables (male gender, low age, and low socioeconomic status) and of the history of arrest. The effect of major mental illness and the effect of low socioeconomic status on violent behavior appeared to be approximately the same size. This breakthrough study thus demonstrated for the first time that the association of major mental disorders with violent behavior is not an artifact due to biases involved in sample selection or in police procedures.

These results were soon confirmed in a study that compared mental patients and never-treated community residents on official records of arrest for violent offenses, self-reported arrests, and four self-reported measures of violent behavior: hitting others, fighting, using a weapon in a fight, and ever hurting someone badly (Link et al. 1992). Mental patients were more violent than the community residents who had never been treated for mental illness. This difference was not attributable to age, gender, or ethnicity. A measure of psychotic symptoms was also obtained. If mental disorders cause people to be violent, one of the possible mechanisms is that psychotic symptoms (such as false beliefs) may induce the individuals to hurt others.

For such a hypothesis to be valid, psychiatric individuals would have to be more dangerous when they are more psychotic. The hypothesis was tested by introducing a psychotic symptom scale score as a covariate into logistic regression analyses of violent behaviors (Link et al. 1992, p. 152, Table 5). Psychotic symptoms were indeed significantly related to violent behavior. More detailed analysis identified 3 of the 13 rated symptoms as being specifically related to violence: delusions of thought control, thought insertion, and delusions of persecution (Link and Stueve 1994). These relationships between symptoms and violent behavior were replicated and expanded in a large epidemiologic study (N=2,741) conducted in Israel (Link et al. 1998). However, they were not replicated in a set of data generated by the MacArthur Violence Risk Assessment Study mentioned previously (Appelbaum et al. 2000) or in a study of aggressive incidents in first-episode psychosis (Milton et al. 2001).

Connections between psychiatric symptoms and violence are intuitively meaningful, but the time link between the violent act and psychotic symptoms is quite loose. The psychotic symptom scale interview was concerned with symptoms occurring during the previous year (Link and Stueve 1994, p. 144, Table 1; Link et al. 1998). The prevalence of violent behaviors was determined for the preceding month and for the preceding year (Link and Stueve 1994), or for the preceding 5 years (Link and Stueve 1994; Link et al. 1998). Thus, the symptoms might have been absent at the time of the violent act. One might even consider the possibility that the symptoms only developed after the violent act. In that case, the symptoms could not have caused the violence. It appears that these researchers did not ask their subjects any questions about the temporal relationship between violent acts and psychotic symptoms.

However, such questions were asked by another researcher investigating the motives of violent crimes (P.J. Taylor 1985). Interviews of mentally ill prisoners indicated that more than 80% of their index violent offenses were committed under the influence of psychosis. Thus, this British study supports the notion of a direct and causal relationship between violent acts and psychotic symptoms, providing crucial evidence of temporal linkage between the two phenomena. Similar evidence of this temporal linkage was reported elsewhere (Martell and Dietz 1992). In general, the prevalence of acting on delusions is an important issue, which was studied by using a special questionnaire (Maudsley Assessment of Delusions Schedule) developed for this purpose. This questionnaire was administered to assess newly admitted British psychiatric (nonforensic) patients selected because they had at least one delusion (Wessely et al. 1993). The patients (N=83) were interviewed regarding their actions in response to the delusions; 18% of the patients hit someone and 19% broke something because of a delusion. In an American study of nonforensic delusional patients (N=54), 17.5% of the patients reported at least one incident that was extremely violent and definitely motivated by a concurrent delusion (Junginger et al. 1998). Thus these two studies, conducted in different countries and using somewhat different methods, yielded consistent estimates. Interestingly, in a forensic sample of German schizophrenic offenders (N=284), 18% of the patients reported that voices ordered them to commit the crime (Hafner and Boker 1982). Is it possible that delusions are related to command hallucinations that lead more directly to violent acts? Similar speculations exist (Junginger and McGuire 2001), but conclusive data addressing this possibility are not yet available.

Command hallucinations to do harm are associated with increased levels of dangerous behavior (Junginger 1995). Among 103 psychiatric patients on a short-term inpatient unit who filled out a questionnaire pertaining to their experiences in the previous year, 30% reported command hallucinations and 22% reported compliance with the commands. Patients who experienced command hallucinations were significantly more violent than others (McNiel et al. 2000).

It is not clear that the command hallucinations or delusions that appear to be related (perhaps causally) to a violent act are affecting the patient's behavior specifically, in the sense that they are unrelated to other psychopathology experienced by the patient at the moment. After the effects of general psychotic symptoms were accounted for statistically, command hallucinations were no longer significantly associated with violence (McNiel et al. 2000). Violent patients have more severe psychotic symptoms than nonviolent ones (Krakowski et al. 1999), and thus there may be an underlying disease process that causes violence and is manifested by command hallucinations and other psychotic symptoms.

To date, all published studies relating delusions and hallucinations to violence are retrospective. It is unlikely that such studies, covering long periods of time and subject to imperfect or distorted recall, can resolve the questions surrounding relationships between symptoms and violence. Temporal relations between psychopathology and violence are better assessed by investigating each violent incident and its attendant symptoms within hours after it occurred; this effort is now in progress at the Nathan Kline Institute.

Scandinavian Epidemiologic Studies

A study of an unselected Swedish birth cohort (Hodgins 1992) confirmed and expanded the relationships reported by the two American teams (Link et al. 1992; Swanson et al. 1990). The cohort consisted of 15,117 persons born in Stockholm in 1953; these subjects were followed up until age 30 years. Criminal records were obtained from the Swedish National Police Register, and mental health records were obtained from the Stockholm County Register and other sources. Major mental disorders (schizophrenia, major affective disorders, paranoid states, and other psychoses) occurred in 1.1% of the subjects. The definition of violent crime was broader than that used in the United States (Maguire et al. 1993): in addition to assault, rape, robbery, and murder, the Swedes included "unlawful threat," "molestation," and perhaps other offenses. Among persons without mental disorders, the conviction rate for violent offenses was 5.7% in the men and 0.5% in the women.

The magnitude of the risk of violence associated with mental illness is typically expressed as the odds ratio (Feinstein 1985, p. 124). If a group of patients with mental illness is compared with another group in terms of violence, an odds ratio greater than 1.0 indicates an increased risk of violence associated with mental illness. An odds ratio of 2, for example, indicates that a person with mental illness is twice as likely to be violent as a person from the comparison (control) group. The 95% confidence interval (95% CI), usually provided in parentheses after the estimated odds ratio, indicates that the true odds ratio in the larger population from which the sample was drawn has a 95% probability of being located in the interval.

In this Swedish study (Hodgins 1992), the odds ratio of violent offense for men with major mental disorders was 4.2 (2.2–7.8), and for women it was 27.5 (9.8–76.9). This is a study based on arrest rates; the limitations of such studies are discussed previously.

More recent epidemiologic investigations based on a large Danish birth cohort (Brennan et al. 2000; Hodgins et al. 1996) avoid many of the problems of the earlier studies. The cohort includes 358,189 individuals born in Denmark between January 1, 1944, and December 31, 1947. Official arrest and conviction data through 1991 were obtained from the Danish National Police Register in Copenhagen. Records of psychiatric hospitalizations (dates and diagnoses) through 1991 were obtained from the Danish Psychiatric Register. Data from these two registers were merged, and the computations that were implemented provided important information about relationships between mental disorders and crime, particularly violent crime.

The data from this Danish cohort are less distorted by sampling and other biases than the earlier studies. Furthermore, the clearance rates for crimes in Denmark are relatively high (e.g., 97% for homicide, compared with 65% in the United States) (Maguire and Pastore 1995, p. 406) (see Chapter 1). Importantly, the police in Denmark do not have the discretionary power of whether to arrest a person suspected of a crime. Mentally ill individuals who commit a crime are first arrested and then transferred. Therefore, the process leading to arrest is unbiased.

A major study using the Danish birth cohort confirmed an increased risk of crime for persons with a history of psychiatric hospitalization in comparison with persons who were never hospitalized (Hodgins et al. 1996). A more recent study of the same cohort focused more specifically on the relationship between arrests for violent crime and individual major mental disorders (schizophrenia, organic brain syndrome, affective psychoses, and other psychoses) (Brennan et al. 2000). Confidence intervals of odds ratios of criminal violence were 2.0–8.8 for men and 3.9–23.2 for women with major mental disorders. The analogous ratios for schizophrenia were 4.6 (3.8–5.6) for men and 23.2 (14.4–37.4) for women. Very importantly, the odds ratios for schizophrenia remained significantly higher in subsets of patients without diagnoses of comorbid personality disorders or substance use disorders, and after controlling for socioeconomic status. Therefore, the authors maintain, this relationship between violent crime and schizophrenia cannot be fully explained by demographic factors or comorbid conditions. However, it must be kept in mind that the diagnostic information relied exclusively on hospital charts. Thus, unless a patient had a discharge diagnosis of substance abuse, he or she was assumed not to have that condition. I believe that the chart diagnoses of substance use disorder were correct in the sense that patients so diagnosed truly had the condition. However, I think that less severe cases of substance use disorders were likely to be missed even though they were meeting the diagnostic criteria. Furthermore, even if the psychiatrists did not miss any diagnoses, a person can do quite a lot of drinking without meeting any diagnostic criteria. For these reasons, it is necessary to view with caution the authors' claim that the risk of violence associated with schizophrenia exists separately from the risk of substance abuse.

Investigations of another Scandinavian birth cohort yielded somewhat similar results. Unlike the Danish cohort, the northern Finland birth cohort ($N=12,058$) was investigated prospectively. The subjects' history of hospitalizations as well as their criminal records were evaluated when they were 26 years old (Rasanen et al. 1998; Tiihonen et al. 1997). The odds ratio of criminal violence was 3.1–15.9 for men with the diagnosis of schizophrenia (overlapping with the analogous Danish estimates of 3.8–5.6; see above).

Another Finnish study investigated the prevalence of mental disorders among homicide offenders (Eronen et al. 1996c). Approximately 95% of homicide cases are solved in Finland; 1,423 homicide offenders were so identified in a 12-year cohort. Schizophrenia or schizophreniform disorder was diagnosed in 86 male and 7 female offenders. These data enabled the computation of odds ratios of homicide that are representative of Finland. The odds ratio for schizophrenia and schizophreniform psychoses in males was 10.0 (8.1–12.5), and in females it was 8.7 (4.1–18.7). The authors estimated that of the 86 male offenders, 38 had comorbid alcoholism and 48 did not. The odds ratio for those without comorbidity was lower than for those with it, but both ratios were significantly elevated; therefore comorbid alcoholism probably cannot fully explain the increased risk of homicidal behavior in schizophrenia in this sample. However, the estimates of comorbid alcoholism are based on North American prevalence data that may not apply in Finland; therefore these results regarding comorbidity must be viewed with caution. Odds ratios of homicidal behavior for other mental disorders are reported in an earlier subset of these homicide offenders; as expected, alcoholism and antisocial personality disorders are associated with very high odds ratios (Eronen et al. 1996b).

The Scandinavian studies clearly demonstrated links between violent behavior in the community and major mental illness. However, Scandinavia is socially very different from the United States. During the period of these studies, Scandinavian countries were relatively prosperous, egalitarian, ethnically homogeneous societies where drug abuse and access to handguns were considerably less widespread than in the United States. Therefore, the criminogenic factors specific to mental illness probably have a smaller effect in the United States than in Sweden (relative to the criminogenic factors affecting the general population).

In summary, the results obtained in the American and Scandinavian populations indicate that major mental disorders increase the risk for violent behavior. The risk increase is greater in females and in patients with comorbid alcoholism and substance use disorders, but the relationship between major mental illness and violent crime cannot be fully explained by these comorbid conditions. The remaining important issues are the magnitude of the added risk and the contribution of that risk to the rate of violent crime in the general population.

The *magnitude of the risk of violence associated with mental illness* was discussed in part in the review of Scandinavian studies. Some American data are available in a study already cited (Link et al. 1992). These authors used six measures of violent behavior (outcomes), and they accounted for sociodemographic variables in determining the relationship between patient status and the outcomes. For each of the six outcome (dependent) variables, the authors computed a logistic regression equation using the following independent variables: patient status (patient versus never treated), age (in years), gender, education (in years), and ethnicity (blacks and Hispanics were separately contrasted against whites). Because they published logistic regression coefficients (Tables 2–4 in Link et al. 1992, pp. 285–287), I was able to compute the odds ratios for each independent variable. (Readers who are interested in checking my calculations should know that I used "repeat-contact" patient status and computed the odds ratios for model 3. The authors computed the odds ratio for 4 years of education because this time period reflected the difference between college and high school; I followed their procedure.) The odds ratios are presented in Table 9–2.

Table 9–2. Violent behaviors and odds ratios

	Independent variables				
Dependent variables	Patient (yes or no)	Age (years)	Gender (male)	Education[a]	Ethnicity (black)
Official arrest record	7.36	NS[b]	21.32	2.08	13.00
Self-reported arrest	2.80	NS	5.58	1.70	1.85
Hitting others	2.42	NS	NS	2.36	NS
Fighting	1.94	—[c]	2.54	NS	NS
Weapon use	3.30	NS	NS	2.32	NS
Ever hurt someone badly	NS	NS	4.49	2.34	6.03

Note. Odds ratios were computed from published logistic regression coefficients (Link et al. 1992). For example, the odds ratio in column 1, row 1, means that patients were 7.36 times more likely than nonpatients to have an official arrest record.
[a]Computed for 4 years of education (see text).
[b]Logistic regression coefficient not statistically significant ($P>0.05$).
[c]Odds ratio was not computed because of unknown age range or class.

Patienthood increased the likelihood of violent behavior. This effect was generally smaller than that of gender but greater than the effects of age or education. (The lack of age effect is surprising; perhaps it is due to the fact that the relationship between age and violence is generally nonlinear, peaking between 15 and 25 years [see Chapter 6]. The logistic regression analyses tested linear relationships.)

The *contribution of major mental disorders to the rate of violent* crime in the general population is generally agreed to be small. Although psychotic symptoms are related to violence, "such symptoms are relatively rare and are in no way as important as the influx of drugs, the breakdown of communities, and similar factors as causes of violent/illegal behavior" (Link et al. 1992, p. 290).

This disclaimer, although not supported by any data provided by the authors (Link et al. 1992), makes intuitive sense. The lifetime prevalences of major mental disorders are low, and the violent crime rates are high. However, the contribution of major mental disorders to violence and violent crime can be amplified by several factors.

First, offenders with major mental disorders may *commit more crimes per individual* than offenders without mental disorders (see "Crime Rates of Individuals" in Chapter 1). The American community studies (Link et al. 1992; Swanson et al. 1990) provide very little information on individual rates, but the Swedish study reported that the average number of convictions among male offenders without mental disorders was 7.6, but among those with major mental disorders it was 13.2 (Hodgins 1992, p. 479). The number of convictions specific for violent offenses was not reported, but the subjects with major mental disorders "have committed many serious offenses throughout their lives" (Hodgins 1992, p. 476). Other authors explained their observation of a slightly higher arrest rate for violent crime among schizophrenic persons as being "a result of high rates of violent crimes perpetrated by a few individuals" (Teplin et al. 1993, p. 97). Thus, it is possible that major mental disorders not only increase the likelihood of participation in violent and illegal behavior but also are associated with higher rates of such behavior among the participants. It is regrettable that little is known about mental patients' criminal careers, although a theoretical framework for the type of research required was provided (Mulvey et al. 1986).

Second, the association between major mental disorders and violent behavior may be strengthened by *comorbidity with substance abuse.* A demonstration of this effect was provided in a longitudinal prospective study of a population-based cohort of 644 individuals with schizophrenia in Sweden (Lindqvist and Allebeck 1990). Thirty-eight of these patients were responsible for 71 violent offenses between 1972 and 1986. Fourteen of these offenders abused alcohol and/or drugs, and another seven were probable abusers. Similar effects were demonstrated in the United States (Swartz et al. 1998b). As discussed elsewhere in this book, alcohol and drug abuse are clearly implicated in the causation of violent behavior. Major mental disorders are associated with an increased risk for substance abuse; the evidence regarding schizophrenia is particularly persuasive.

The ECA study reports that 47.0% of persons with a lifetime diagnosis of schizophrenia or schizophreniform disorder also met diagnostic criteria for substance abuse or dependence (33.7% for an alcohol abuse disorder and 27.5% for another drug abuse disorder) (Regier et al. 1990). The odds ratio of a substance abuse diagnosis in persons with schizophrenia or schizophreniform disorder is 4.6 (i.e., the odds are 4.6 times higher in persons with schizophrenia than in the rest of the population). The analogous odds ratio in persons with mood disorders was 2.6 (Regier et al. 1990). It should be noted that the ECA substance abuse diagnoses were based only on interviews; this limitation might have resulted in underestimates of prevalence. Even when a systematic effort to diagnose substance abuse is made, a proportion of individuals whose urine samples contain cocaine will deny its use (Shaner et al. 1993). Covert abuse of other substances is also likely.

The rates of comorbidity of schizophrenia and substance abuse (specifically, abuse of alcohol and stimulants) have probably been rising over past decades (Cuffel 1992). Cuffel's evidence for this rise has been disputed (Alterman 1992), but I think that experienced clinicians practicing psychiatry in the public sector agree with Cuffel.

The relative magnitude of the contribution of mental illness to violent crime probably varies across societies. The prevalence of major mental disorders shows only slight variations among different countries, but the variations in the rates of violent crime are quite large. Therefore, the absolute contribution of mental illness to violent crimes probably remains stable across societies, but its relative contribution varies. For example, the elevation of the violent crime rate in the United States compared with other countries is not attributable to mental illness but to societal factors. Formal comparisons of the relative contributions of mental illness to violence in various countries are difficult because there are many differences in the definitions, detection, and registration of violent behaviors, violent crimes, and mental illnesses. Nevertheless, at least one such study compiled and compared national statistics comparing rates of homicide committed by mentally ill ("abnormal") offenders with overall homicide rates (Coid 1983). The results are presented in Figure 9–1.

The rates of homicides committed by mentally ill offenders are approximately equal in all countries and in all time periods examined. The

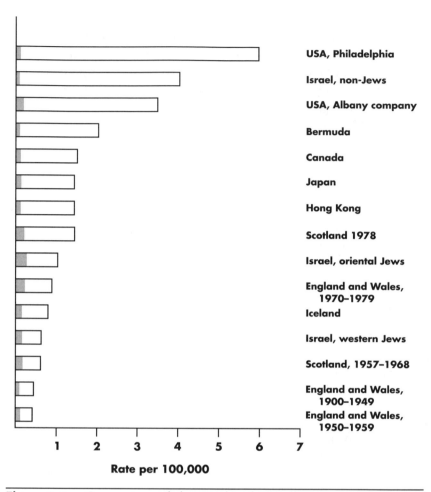

Figure 9–1.   Comparison of abnormal and overall rates of homicide.

Source.   Reprinted from Coid J: "The Epidemiology of Abnormal Homicide and Murder Followed by Suicide." *Psychological Medicine* 13:855–860, 1983. Reprinted with the permission of Cambridge University Press.

wide variation of overall homicide rates is attributable to the "normal" offenders. Thus, the relative contribution of major mental disorders (or "abnormality") to homicide is smaller in the United States than in other countries. These findings on homicide may not generalize to other crimes such as assault. The rate of assault in schizophrenia patients in the developing countries is approximately three times higher than in the developed countries (Volavka et al. 1997). This would further increase the relative contribution of major mental disorders to criminality in developing countries in comparison with the United States.

Major Mental Disorders Among
Persons Exhibiting Violent Behavior

Prevalence of Major Mental Disorders Among
Identified Violent Criminal Offenders

Numerous studies estimate the prevalence of major mental disorders among incarcerated offenders; 18 studies published between 1976 and 1986 were critically reviewed elsewhere (Teplin 1990). These studies showed increased prevalences of major mental disorders among inmates, but otherwise the results were inconsistent; the studies shared serious methodological flaws that I do not review here.

Probably the most sophisticated study of this subject determined the current and lifetime prevalence rates of schizophrenia and major mood disorders in a random sample of male jail detainees (Teplin 1990). Using a standard diagnostic interview (Diagnostic Interview Schedule) (Robins et al. 1981), Teplin determined that the current prevalence of schizophrenia was 2.7% and that of any severe disorder was 6.4%. The rates were generally two to three times higher than those detected in the general population in the ECA study (Regier et al. 1988; Robins et al. 1984). Similar unpublished data obtained in California prisons are quoted elsewhere (Monahan 1992, Table 4, p. 518).

A privately sponsored nationwide questionnaire survey of 1,391 jails indicated that 7.2% of jail inmates in the United States have "serious mental illness" defined as "schizophrenia, manic-depressive illness and related conditions" (Torrey et al. 1992, Table 2.1, p. 15). The diagnosis of serious mental illness was apparently made by jail officials, based on brief descriptions of typical symptoms included in the questionnaire; nevertheless, the average result was close to Teplin's estimate of 6.4% (see above).

Unfortunately, it is not known whether the rates of major mental disorders among jail and prison inmates are specifically related to violent offending—in terms of either current offense or criminal careers. The risk of violence among male inmates with schizophrenia was reported to be high (P.J. Taylor and Gunn 1984), but my calculation (based on Tables 4 and 5 in P.J. Taylor and Gunn 1984) indicates that the relationship between conviction for violent crime and schizophrenia was not statistically significant (χ^2=0.217, df=1). A similar nonsignificant association between violent crime and major mental disorders was reported elsewhere (Ashford 1989). Opposite results (i.e., less violent crime in psychotic prisoners) were also published (Valdiserri et al. 1986).

In a jail survey, the most common offense leading to arrests of seriously mentally ill persons was assault and/or battery, followed by theft and disorderly conduct (Torrey et al. 1992, p. 19, Table 2.3). Many trivial offenses were listed, supporting the notion that in some cases serious mental illness is being criminalized. The survey, unfortunately, did not inquire about the most common offenses among the mentally healthy inmates; it is therefore difficult to evaluate the meaning of the data on the offenses of mentally ill persons. However, a jail survey conducted by the U.S. Department of Justice indicates that assault is less frequent than theft, burglary, drug possession, drug trafficking, driving while intoxicated, and traffic offenses (Maguire et al. 1993, p. 600, Table 6.45). This survey did not address the inmates' mental status. If these two surveys are otherwise comparable, and if both yielded reliable data, one would conclude that seriously mentally ill inmates were overrepresented among the criminals committing assault.

A large survey of mental illness among violent criminal offenders was conducted in Germany (Hafner and Boker 1982). The survey had a different focus than most American studies. The authors identified criminal offenders (*N*=533) who were charged with homicide or attempted homicide, committed the alleged offense between 1955 and 1964, and were found "mentally ill or mentally defective." Diagnoses of schizophrenia, affective psychoses, exogenous psychoses (organic), dementia, or mental deficiency (retardation) were apparently abstracted from charts; no diagnostic criteria are offered. Four comparison groups were used: the general population, mentally normal violent offenders convicted between 1955 and 1964, mentally abnormal persons in the general population, and mentally abnormal nonoffenders.

The results indicated an overrepresentation of the diagnoses of schizophrenia (particularly the paranoid type) and mental retardation in the homicide group (compared with nonoffenders with mental disorders). The opposite was true for affective psychoses and dementias. Epilepsy was equally represented in these two groups. The schizophrenic offenders were older (peak of the age distribution, 30–40 years) than the mentally normal offenders (peak of the age distribution, 21–25 years). Onset of schizophrenia preceded the crime by 1–5 years in 35% of these offenders and by 5–10 years in 24% of the offenders. (Note similar data in Figure 5–6 in Chapter 5 of this volume.) This study has methodological problems that make it unsuitable for deriving prevalence estimates of mental illness, but it contains interesting information on psychopathology.

In summary, major mental disorders are two to three times more prevalent among jail inmates than among the general population. The implications of this consistent finding for violence research are unclear because several attempts to find a specific relationship between violent criminal offenses and mental illness among inmates yielded equivocal results.

Prevalence of Major Mental Disorders Among Violent Persons in Community Samples

Very little is known about the prevalence of major mental disorders among violent persons in the community. The ECA survey yielded a categorical classification of community respondents as "violent" or "nonviolent" on the basis of their self-reports. The prevalence of mood disorders was approximately three times higher among the violent respondents than among the nonviolent respondents; a similar ratio was obtained for schizophrenia (Swanson et al. 1990, p. 765). The extent of comorbidity with substance abuse and potential inflation of these ratios by such comorbidity were not discussed. Nevertheless, the results indicate that major mental disorders occur more frequently among violent people.

RISK ASSESSMENT

Regardless of the arguments and theories about the prevalence of violence among mentally ill persons, psychiatrists and other health professionals must make practical decisions that are implicitly or explicitly based on assessments of individual patients' potential for violent behavior. Decisions involving predominantly *implicit* assessment as one of the factors in clinical management must be made quite frequently; they involve patients' admissions and discharges, psychopharmacological and other treatment, and various security arrangements, including those for the professionals' own safety.

Furthermore, whether they like it or not, psychiatrists must interact with a criminal justice system that demands *explicit* predictions of "dangerousness" (Monahan 1993). Such predictions are required for many legal purposes, including commitment and release of "dangerous" persons, sentencing, bail, and so forth (Monahan 1981, pp. 22–23). The explicit predictions provided for legal purposes are the ones most visible to the general public, particularly when they fail, which they do frequently. Most research studies are concerned with explicit prediction.

Dangerousness, Prediction, Risk, and Harm

Dangerousness may mean either that someone would commit a violent act or that he or she would be likely to do so under some conditions (e.g., if intoxicated). The "if" is important because, for example, people may remain dangerous in this sense for the rest of their lives, even if they never commit a violent act. Thus, this vague term should be avoided.

Instead of dangerousness, psychiatrists should specify harm, risk, and predictors (risk factors) (Monahan and Steadman 1994). *Harm* indicates the type and seriousness of violence (e.g., assault resulting in injuries requiring hospitalization). *Risk* is an estimate of the probability of harm; that estimate is conditional on circumstances (e.g., the risk of violence among discharged schizophrenic patients depends on the patients' compliance with antipsychotic drug treatment). Risk changes over time; ongoing risk assessments adjusting to changing circumstances are more likely to be useful in future research and practice than the one-time predictions that have been customary until now. *Risk factors* are the variables that affect the risk; therefore, they are used to predict violence (gender, age, and drug abuse are typical examples). Obviously, risk factors that are amenable to change (e.g., drug abuse) are potential foci of prevention strategies.

Methods Used for Risk Assessment

Independent Variables (Risk Factors or Predictors)

The clinical or actuarial method is used to manage independent variables. The clinical method is based on the skill of the clinician who interviews the patient, reads the patient's records, elicits the information he or she considers important for the prediction of violence, evaluates the information within the framework of his or her experience with risk assessment in similar patients, and then usually makes a categorical (yes or no) statement regarding the patient's risk for violent behavior. A classic study of this type provides an illustrative list of data elicited from patients for the prediction of dangerousness, for example: "What is his conception of an ideal person?" "Does he have sympathetic identification with others?" "How did he get along with his peers?" "Did the patient feel loved, supported, encouraged by either or both parents?" (Kozol et al. 1972, p. 385).

This approach has several strengths. One lies in its proximity to real-life clinical case conferences. Clinicians can understand and identify with this approach. Furthermore, this procedure is based on clinicians' training, leaving open the possibility for judgments based on intuition. Importantly, it enables the clinician to use any information available. Most actuarial studies rely on preprinted (or preprogrammed) data entry forms; usually that makes it impossible to use data that were not foreseen as important. Therefore, one advantage of the clinical approach is the possibility of tailor-made, specific risk assessment for individual patients.

Unfortunately, these strengths may also be seen as weaknesses. Let us examine the individual components of the clinical prediction procedure. The entire procedure depends on the clinician's skill and experience. These attributes are hard to define or measure, but we know that clinicians vary widely in skill and experience. Variables considered important by one clinician may not be important to another, and this difference in variable selection may occur in some patients but not in others. Thus, we have a situation where the variables selected for risk assessment depend on the clinician as well as the patient. To make matters even more confusing, the variables may be inadequately defined. To illustrate, "sympathetic identification with others" may depend on many factors, for example on who the "others" are. Finally, no method for integrating information and using it for the prediction is offered by most authors.

These problems make the clinical risk assessment process unreliable. It is surprising, therefore, that at one institution, clinicians showed moderately good interrater reliability when using a scale to assess emergency room patients' potential for violence toward others in the next 6 months (score, 0–10; $r=0.68$) (Lidz et al. 1993). The ratings were done independently, but they were performed after the patient's disposition was decided by the raters. This arrangement might have inflated the interrater agreement on the scale; for example, if the clinicians decided after a discussion not to admit a patient, it is reasonable to assume that they both thought that the patient was not very dangerous and that they shared that opinion with each other during that discussion, implicitly or explicitly.

The actuarial method differs from the clinical method primarily in the way the information on individual patients is integrated and used for prediction. Instead of the intuitive integration focusing on an individual, the actuarial approach uses various statistical methods applied to groups of individuals. The actuarial method may use variables that are defined with varying degrees of precision; it can use, for example, a loosely defined variable such as "sympathetic identification with others" (present or absent) as one of the predictors of violent behavior. However, researchers using the actuarial approach typically define their variables more explicitly and quantitatively than this example. A statistical explanation of the actuarial method is provided in the appendix.

Dependent Variables (Measures of Violence)

Typical dependent (or criterion) variables are arrest for violent crime, hospital admission for violent behavior, and self-reported violent behavior. Most risk assessment studies report only a dichotomous classification (violent or nonviolent) to describe behavior during the follow-up period. This is unfortunate, because valuable information about the number and seriousness of episodes of violent behavior is lost.

The dependent variables are obtained during a specified time period (follow-up period). This period should be explicitly specified in advance, at the time the prediction is made. Furthermore, the results should be adjusted for the time at risk. For example, if the dependent measure is the number of arrests, it should be adjusted as the number of arrests per year or per month the subject spends out of prison or hospital (and is therefore at risk for arrest) during the follow-up period.

Assessing Accuracy of Risk Assessment

Clinical and actuarial methods usually yield a categorical prediction: the patient either will or will not be violent. To assess the accuracy of the prediction, one may utilize the diagnostic marker approach (Feinstein 1985, pp. 434–435). Using this approach, the predicted outcome (violence) is considered a disease, and the predictor (or a set of predictors used in an equation) is the diagnostic marker. One then constructs a fourfold table showing hypothetical data in a violence prediction study (Table 9–3).

In Table 9–3, cell a contains true-positive; cell b, false-positive; cell c, false-negative; and cell d, true-negative results of the prediction. To assess the performance of the prediction, one can estimate its nosologic and diagnostic accuracy; sensitivity and specificity are computed for each of these measures of accuracy. *Nosologic sensitivity* is $g = a/n_1$: the proportion of subjects, among those who actually turn out to be violent, who were predicted to be so. *Nosologic specificity* is $f = d/n_2$: the proportion of subjects, among those who turned out to be nonviolent, who were predicted to be so. *Diagnostic sensitivity* is $v = a/m_1$: the proportion of subjects, among those predicted to be violent, who actually turn out to be violent. This index reflects the predictive accuracy of a positive prediction. Thus, low diagnostic sensitivity indicates overprediction of violence, which is a common problem (see below). *Diagnostic specificity* is $u = d/m_2$: the proportion of subjects, among those predicted not to be violent, who turn out not to be violent. This index reflects the predictive accuracy of a negative prediction. Low specificity indicates underprediction.

Table 9–3. Fourfold table showing hypothetical data in a violence prediction study

Violence predicted to occur	Violence occurred	Violence did not occur	Total
Yes	a (true positives)	b (false positives)	m_1
No	c (false negatives)	d (true negatives)	m_2
Total	n_1	n_2	N

Diagnostic accuracy is influenced by the prevalence or "base rate" of the disease (in this application, violent behavior) among the persons being studied. Diagnostic sensitivity and specificity decrease as prevalence decreases. These relationships follow from the Bayes theorem (see appendix).

Violent events, particularly serious ones, are rare. This low base rate has resulted in reduction of diagnostic accuracy (diagnostic sensitivity in particular), which has hindered the efforts to make predictions that have practical usefulness. One can mitigate the problem by deliberately selecting subjects who are at particularly high risk for violence and are therefore expected to have high base rates (Klassen and O'Connor 1988b) or by using other methods (Quinsey 1980).

Results of Prediction Studies of Violence in the Community

Before reviewing this research, it is important to point out that no truly representative samples could be studied. In forensic practice, patients who are thought to pose a clear danger of violence are not released; therefore, their behavior in the community cannot be studied. This practice is appropriate from the ethical and legal standpoints, but it confounds the research on prediction of violence: how can one test the accuracy of prediction when the most violent patients are systematically excluded from the samples (Litwack et al. 1993)? To circumvent this limitation, researchers studied samples of patients who were assessed as dangerous by clinicians and then released for administrative or legal reasons despite that assessment (Steadman and Cocozza 1974). Such samples of opportunity are valuable but are not representative. This problem of biased subject selection cannot be resolved by improvements in the definition of risk factors or by sophisticated statistics; it is an inherent flaw that will always limit the validity of research in this area.

Clinical Prediction

Early studies have demonstrated poor reliability of clinical prediction (Cocozza and Steadman 1976; Steadman and Cocozza 1974; Steadman and Keveles 1972; Thornberry and Jacoby 1979). Attempts to predict violence were hampered by problems in the theory and practice of clinical risk assessment.

After the publication of a landmark book on the prediction of violence (Monahan 1981), research on clinical prediction was better informed. Somewhat encouraging results of clinical prediction were based on a pretrial assessment of dangerousness and a 2-year follow-up for violent behavior, using official records of the criminal justice and mental health systems in the province of Ontario, Canada. Psychiatrists evaluated 364 subjects. A fourfold table (prediction versus outcome) was presented (Sepejak et al. 1983, p. 176). Unlike the predictions in the previous article (Cocozza and Steadman 1976), these were significantly better than chance ($\chi^2=12.9$, $df=1$, $P=0.003$). Using the same table in that publication (Sepejak et al. 1983), I calculated four indexes of prediction accuracy (diagnostic and nosologic specificities and sensitivities). These indexes ranged between 56% and 63%, indicating a very modest accuracy of the prediction.

A most sophisticated study of clinical prediction data used a sample of 357 emergency room patients whom clinicians assessed as likely to be violent and a sample of control patients matched on gender, race, and age. Patients were followed up for 6 months (Lidz et al. 1993). The follow-up data on violent behavior were collected during repeated interviews with the patients and collateral informants; police, court, and hospital records were also used. Because the patients were matched on demographic characteristics, the clinicians' predictive accuracy was over and above what would be achievable if those demographic features had been considered.

The accuracy of the clinical prediction was better than chance, but still very modest. Nosologic sensitivity and specificity were 60% and 58%, respectively. Diagnostic sensitivity and specificity were 53% and 64%. Violence during the follow-up period was reported in 36% of the comparison group and in 53% of the patients predicted to be violent. Predictive accuracy was better for men than for women (among women, it was not better than chance).

These results were obtained by experienced researchers using a sophisticated design at a university-affiliated site; the research was financially supported by multiple grants. I see a disparity between the resources deployed and the marginal accuracy of the prediction. Contrary to the authors, I do not think that the long-term clinical prediction of violence in the community can be much improved; if these researchers, with their experience and support, could not do it, probably nobody can.

In summary, the clinical prediction of violence for 6 months or more among mentally ill persons in the community may not be feasible without a major expansion of the knowledge concerning causes of violence. The results of current studies may be statistically significant, but the predictions remain too inaccurate for practical use. Perhaps the method has "hit the forensic sound barrier" (Menzies et al. 1985): improving this technology while keeping its basic idea intact will be like trying to cross the sound barrier with an improved, but still propeller-driven, airplane.

Predictions for shorter periods of time and for explicitly described environmental conditions are likely to be more accurate.

Actuarial Prediction

The design for actuarial risk assessment was first applied in retrospective studies that simulated prediction of violence (Steadman and Morrissey 1981). These methodological advances informed the development of a systematic, truly prospective program for actuarial predictions of violence among mentally ill persons by Klassen and O'Connor.

The prospective longitudinal design used by Klassen and O'Connor included a calibration sample of subjects to develop their prediction method and a cross-validation sample to test it.

The *calibration sample* (N=304) was selected among patients admitted to a community mental health facility in Kansas City, Missouri. To maximize the base rate of future violence (see previous "Assessing Accuracy of Risk Assessment" section), subjects with increased potential for violence were selected for this study (Klassen and O'Connor 1988b). The predictor variables used in the calibration sample covered demographic characteristics, living arrangements, and family background; current marriage, family, friendships, and employment over the past 3 months; history of arrests, psychiatric admissions, and violent incidents; and drug and alcohol use.

Two preliminary reports on the calibration sample alone were published (Klassen and O'Connor 1988a, 1988b). The important purposes of the discriminant analysis were the screening of predictor variables and the computations of beta weights to be used for the prediction of violence in the cross-validation study (see previous "Methods Used for Risk Assessment" section and appendix).

The *cross-validation sample* (N=256) was selected at the same facility; all men (irrespective of their estimated propensity for violence) were invited to participate as subjects. The methods of data collection were similar to those used for the calibration sample. On the basis of analyses of the calibration sample data, five predictor variables were selected: early family quality, current intimate relationship, arrest history, admission history, and assault as a presenting problem. The beta weights determined in the calibration sample for these five variables were used to compute a score for each subject; the score was used as an estimate of that individual's risk for violence. The cutoff point derived from the calibration sample was used to classify these scores as predictive of either violence or nonviolence.

With this procedure, 63 men were predicted to be violent, but only 33 of them behaved accordingly (Table 9–4). The prediction accuracy was

Table 9–4.   Cross-validation of risk assessment

Violence predicted to occur	Violence occurred	Violence did not occur	Total
Yes	33	30	63
No	34	168	202
Total	67	198	265

Note. $P < 0.0001$.

Source.   Adapted from Klassen D, O'Connor WA: "Assessing the Risk of Violence in Released Mental Patients: A Cross-Validation Study." *Psychological Assessment: A Journal of Consulting and Clinical Psychology* 1:75–81, 1989. Copyright 1989 by the American Psychological Association. Used with permission.

significantly better than chance, but the improvement over chance was only 13%. Using the data presented in Table 9–4, I computed nosologic sensitivity, nosologic specificity, diagnostic sensitivity, and diagnostic specificity. The results were 49%, 85%, 52%, and 83%, respectively. Thus, the positive prediction was less accurate than the negative one (there were relatively more false positives than false negatives). Compared with the accuracy of the clinical predictions reviewed previously, this actuarial prediction has improved specificity but not sensitivity.

There was an indication that schizophrenic patients were overrepresented among the violent subjects. However, clinical features such as symptoms or diagnoses were not selected as predictors in the cross-validation study, although substance abuse was strongly related to violence in the calibration sample (Klassen and O'Connor 1988a, p. 309, Table 3).

The actuarial method was used to examine the relationship between violent acts and threats by patients with serious mental illness, their social networks, and the social support they received (Estroff and Zimmer 1994; Estroff et al. 1994). A group of 169 patients and 59 of their significant others were interviewed. Data on acts and threats of violence by the patients over an 18-month period were collected from interviews and court records. Patients in larger networks, those with networks composed primarily of relatives, and those who lived with unrelated persons were more likely to threaten violence. More than half of the targets of violence were patients' relatives, particularly mothers living with a patient.

A longitudinal prospective study of arrest rates for violent crime among released jail detainees has not detected any significant effect of major mental disorders on the rates (Teplin et al. 1993). Nevertheless, the average number of arrests for violent crime during the 3-year follow-up period in schizophrenic persons ($n=23$) was 1.42; the average was 0.79 for the detainees with no mental disorder ($n=240$). As the authors point out, the lack of statistical significance of the difference (P=0.08) might be explained by the small number of schizophrenic persons in their sample.

A group of Finnish-American investigators (Virkkunen et al. 1989b) studied biological predictors of criminal recidivism in a group of released violent offenders. Their first report indicated that the combination of blood glucose nadir in the glucose tolerance test (see "Insulin" in Chapter 3) and the 5-hydroxyindoleacetic acid (5-HIAA) level in the cerebrospinal fluid successfully predicted recidivistic offending in a small sample (N=58) composed of violent offenders and arsonists. However, the glucose nadir failed to predict violent recidivism in a larger sample (DeJong et al. 1992). The sample consisted of 248 murderers and 100 arsonists. It included the 58 subjects from the previous study by the same group of investigators (Virkkunen et al. 1989b). Discriminant analyses yielded two principal predictors of violent recidivism among the murderers: the impulsivity of the index crime and the diagnosis of antisocial or conduct disorder (DeJong et al. 1992). The determination of impulsiveness was based on police reports describing the following characteristics of the index crime: victim unknown to offender, no or minor provocation, no premeditation, and no financial gain (impulsiveness is discussed in Chapter 7). These predictors of violent recidivism (impulsive crime and antisocial personality) should be viewed as provisional until they are cross-validated.

An actuarial method called Iterative Classification Tree (Monahan et al. 2000) was developed and applied in a subset of patients (N=939) enrolled in the MacArthur Violence Risk Assessment Study described previously (Steadman et al. 1998). While in the hospital, the patients were assessed on 106 risk factors. They were monitored for violent behavior for the first 20 weeks after discharge. The classification was based on two cutoff points that defined three categories: high risk, low risk, and unclassified. A more usual practice is to define two categories using a single cutoff point. Their procedure left 27.4% of the sample unclassified, and the remaining patients were classified as high risk or low risk. This approach is less ambitious and more realistic than trying to classify all patients. An iterative procedure was used to prune the risk factors from 106 to 15; this resulted in an actuarial instrument that is feasible to administer under clinical conditions. The 15 factors yielded diagnostic sensitivity of 45% and diagnostic specificity of 95% (calculated from Table 2 of Monahan et al. 2000) in subjects who could be classified. Thus, similar to other actuarial instruments, positive prediction was less accurate than the negative one. Information on other actuarial instruments, particularly on the Violence Risk Appraisal Guide, can be found elsewhere (Harris and Rice 1997).

In summary, actuarial assessment of risk for violent behavior in the community has not yet yielded sufficiently accurate predictions. Successful cross-validation presents problems.

SUMMARY AND CONCLUSIONS

Prevalence studies indicate that most psychiatric patients are not violent. However, patients with major mental disorders who were discharged from psychiatric hospitals, those who are about to be admitted to such hospitals, and those who are treated as outpatients show higher rates of violent behavior compared with the general population. Arrests for violent crimes constitute one of the measures of such behaviors in discharged patients; such arrests have been increasing over the past several decades. Furthermore, major mental disorders are two to three times more prevalent among jail and prison inmates than in the general population.

These data are generally consistent with the notion that major mental disorders are associated with violent behavior. However, alternative explanations of the data include the biased selection of patients, biased or inconsistent procedures leading to arrest, and more generally, changing relationships between the criminal justice and the mental health systems. Until approximately 1990, these alternative explanations were believed to account for the reports of violent behavior by identified mental patients. In other words, the relationship between major mental illness and violence was seen as spurious.

Criminalization of mental illness, psychiatrization of criminal behavior, and other phenomena confound the arrest rates among discharged psychiatric patients. However, these phenomena cannot explain the association between violence and mental disorder documented in recent studies of representative community samples. The bias in subject selection that had been invoked to explain the results of previous studies was not present in the community samples. Furthermore, these new findings were partly based on self-reports, obviating the potential biases of arrest rates. Specific psychotic symptoms were related to violent behaviors; this finding suggests a direct, and possibly causal, relationship between mental illness and violence in the community.

The recent studies of community samples not only confirmed the relationship between mental illness and violence but also estimated the magnitude of the contribution of mental illness to the risk of violence. Future research focused on particular risk factors may yield powerful strategies for risk assessment and ultimately for risk management.

Clearly, comorbid substance use disorders as well as nonadherence to continued treatment regimens are the major risk factors for violence in the mentally ill. Some studies even suggest that the risk for violence in the mentally ill who do not abuse substances is not increased in comparison with healthy community residents. However, the preponderance of evidence indicates that major mental disorders such as schizophrenia increase the risk for violence even in the absence of comorbid substance use. Nevertheless, preventing and treating comorbid substance use disorders and providing continued pharmacologic and social treatment are useful strategies to reduce the risk of violent behavior in patients with major mental illness.

Despite recent advances, neither clinical nor actuarial risk assessment studies have yet yielded accurate or practical predictions. Future studies of this type could be enhanced by acquiring independent (predictor) variables not only before patients' discharge, but also during the follow-up period. Thus, predictions developed on the basis of the predischarge data could be repeatedly updated. Such variables would include compliance with psychopharmacologic treatment; discontinuation of antipsychotics is a typical cause of relapse that may be associated with assault and other illegal behavior. The subjects' utilization of outpatient mental health services would be the logical starting point for the study of risk management; outpatient clinic records of patients' appointments and attendance are usually easy to obtain and abstract. If these factors are included in future studies, one might expect assessments of risk conditional on patients' keeping their next outpatient appointment and on their adherence to medication regimens. Plasma levels of antipsychotic medications are useful for the assessment of short-term adherence; levels in the patients' hairs can provide information about medication intake over a period of weeks or months. Development of, or an increase in, substance abuse during the follow-up period is another variable that would be potentially useful for updating prediction. Design and implementation of such studies would require interdisciplinary research teams.

10 | Violent Behavior of Psychiatric Inpatients

Violent behavior is a principal reason for psychiatric hospital admission. This connection is reflected by many studies indicating that violence frequently occurs immediately preceding admission; these studies are reviewed in Chapter 9 (Craig 1982; Lagos et al. 1977; McNiel et al. 1988; Rossi et al. 1986; Tardiff and Sweillam 1980). Continuity of violence is one of the most replicated observations; prior violence is usually a very good predictor of future violence. Therefore, it is not surprising that some patients continue to be violent after they are admitted to the hospital. However, not all inpatient violence can be seen as simple persistence of preadmission behavior. Violent behavior will fluctuate with changes in the type and severity of patients' symptoms. It can be suppressed or augmented by medication as well as by behaviors of caregivers and fellow patients. Public hospital wards are frequently crowded, noisy, and chaotic; these factors may contribute to conflicts and overt aggression. The necessity to share limited facilities with others calls for patience, tolerance, and social skills; these assets are frequently affected by mental illness. Thus, institutionalization may aggravate or even elicit the violent behavior it is assumed to treat.

PREVALENCE STUDIES

The reported prevalence of violence depends to an extent on the definition and detection of violent behavior (see Chapter 1). Detection methods include continuous videotaping, making direct visual observations, interviewing staff members, reviewing charts and ward journals, and examining official incident reports. There is an increasing loss of information as one progresses from videotaping to the official incident report.

The loss of information (or underreporting) is greatest for the assaults that result in no injuries or in only very minor ones (see Chapter 1).

Restraint and seclusion are sometimes used as measures of dangerous behavior, but these measures are indirect and are not specific for violence; for example, patients may be restrained or secluded for agitation or self-injurious behavior. Restraint and seclusion are used to prevent violence in patients who induce fear by threats or other means. These interventions are clinically useful and ethically necessary, but they may confound results of prevalence and prediction studies: patients predicted to be violent would have been violent without the intervention. This spuriously inflates the rate of false-positive predictions.

Prevalence studies typically report the number (or proportion) of assaultive patients in a defined sample. This proportion is important, but it does not tell us anything about rates of assault by individual patients. Similarly to the individual crime rates discussed in Chapter 1, individual assault rates can be determined for hospitalized psychiatric patients. One practical reason for studying individual rates is to focus preventive measures on the individuals who commit the most assaults. Furthermore, recidivistic and nonrecidivistic violence may have different psychobiological bases; I return to this issue later.

I define *generic assaultiveness* as a characteristic of patients who assault another person at least once during a given time period. *Recidivistic assaultiveness* describes patients who commit assault at least twice during that period. Arbitrarily, some authors define recidivistic patients as those who commit assault at least three times (Convit et al. 1990a; Shader et al. 1977). There are nonrecidivistic violent patients who commit assault only once (or twice) during that period; these patients demonstrate *nonrecidivistic assaultiveness*. When I speak of assaultive patients in the subsequent text, I mean generic assaultiveness (patients who commit assault at least once in a given period) unless otherwise specified.

The proportion of assaultive patients is maximal in the short time period immediately after admission. A proportion of patients respond to treatment, and that proportion gradually increases over several weeks. Most schizophrenic patients who will respond to typical neuroleptics such as haloperidol will do so within approximately 6 weeks, and the most pronounced improvement of positive symptoms occurs within the first 2 weeks of treatment (Volavka et al. 1992a). Patients who are assaultive primarily because of their psychosis will stop being violent as their psychosis improves. This mechanism will thus reduce the proportion of inpatients who are currently violent.

However, a countervailing mechanism will tend to increase the proportion of recidivistically assaultive inpatients with the length of stay. The patients who improve will be discharged, and the patients who do not improve will stay. Thus, the proportion of nonresponders increases with the length of stay; some of these nonresponders are violent. As the pressure to discharge patients increases, the patients who are considered less dangerous leave the hospital, thereby increasing the proportion of recidivistically violent patients among those who stay. This phenomenon is particularly pronounced in long-term-care state hospitals. Violent behavior was associated with longer hospital stay in schizophrenic patients in some reports (Greenfield et al. 1989; Shader et al. 1977), but no such association was found by others (Karson and Bigelow 1987). Thus, diagnosis, treatment, and course of illness interact with each other in their effects on assaultiveness in complex ways that are poorly understood. It is clear, however, that short-term hospitalization and long-term hospitalization present different patterns of violence.

Short-Term Hospitalization

Within the first 3 days of hospitalization, 44 of 253 (17.4%) newly admitted patients physically attacked another person at a short-term psychiatric facility (Binder and McNiel 1990, p. 111). The percentage was lower for males (13.6%) than for females (21.5%). Another sample was restricted to newly admitted male schizophrenic and schizoaffective patients whose behavior was observed during the first 8 days of hospitalization; 25 of 289 patients (8.7%) assaulted another person at least once (Tanke and Yesavage 1985, p. 1410).

Long-Term Hospitalization

Using a special reporting instrument developed for their project, Tardiff and Sweillam (1982) studied the proportion of assaultive persons among 5,164 patients who were hospitalized for at least 1 month in two large public (state) hospitals. They found that 7% of these patients had physically assaulted other persons in the hospital at least once during the preceding 3 months. Similar rates of assaultiveness were reported in private hospitals (Tardiff 1984). Other reports were published, but either assault rates could not be inferred from them (Fottrell 1980) or they were outdated; the older literature is reviewed elsewhere (Tardiff 1992).

In summary, the results of prevalence studies depend to a large extent on the methods used to define and detect violence, the type of facility, and the patients' stage of illness. The proportion of assaultive patients (but not individual assault rates) was determined in short- and long-term facilities. The prevalence is maximal during the first several days after admission, and then it decreases. In long-term psychiatric hospitals, the 3-month prevalence is approximately 7%.

CORRELATES AND PREDICTORS OF VIOLENCE

The correlates can be classified into two major groups: those inherent in the violent individual and those imparted by the environment in which the violent incident occurs. Much more is known about the individual than about the environmental correlates.

The individual-related correlates include gender, race, age, and genetic and developmental factors that are considered in Chapter 5; these variables need not be discussed in detail here. Briefly, males are overrepresented among violent patients in the community, but that gender difference disappears (or may even be reversed) once the patients are hospitalized. Racial differences in violence were not detected among inpatients. Assaultiveness among inpatients is greatly reduced after age 30 years, but there is a slight increase in assaultiveness in women after age 65 years.

A history of violent behavior is an important correlate and predictor; I discussed the continuity of violence in Chapter 6. A history of substance abuse is related to inpatient violence; the relationship may be mediated in part through personality disorders. Clinical factors such as the Axis I diagnosis, current symptoms, and response to treatment are considered in greater detail here.

The environmental and social correlates considered include the time of day, ward characteristics such as staffing, and (more recently) behavior of the victims.

Short-Term Hospitalization

Correlates of Violence

Violent behavior in the community during the 2 weeks preceding admission was associated with violence during the first 3 days of hospitalization (McNiel et al. 1988); a similar relationship was found for preadmission threats (McNiel and Binder 1989) (see also Chapter 9).

Diagnosis may be a variable correlated with assaultiveness among hospitalized patients, but the correlation may vary as a function of postadmission time. During the first 24 hours of hospitalization, manic patients were more violent than schizophrenic and other patients (Binder and McNiel 1988). However, it is not known how long this situation persisted.

Manic patients may respond faster and more uniformly to treatment than schizophrenic patients (treatment resistance is less prevalent in patients with mania). Therefore, it is possible that violence related to psychosis abates faster in manic patients than in schizophrenic patients. Bipolar patients are more likely to be violent when manic than when depressed (Yesavage 1983a). Schizophrenia and mania were overrepresented among assaultive patients in private hospitals (Tardiff 1984).

In schizophrenic patients, violent behavior within the first 8 days of hospitalization was associated with a history of blackout episodes and assaultiveness while drinking and of being "loud" under the influence of illicit drugs (Yesavage and Zarcone 1983). A history of substance abuse was related to assaultiveness on other acute-care wards (Myers and Dunner 1984; Walker and Seifert 1994).

Symptoms recorded on admission are related to assaultiveness in the subsequent days or weeks. Such relationships were studied particularly in patients with schizophrenia or schizoaffective disorder. The Brief Psychiatric Rating Scale (BPRS) (Guy 1976) was administered on admission to 207 such patients, whose assaultive behavior was then observed for the first 8 days of hospitalization (Yesavage 1983b). A principal-component analysis was used to reduce the 18 BPRS items to five factors. Two of these factors were positively related to assaultiveness; one of them reflected conceptual disorganization, hallucinations, and unusual thought content; the other described suspiciousness, uncooperativeness, and hostility. One factor (blunted affect) was negatively related to assaultiveness.

Association between positive symptoms on admission and violence during the first several weeks of hospitalization has been confirmed in a study that focused, I think rather uniquely, on the relationship between several aspects of patients' insight on admission and later violence. Insight of mental illness, need for treatment, social consequences of the disorder, and signs and symptoms were all impaired in violent patients in comparison with nonviolent counterparts (Arango et al. 1999, Table 3, p. 498).

Verbal hostility was related to physical assaultiveness (P.D. Werner et al. 1983) in what appeared to be a subset of the patients described elsewhere (Yesavage 1983b). Relationships between verbal cues and assault were further pursued in a subsequent report (Tanke and Yesavage 1985), which apparently included the data published earlier (P.D. Werner et al. 1983; Yesavage 1983b). Assaultive patients who issued verbal threats before their assault ("high-visibility" patients, $n=12$) were compared with those who did not threaten before assaulting ("low-visibility" patients, $n=13$) and with patients who did not assault during the first 8 days of hospitalization ($n=253$). The low-visibility patients were more withdrawn and slightly less hostile than the high-visibility ones. These results (Tanke and Yesavage 1985) await replication in a larger sample. Because verbal threats occurred in fewer than 50% of the cases of assault, one may conclude that they have low nosologic sensitivity if used as a marker or predictor (Feinstein 1985, p. 434) (see also Chapter 9).

Similarly to findings in schizophrenic and schizoaffective patients, positive symptoms on the BPRS on admission were related to assaultiveness during the first 8 days of hospitalization among patients with bipolar mood disorders (Yesavage 1983a).

Risk Assessment During Short-Term Hospitalization

Several groups used emergency involuntary commitment as a setting for studies of risk assessment. The procedures for such commitment vary somewhat among jurisdictions and in time. In principle, a clinician is required to justify commitment by stating that the patient poses a substantial risk of harm to himself or herself or others. The patients who are committed because of the risk of harm to others are then observed for manifestations of such risks (such as assaultive behavior) in the hospital. They are then compared with other control patients who were admitted under different circumstances.

Two problems are inherent in the use of this situation for research. First, the clinicians usually make no explicit risk assessment of the control patients. Second, the risk assessment that forms the basis of the commitment is implicitly made for the patient's continued stay in the community: unless the patient is immediately hospitalized, he or she might attack someone, and therefore he or she must be hospitalized. It is understood that hospitalization is intended and expected to prevent, or at least mitigate, the behavior that is being predicted. A similar point was raised elsewhere (Litwack et al. 1993).

A study of dangerous behavior after admission compared 59 patients admitted via emergency civil commitment with 59 control subjects (Rofman et al. 1980). The committed group caused significantly more assaultive incidents than the control subjects (not all of these incidents were physical assaults). The difference was mainly accounted for by incidents that occurred during the first 10 days of hospitalization. A similar study failed to find the expected difference in rates of hospital assaultiveness; this failure was attributed to a different method used to select the control group (Yesavage et al. 1982). The follow-up period was 1 week.

Patients admitted because they were perceived to be dangerous to others ($n=47$) were compared with other involuntary patients (control subjects; $n=54$) on the number of physical assaults and on seclusion or restraint for dangerousness after admission (McNiel and Binder 1987). The patients were admitted on the basis of California's Lanterman-Petris-

Short Act, which provides for the emergency involuntary commitment of mentally ill patients for up to 72 hours; accordingly, the patients were followed up for 72 hours after admission. As expected, the patients admitted because of perceived danger to others were significantly more likely than control subjects to assault others and to be restrained or secluded during the follow-up period. The differences in violent behavior between the two patient groups, which were most clearly expressed during the first 24 hours, began to fade in the second 24 hours and lost statistical significance in the third 24-hour period after admission. During the first 24 hours, 64% of the patients admitted because of perceived danger to others were involved in an assaultive incident (i.e., a 36% false-positive rate).

It is not entirely clear who made the judgment of danger to others—the basis for the commitment. Perhaps it was "an authorized mental health professional or a peace officer" (McNiel and Binder 1987, p. 198). One might therefore assume that the judgment was based more on recent violent behavior than on psychopathology.

Taken together, these three studies (McNiel and Binder 1987; Rofman et al. 1980; Yesavage et al. 1982) suggest that the assessment of danger to other persons may be relatively reliable for approximately 48 hours after the emergency commitment. The 36% false-positive rate was perhaps inflated by hospital treatment intended to reduce assaultiveness; had the patients remained untreated and unsupervised in the community, they would probably have committed more assaults than they did in the hospital (thus, some patients who were false-positive cases in the hospital would have been true-positive cases in the community). The speedy effectiveness of psychopharmacologic treatment of violence may be inferred from the negative correlation between the plasma level of thiothixene (measured within the first 3 days of treatment) and assaultiveness during the first 8 days after the start of treatment or after admission (Yesavage 1982); patients with plasma levels above the average (13 ng/mL) were generally not assaultive.

Various aspects of the hospital environment actually promote aggression; however, in my opinion, the great reduction of positive symptoms in schizophrenic and manic patients within the first days and weeks of antipsychotic treatment outweighs the potential negative effects of the hospital environment. Hospitalization obviously cannot prevent all assaults, but I think that it probably mitigates the risk of serious injury experienced by participants in assaults that occur: patients are usually unarmed, and combatants can be separated by staff members before serious injuries occur. All these considerations suggest that short-term emergency commitment is justified in principle because it protects both society and the patients themselves.

A different approach used a more formal and explicit clinical assessment of the risk of violence among newly admitted psychiatric inpatients (McNiel and Binder 1991). It appears that the 149 patients assessed were consecutively admitted; only 30% of these patients were admitted involuntarily because of danger to others. At admission, nurses and physicians independently estimated the probability that each of 149 patients would physically attack someone during the first week of hospitalization. They used all information available at the time of admission. The Overt Aggression Scale (Yudofsky et al. 1986) was used to rate the patients' behavior for 1 week.

The nurses' ratings showed modest agreement with those of the physicians (intraclass correlation coefficient $r=0.46$). The nurses' and the physicians' predictions were better than chance, but overprediction of physical attacks was a problem: the false-positive rates were 60% for the nurses and 78% for the physicians. To the extent that these studies (McNiel and Binder 1987, 1991) are comparable, it seems that the judgment of a health professional or a police officer that a patient must be admitted because of danger to others results in less overprediction of violence than a judgment by health professionals about unselected patients. This conclusion suggests that the accuracy of a positive prediction of imminent violence depends on the type of patient assessed: the more violent or fear-inducing the patient is before admission, the more accurate the positive prediction.

Thus, patients differ in their predictability. Furthermore, patients differ in the extent to which raters trying to predict their violent behavior agree with each other. Consensus (or interrater reliability) in risk assessment was addressed in a small study that suggested that clinical symptoms affect consensus and that certain aspects of prediction accuracy (or validity) are related to consensus (P.D. Werner et al. 1990). Another study of interrater reliability involved evaluations of 411 patients by 96 different clinicians (Lidz et al. 1989). The intraclass correlation coefficient ($r=0.67$) among clinicians indicated a moderately reliable assessment of the item estimating the current dangerousness of these patients.

In summary, the most important correlates of assaultiveness during the first several days or weeks after the admission include a history of violent behavior or threats occurring in the community during the 2 weeks preceding the admission and patients' positive symptoms on admission. Patients judged dangerous to others and admitted under the provision of short-term emergency involuntary commitment have higher levels of assaultiveness for several days after the admission than patients admitted under different conditions. This outcome can be seen as a justification of the short-term commitment in principle.

Long-Term Hospitalization

Individual-Related Correlates of Violence

Generic and recidivistic assaultiveness are reviewed in separate sections.

Generic assaultiveness. Generically assaultive patients were defined as those who "assaulted other persons in the hospital at least once within the preceding 3 months" in a classic study (Tardiff and Sweillam 1982, p. 212). That study, which yielded the 3-month prevalence of violence among 5,164 patients in public hospitals (see "Prevalence Studies" above), also assessed correlates of assaultive behavior (Tardiff and Sweillam 1982). Assaultive patients were younger than nonassaultive ones and had a greater likelihood of suicide attempts. They were more likely to have primary diagnoses of nonparanoid schizophrenia, organic brain syndrome, or mental retardation; the nonassaultive patients were more frequently diagnosed with paranoid schizophrenia. Furthermore, the assaultive patients were more likely to have a seizure disorder. The psychiatric diagnoses (DSM-II) (American Psychiatric Association 1968) were made by trained surveyors (Tardiff and Deane 1980).

Schizophrenia was the most common diagnosis among violent patients in three British hospitals (Fottrell 1980), but this report is difficult to evaluate because the prevalence of schizophrenia among the nonviolent patients was not given. A retrospective survey of 140 patients admitted to the research wards of the National Institute of Mental Health revealed that 44 of them assaulted another person at least once during their hospitalization (Karson and Bigelow 1987). Compared with the nonassaultive patients, the assaultive patients were more likely to be younger and to have the diagnosis of schizophrenia. The authors noted that history of violence before entering the research program was associated with a high number of prior hospitalizations; this finding led them to infer that violent behavior might be associated with a poor prognosis. I think that recidivistic violent behavior may lead to recidivistic hospitalizations simply because it induces fear; nevertheless, their point about poor prognosis is interesting, and I will return to it. As the authors point out, only patients with treatment-resistant disorders were selected to enter their program; this bias limits the ability to generalize from their findings.

A retrospective survey of incident reports at a large state hospital revealed that the diagnoses of organic brain syndrome and personality disorders (but not schizophrenia) were overrepresented among assaultive patients (Evenson et al. 1974).

Recidivistic assaultiveness. A small group (*N*=13) of recidivistically assaultive schizophrenic and schizoaffective patients were identified in an early study (Shader et al. 1977). Soon thereafter, a large study involving three hospitals (N=2,822) indicated that a small group (1%–4%) of patients were involved in a large percentage (41%–70%) of incidents (Fottrell 1980, Table VII, p. 220). The recidivists tended to be psychotic females under age 50 years with a prominent history of violence.

In a study of 1,552 inpatients, 576 violent incidents (assaults or fights) were identified during a 6-month period; 5% of the patients were responsible for 53% of the incidents (Convit et al. 1990a). Furthermore, recidivist men inflicted serious injuries (joint dislocation, fracture or possible fracture, burn, or severe laceration) at a rate 10 times higher than that for all the other violent patients. The group of recidivists consisted of 31 males and 39 females whose average age was lower than that of nonrecidivist assaulters. Personality and impulse disorder diagnoses tended to be overrepresented among the male and female recidivists; a slight overrepresentation of schizophrenia was limited to the males. These patients' disorders were—almost by definition—resistant to treatment.

A case-control study compared 69 recidivistically violent patients with 40 nonviolent control patients (Convit et al. 1988a). The data included scores on a quantified neurological examination scale, visual electroencephalographic assessment, history of deviant family environment (based on parents' psychiatric hospitalizations, their substance abuse, absence of intact family, and the patient's physical abuse as a child), suicide attempts, and criminal history. All historical data were self-reported. The results are summarized in Table 10–1.

Self-reports of arrests and convictions for violent (but not for nonviolent) crime were the strongest discriminators between the violent and nonviolent patients in the hospital. A history of family deviance and the current neurological abnormality score also discriminated between the patient sets.

A companion study investigated the neurological status of 28 recidivistically violent schizophrenic inpatients compared with two groups characterized by either nonrecidivistic violence or no violence (Krakowski et al. 1989). Neurological and neuropsychological abnormalities differed among the groups: the recidivists showed more abnormalities than the other two groups in the areas of integrative sensory and motor functions. These differences might have been a consequence of repeated head injuries sustained in fights, but reports of head trauma were not different among the groups. A history of violent crime was more prevalent among both violent groups compared with the nonviolent group. Taken together, these results suggest that recidivistically violent schizophrenic patients have a more severe (or perhaps an entirely different) form of the disease.

Table 10–1. Historical and biological characteristics of violent and nonviolent patients

Characteristic	Violent ($n=69$)	Nonviolent ($n=40$)	P
Arrested for nonviolent crimes	50.7%	50.0%	NS
Convicted for nonviolent crimes	24.6%	17.5%	NS
Arrested for violent crimes	46.4%	7.5%	0.002[a]
Convicted for violent crimes	34.8%	5.0%	0.002[a]
History of nonviolent suicide attempts	22.2%	16.7%	NS
History of violent suicide attempts	39.1%	19.4%	0.08[a]
Mean deviance of family environment	0.25	0.18	0.05[b]
Mean neurological abnormality score	0.08	0.04	0.01[b]

Note. NS=not significant.
[a]χ^2 test.
[b]t test.

Source. Reprinted from Convit A, Jaeger J, Lin SP, et al.: "Predicting Assaultiveness in Psychiatric Inpatients: A Pilot Study." *Hospital and Community Psychiatry* 39:429–434, 1988. Copyright 1988 American Psychiatric Association. Used with permission.

Numerous neurological abnormalities were reported in patients with treatment-resistant chronic schizophrenia (D.W. Heinrichs and Buchanan 1988; Weinberger et al. 1980), in schizophrenic patients with premorbid asociality (Quitkin et al. 1976), and in violent patients with various diagnoses (see Chapter 4).

In summary, studies of large patient samples in long-term facilities indicate that young patients with the diagnosis of nonparanoid schizophrenia are overrepresented among the generically assaultive patients. Diagnoses of organic brain syndrome and personality disorders may also be associated with assaultiveness.

Studies of recidivistic assaultiveness indicate that a small group of patients are responsible for a disproportionate number of assaults and that these assaults cause serious injuries. Recidivistic assaultiveness among patients unselected for diagnosis is associated with a history of deviant family (rearing) environment, violent crime, and current neurological impairment. Recidivistically violent schizophrenic patients have abnormalities of integrative sensory and motor functions.

Environmental and Social Correlates of Violence

The number and behavior of staff members may be related to violence (Tardiff 1992, p. 17), but it is difficult to find consistent evidence to support these intuitively plausible effects. The number of patients per physician was positively related to the number of incidents involving physical aggression at a forensic hospital (Carmel et al. 1991). Other incidents including verbal aggression, seclusion, and restraint increased with the relative number of psychiatrists available; thus, it is possible that the psychiatrists were able to prevent some of the lesser incidents from developing into physical aggression.

However, when one examines the nursing staff levels in the specific wards at the times when assaults occurred, it seems that more assaults take place when the staffing levels are higher (Depp 1983, p. 31). One of the reasons for an increase in incidents with increased staff is that staff members demand patient activity; for example, patients are asked to get out of bed, shower, dress, or go to the dining room. Such activities are frequently demanded in the morning; accordingly, assault frequency peaks between 6:00 and 8:00 A.M.; smaller peaks occur around lunch and dinner times (Depp 1983; Dietz and Rada 1982). Mealtime aggressive incidents can be substantially reduced by simple adjustments of ward procedures during meals (Hunter and Love 1996).

Another possible reason for the apparent increase in incidents when more staff members are around is that in at least some hospitals, additional staff members are made available on a short-term basis to a ward that has patients who are currently violent. One of the mechanisms for this short-term availability is that the ward psychiatrist prescribes "close observation," "constant observation," or "one-to-one" observation for a fear-inducing patient; additional staff members are then requested from the nursing supervisor who controls staffing on several wards or in the entire hospital. Thus, violence or fear may lead to higher staffing.

Ward crowding reduces the patients' personal space, increases the competition for the use of shared facilities such as television and bathrooms, increases the volume of noise on the ward, reduces the time that is available for treating individual patients, and generally tends to make the wards more chaotic. It is therefore not surprising that it also increases the likelihood of violent incidents (B. Ng et al. 2001; Palmstierna et al. 1991).

The organization of the wards and the behavior of staff members exert considerable effects on patient assaultiveness (Armond 1982). These effects are difficult to study. Many violent patients appear to respond positively to the structured environment and close supervision offered in units that specialize in the management of violent patients. After these patients are transferred to such a unit, their violent behavior significantly decreases (Krakowski et al. 1988b). Unfortunately, it is not clear how to interpret such results. Because it is ethically and practically impossible to transfer only a randomly assigned subset of all the violent patients deemed to need the transfer, there is no control for the effects of time:

some of the patients might have improved without the transfer. Furthermore, it is extremely difficult to implement any research-oriented procedure concerning the pharmacotherapy of these fear-inducing patients, including attempts to hold the medication constant (see Chapter 11). The effect of the changed environment due to the transfer is therefore uncontrollably confounded by the effects of changes in medication. These reservations do not mean that the specialized units are not effective; I am merely discussing the difficulties involved in demonstrating and understanding these effects.

Unpublished impressions suggest that consistent differences exist in the levels of violence among wards that have the same staffing levels, have the same organization (at least officially), and serve the same type of patients. These differences may be attributable to staff training and attitude; these factors probably play an important role in creating a therapeutic environment conducive to the reduction in patients' violent behavior. An active and optimistic staff that takes an interest in patients can prevent violent incidents more effectively than employees who have given up on patients and spend much of their time talking to each other in offices that are not accessible to patients. Similar impressions were published by others (Depp 1983). Such impressions are difficult to transform into practically testable hypotheses. Nevertheless, common sense, informal discussion with staff members, and empirical observations argue that staff training and attitudes are perhaps more important than the number of staff available.

Patient victims tend to be older, to weigh less than the assaulters, and to be intrusive or meddlesome. Furthermore, the victims' position in the ward's social hierarchy tends to be lower than that of the assaulters (Depp 1983). The hierarchy was established by asking staff members to rank patients in terms of rights, privileges, and status; it is not clear whether the staff members used the assaults and their outcomes to determine the patients' positions in the hierarchy. Neither the reliability of the determination of patients' positions nor the stability of those positions in time was reported. Research on social hierarchy and aggression in animals has been very fruitful (see Chapter 2); it is not clear why analogous research in patients has not been pursued more vigorously.

Although much has been learned about assaulters and their victims, very little reliable information is available about the assaults. When staff members at a forensic psychiatric unit were asked to provide an explanation for patients' assaultive behaviors, the most frequent reason given was that the patient was ordered to do something. However, when the patients were asked to explain the same behavior, their most frequently offered reasons were that they were teased or that they were provoked by staff (Harris and Varney 1986) (Table 10–2). In another study, assailants claimed to have been playing with the victim, complained of verbal abuse, or said they wanted to stop objectionable behaviors by the victim. The results suggest that assailants may perceive some behaviors by victims as provocations (Crowner et al. 1995). A review of incident reports at a psychiatric unit of a university hospital suggested different contexts in which assaults occur: a seclusion procedure, an argument, or the verbal denial of a privilege (e.g., smoking) by staff (Conn and Lion 1983).

Table 10–2. Reasons given for assaultive behavior ($n=1,172$)

Reason	Ward staff (%)	Assaulter (%)
None provided/no response	0.4	23.8
Ordered to do something	16.8	4.8
Request refused	4.7	3.5
Teased or "bugged"	6.4	20.5
Crowded	1.0	2.6
Voices, delusional orders	2.6	3.1
Reaction to sexual approach	0.3	0.5
Angry at ward rules	5.5	2.2
Provoked by staff	0.2	12.0
Building tension, upset	1.2	5.3
Other specified	2.3	6.2
No reason/unknown	58.6	15.4

Source. Reprinted from Harris GT, Varney GW: "A Ten-Year Study of Assaults and Assaulters on a Maximum Security Psychiatric Unit." *Journal of Interpersonal Violence* 1:173–191, 1986. Copyright Sage Publications, Inc. Reprinted by permission of Sage Publications, Inc.

Thus, interviews of participants and witnesses provide various points of view and justifications. This information is interesting, but it does not describe what actually happened. Continued video recording is the most reliable way to capture that information. A recording system is described in Chapter 1. Preliminary data indicate that approximately 50% of assaults are preceded by various "warnings" (by the assailant) and/or by "provocations" (by the victim) (Crowner et al. 1991). Environmental correlates of psychiatric inpatient violence were reviewed in greater detail elsewhere (Crowner 1989). A review of 155 videotaped assaults resulted in a new typology of these incidents (Crowner et al. 1994). Videotape analyses of assaults are continuing at the Nathan Kline Institute.

In summary, not enough is known about environmental and social correlates of inpatient violence. Some of the violence is triggered in interactions with staff members when the patient is asked to do something (generally to conform) that he or she refuses to do, or when the patient asks a staff member to do something (generally to grant a privilege) that is refused. Emerging research using video recordings of assaults is beginning to define the behavioral cues emitted by the assaulters and their victims.

Risk Assessment During Long-Term Hospitalization

The largest risk assessment study during long-term hospitalization used 5,525 patients (Hedlund et al. 1973). All evaluations were retrospective; this was thus a "postdiction" rather than a prediction study. Patients were randomly assigned either to a calibration sample ($n=2,763$) or to a cross-validation sample ($n=2,762$). Linear discriminant equations for three measures of violence as the dependent variables were computed in the calibration sample (see appendix for technical details). The measure that was most comparable with other reports was "has harmed others." The equation for this measure was used in the cross-validation sample. The diagnostic sensitivity on cross-validation (calculated from Table 1 of Hedlund et al. 1973, p. 444) was only 25% (a very low predictive accuracy of positive prediction); the diagnostic specificity was 96%. The base rate of "has harmed others" was 5%, and it appears that no adjustment for the base rate was made (see Bayes function in appendix).

In another study, a subset of patients ($n=51$) observed in the retrospective case-control study mentioned above (Table 10–1) (Convit et al. 1988a) were used to develop a logistic regression model for a prospective risk assessment study of a cross-validation sample ($N=79$) (Convit et al. 1988a, 1988b, 1989). Four risk factors were used: convictions for violent crime, neurological abnormality score, deviance of the family environment, and history of violent suicide attempts. After a base-rate correction, the diagnostic sensitivity was 46%, and the diagnostic specificity was 78%. These measures of accuracy compare favorably with those obtained in similar projects (see above and Chapter 9).

SUMMARY AND CONCLUSIONS

Most published research on violence in psychiatric facilities deals with *assaultiveness* as a generic term defined as the proportion (prevalence) of patients who commit assault at least once during an observation period. I defined the subtypes of recidivistic and nonrecidivistic assaultiveness. These subtypes can be reliably determined and may have different underlying mechanisms.

Generic assaultiveness is maximal during the first several days after admission, and then it decreases. In long-term psychiatric hospitals, the 3-month prevalence is approximately 7%.

Correlates of assaultiveness during the first days after the admission include violence preceding the admission and patients' positive symptoms on admission. Compared with other patients, those judged to be dangerous to others have higher levels of assaultiveness for several days. This can be seen as an example of successful short-term risk assessment.

Young patients with the diagnosis of nonparanoid schizophrenia are overrepresented among generically assaultive patients in long-term facilities. A small group of recidivistic patients is responsible for a large number of assaults that are particularly serious. Recidivistic assaultiveness is associated with a history of deviant family environment, violent crime, and current neurological impairment.

Environmental and social correlates of inpatient violence are poorly understood. Some of the violence is triggered in interactions with staff members. Researchers are beginning to understand the interactions between victims and assaulters by studying videotape recordings of assaults and their immediate antecedents.

Summarizing and interpreting the information on violence in schizophrenic patients presented in this chapter and in the preceding one, one can hypothesize that there are two subtypes of violence associated with the illness. Subtype I is characterized by transient violence, and subtype II is characterized by persistent violence. The subtypes are summarized in Table 10–3. Recent work has confirmed the distinctive character of these subtypes (Krakowski et al. 1999).

Table 10–3. Two hypothetical subtypes of violent behavior in schizophrenic patients

Characteristic	Type I	Type II
Diagnostic subtype	Paranoid	Nonparanoid
Time course of violence	Prior to and early after admission	No clear time course
Recidivistic assault	No	Yes
Response to typical antipsychotics	Better	Worse
Neurological impairment	Less	More

Source. Adapted from Volavka J, Krakowski M: "Schizophrenia and Violence." *Psychological Medicine* 19:559–562, 1989. Copyright 1989 Cambridge University Press. Reprinted with the permission of Cambridge University Press.

11

Biological Treatment of Violence

There is no specific biological treatment for violence or aggression. Given at a sufficiently high dose, many drugs will temporarily reduce or eliminate violent or aggressive behavior. High doses of hypnotics, antipsychotics, anticonvulsants, or general anesthetics will make it difficult or impossible to exhibit violent behavior. Such doses will also make it difficult or impossible to exhibit any other behavior; the effect is nonspecific sedation. The goal is to reduce or eliminate aggressive behavior in a safe manner and without interfering with other aspects of the patient's functioning.

EMERGENCY TREATMENT

Acute agitation that may be accompanied by violent behavior requires rapid treatment. Benzodiazepines provide a rapid calming effect. The effect is nonspecific in the sense that it does not depend on the underlying cause of agitation, and the treatment is relatively safe. If psychosis is the underlying cause, an antipsychotic is indicated to treat the symptoms that may be driving the agitated behavior. It is common practice to co-administer a benzodiazepine and an antipsychotic under these circumstances; either one or both may be administered in an intramuscular form. As the agitation subsides, the benzodiazepine is tapered off and the antipsychotic is switched to an oral form.

However, benzodiazepines and antipsychotics may have adverse interactions when combined. Monotherapy of acute agitation and aggression can be quite effective. A retrospective, open study compared the antiaggressive effects of a single dose of haloperidol (10 mg im) with a single dose of lorazepam (2 mg im) in violent psychiatric patients at a crisis unit

(Bick and Hannah 1986). Lorazepam was at least as effective as haloperidol in controlling violent behavior. In a prospective double-blind study, patients diagnosed with schizophrenia, schizoaffective disorder, or bipolar disorder who were experiencing an acute aggressive outburst were randomly assigned to receive a dose of either flunitrazepam (1 mg im) or haloperidol (5 mg im) (Dorevitch et al. 1998). Both treatments were associated with a decrease of aggression. The effect of flunitrazepam lasted longer than that of haloperidol, but otherwise there were no appreciable differences between the treatments. (Because of its abuse potential, flunitrazepam has not been approved for medical use in the United States; see Chapter 8.)

The intramuscular use of typical antipsychotics, particularly haloperidol, may lead to acute dystonic reactions and akathisia, whereas intramuscular benzodiazepines may lead to respiratory depression and confusion. Atypical antipsychotics are less likely to cause these problems, and some of them are becoming available for intramuscular use. Intramuscular olanzapine in doses of 2.5 mg, 5 mg, 7.5 mg, and 10 mg was compared with intramuscular haloperidol 7.5 mg and with intramuscular placebo in acutely agitated patients with schizophrenia. Olanzapine showed a dose-response relationship for reduction of agitation and superiority over placebo. The effect of olanzapine on agitation was not superior to that of haloperidol, but its safety profile was (Breier et al. 2002).

Intramuscular ziprasidone was compared with intramuscular haloperidol in agitated psychotic patients (Brook et al. 2000). In this open-label study, ziprasidone was more effective and elicited fewer extrapyramidal side effects than haloperidol. The effective dose of ziprasidone for psychotic agitation is 10–20 mg im (Lesem et al. 2001). In general, the use of intramuscular forms of atypical antipsychotics for the initial treatment will facilitate the transition to oral maintenance therapy with the same atypical medication.

LONG-TERM TREATMENT

Antipsychotics

Typical Antipsychotics

Antipsychotic drugs have antiaggressive effects in most animal models, but the effect is usually apparent only if the doses are high enough to sedate the animal and suppress general motor activity (Miczek 1987, p. 208). Like animals, humans are sedated after acute doses of antipsychotics; the sedation may reduce violent behavior. The antiaggressive effects of typical antipsychotics are generally nonspecific and have been reported for most disorders listed in DSM-IV (American Psychiatric Association 1994).

Aggression may abate as the patient's psychosis is successfully treated, but many aggressive patients do not respond to typical antipsychotics. It is sometimes believed that the patients do not respond properly because the dose of the antipsychotic medication is not high enough. This belief may explain why chronically violent schizophrenic patients are frequently given very high doses of medications for very long periods. We surveyed patients who were prescribed high doses of antipsychotics (Krakowski et al. 1993); history of violence was a principal reason for the high-dose regimen, without evidence that the incidence of violent behavior was reduced.

In some patients, the rigidity and akinesia caused by typical antipsychotics may perhaps reduce the likelihood of an assault. However, akathisia increases irritability, and it was reported to be associated with violence in several cases (Keckich 1978; Siris 1985). High-dose haloperidol treatment of chronic schizophrenia has been associated with violence (Herrera et al. 1988); akathisia might have been the mediating variable. It is possible that some of the antiaggressive effects of β-adrenergic antagonists added to antipsychotics (see "β-Adrenergic Blockers" below) may actually be due to a reduction of akathisia (Lipinski et al. 1988). In general, recent studies of atypical antipsychotics have demonstrated equivalence or superiority over haloperidol in antiaggressive effects, but with less severe side effects.

Atypical Antipsychotics

Clozapine. Clozapine was the first atypical drug available, and a considerable amount of research to assess its antiaggressive effects has now been published (Table 11–1). The prevailing evidence clearly suggests that clozapine has antiaggressive effects; however, most of the studies have serious methodological problems, which are discussed in detail later. The selection of subjects for clozapine treatment was vaguely defined, and the studies were open and largely uncontrolled.

Only one randomized, double-blind, controlled study is available to date (Citrome et al. 2001b). Inpatients ($N=157$) with treatment-resistant chronic schizophrenia or schizoaffective disorder were assigned to clozapine, olanzapine, risperidone, or haloperidol in a randomized 14-week trial. The Positive and Negative Symptom Scale (PANSS) (Kay et al. 1989) total score was the principal outcome measure; the hostility item

Table 11–1. Studies of the effects of clozapine on hostile and aggressive behavior in patients with major mental disorders

Author, year	N^a	Diagnosis	Study type	Control group	Drug assignment	Measure of effect	Results
Michals et al. 1993	9	Brain injury	Open; retrospective record review	None	Clinical	Incidents of verbal and physical aggression	Reduced aggression in 3 patients
Maier 1992	25	Schizophrenia, schizoaffective disorder	Open; retrospective record review	None	Clinical	Security level, discharge	13 (52%) patients improved
Mallya et al. 1992	107	"Chronic" patients	Open; retrospective record review	None	Clinical	Seclusion and restraint	Reduced seclusion and restraint
Ratey et al. 1993	5	Schizophrenia	Open; retrospective record review	None	Clinical	Seclusion and restraint, aggressive incidents, BPRS	Assaults and seclusions reduced
Volavka et al. 1993	223	Schizophrenia	Open; retrospective record review	None	Clinical	BPRS hostility item	Significant reduction of hostility
Ebrahim et al. 1994	27	Schizophrenia, schizoaffective disorder	Open; retrospective record review	None	Clinical	Seclusion and restraint, BPRS, level of privileges	Significant improvements
Chiles et al. 1994	139	Schizophrenia, schizoaffective disorder	Open; retrospective record review	None	Clinical	Seclusion and restraint, NOSIE	Significant improvements

Table 11–1. Studies of the effects of clozapine on hostile and aggressive behavior in patients with major mental disorders *(continued)*

Author, year	N^a	Diagnosis	Study type	Control group	Drug assignment	Measure of effect	Results
Buckley et al. 1995	30	Schizophrenia	Open; retrospective record review	None	Clinical	Seclusion and restraint, BPRS	Significant reduction of seclusion and restraint
W. H. Wilson and Claussen 1995[b]	100	Chronic psychosis	Open; retrospective record review	None	Clinical	Incidents of aggression	Reduced incidents
Mendito et al. 1996	22	Chronic schizophrenia	Open, case-control	Typical antipsychotics	Clinical	Assaults and threats	Decreased assaults, but no superiority over control group
Rabinowitz et al. 1996	75	Schizophrenia	Open; retrospective record review	None	Clinical	Incidents of aggression, restraint, BPRS hostility item	Significant improvements on all measures
Spivak et al. 1998	60	Schizophrenia	Open, retrospective record review	Typical antipsychotics	Clinical	Incidents of aggression	Superiority over control group
Citrome et al. 2001b	157	Schizophrenia, schizoaffective disorder	Double-blind	Risperidone, olanzapine, haloperidol	Random	PANSS hostility item	Clozapine superior to haloperidol

[a]Total number of subjects, including control groups.
[b]Includes data from an earlier publication (W. H. Wilson 1992).
Note. BPRS=Brief Psychiatric Rating Scale (Guy 1986); NOSIE=Nurses' Observation Scale for Inpatient Evaluation (Honigfeld et al. 1966); PANSS=Positive and Negative Symptom Scale (Kay et al. 1989).

was subjected to post hoc analyses to assess the antiaggressive/antihostility effects of clozapine. In these analyses, covariates included the PANSS items that reflect positive symptoms of schizophrenia (delusions, suspiciousness/persecution, grandiosity, unusual thought content, conceptual disorganization, and hallucinatory behavior), and the Nurses' Observation Scale for Inpatient Evaluation (NOSIE) (Honigfeld et al. 1966) sedation item. Hierarchical linear model analysis was used. The results are summarized in Table 11–2.

Table 11–2. Positive and Negative Symptom Scale hostility item—averages and standard deviations

Drug	N	Baseline	14 weeks[a]
Clozapine	40	2.68±1.58	2.24±1.34[b, c]
Olanzapine	39	2.35±1.47	2.24±1.73
Risperidone	41	2.40±1.19	2.49±1.61
Haloperidol	37	2.42±1.26	2.95±1.51

[a]Or last rating completed for those subjects who did not finish the 14 weeks.
[b]Significant improvement compared with baseline ($P=0.019$)
[c]Significant superiority in improvement compared with haloperidol ($P=0.021$) or risperidone ($P=0.012$)
Source. Citrome L, Volavka J, Czobor P et al.: "Effects of Clozapine, Olanzapine, Risperidone, and Haloperidol on Hostility Among Patients With Schizophrenia." *Psychiatric Services* 52:1510–1514, 2001. Copyright 2001 American Psychiatric Association. Used with permission.

The four treatment arms differed in their effect on the hostility item of the PANSS. Clozapine had significantly greater antihostility effect than haloperidol or risperidone. The effect on hostility appears to be independent of antipsychotic effect on other PANSS items that reflect delusional thinking, disorganized behavior, or hallucinations, and independent of sedation as measured by the NOSIE. Neither risperidone nor olanzapine showed superiority over haloperidol. Thus, clozapine had an advantage over other antipsychotics as a specific antihostility agent. Clozapine also appeared to have a superior antiaggressive effect in comparison with risperidone in an uncontrolled retrospective study of 24 patients who received, at different times, both medications (Sharif et al. 2000).

Patients with schizophrenia are at increased risk for substance abuse, and overwhelming evidence indicates that comorbid substance abuse is associated with violent behavior (see Chapter 10). It is therefore important that clozapine may reduce drug craving and drug use in schizophrenic patients (Albanese et al. 1994; Buckley et al. 1999, 2000; McCarthy et al. 1999) and that the antipsychotic effectiveness of clozapine is maintained in patients with comorbid substance abuse (Buckley et al. 1994).

Other atypical antipsychotics. The results of risperidone studies are summarized in Table 11–3. The results in schizophrenia patients are mixed. The double-blind studies using rating scale items as the outcome measures in large numbers of patients not selected for aggressive behavior show that risperidone had superior effect. It should be noted that the two double-blind studies (Czobor et al. 1995; Marder et al. 1997) were based on (post hoc) analyses of the same data set (Marder and Meibach 1994), and thus the second study (Marder et al. 1997) cannot be seen as a replication.

In contrast, the two small open studies using overt aggression or the staff response to it as the outcome measures did not show superiority for risperidone. It is likely that these studies used patients who were more aggressive than those recruited for the double-blind risperidone trial (Marder and Meibach 1994); this is almost certainly true of the study that used forensic patients (Beck et al. 1997). Thus, it is possible that risperidone is effective against hostility in patients who display relatively low levels of overt physical aggression, but its efficacy in more aggressive patients remains to be determined.

Regarding quetiapine, preliminary data suggest the possibility of antiaggressive effects. Data acquired in a pivotal quetiapine trial (Arvanitis et al. 1997) were subjected to post hoc analyses that used the hostility item on the Brief Psychiatric Rating Scale (BPRS) (Guy 1986) and various combinations of positive symptoms, including that item, as outcome measures (Cantillon et al. 1997). The results showed that quetiapine had antiaggressive effects. Except for an encouraging case report (Citrome et al. 2001a), there is no published study of quetiapine using incidents of overt physical aggression (rather than a BPRS scale item) as the outcome measure.

Olanzapine has not been tested for antiaggressive effects. Aggressive behavior was alleviated by high doses (50 mg/day) of olanzapine in one of two patients. However, there was an *increase* of aggression after administration of olanzapine in one patient (V. John et al. 1998), and "rage attacks" were reported in two of five patients switched to olanzapine from clozapine (Millson and Delva 1999). In a double-blind study described above, post hoc analyses of the PANSS hostility item for olanzapine showed a nonsignificant improvement and no superiority to haloperidol (Table 11–2).

Table 11–3. Studies of the effects of risperidone on hostile and aggressive behavior in patients with major mental disorders

Author, year	N^a	Diagnosis	Study type	Control group	Drug assignment	Measure of effect	Results
Czobor et al. 1995	139	Schizophrenia	Double-blind	Haloperidol, placebo	Random	PANSS hostility item	Superiority of risperidone over haloperidol and placebo
Marder et al. 1997[b]	513	Schizophrenia	Double-blind	Haloperidol, placebo	Random	BPRS Factor 4 (uncontrolled hostility/ excitement)	Superiority of risperidone over haloperidol and placebo
Beck et al. 1997	20	Schizophrenia	Open, case-control	Conventional antipsychotics	Clinical	Assaults, threats	No antiaggressive effect
Buckley et al. 1997	27	Schizophrenia, schizoaffective disorder	Open, case-control	Conventional antipsychotics	Clinical	Seclusion and restraint	No superiority to control group
Sandor and Stephens 2000	28	Tourette syndrome	Open, retrospective	None	Clinical	Assaults	Reduced aggression in 22 subjects

[a]Total number of subjects, including control groups.
[b]Subset of this data base used by Czobor et al. 1995.
Note. PANSS=Positive and Negative Symptom Scale (Kay et al. 1989); BPRS=Brief Psychiatric Rating Scale (Guy 1986).

Methodology of the Studies of Antipsychotics in Aggressive Patients

Overall trial designs of these studies can be classified into two groups.

Group 1 studies are characterized by an open-label design (see Tables 11–1 and 11–3). This introduces the possibility that the doctors' and patients' expectations of positive treatment effects may have confounded the results. With one exception (Volavka et al. 1993), Group 1 studies used incidents of overt aggression (or seclusion and restraint—staff responses to such aggression) as principal outcome measures. The subject selection was usually "clinical"—a doctor believed that the patient needed the treatment. In some studies, the subjects showed a substantial increase in the number of aggressive incidents during the month preceding the start of clozapine treatment (Rabinowitz et al. 1996; W. H. Wilson and Claussen 1995). These data suggest that the patients were selected after (and perhaps because) their aggressive incidents became more frequent. Such accumulation of incidents in a cluster may be a random deviation from the mean, and subsequent incidents may follow with lower frequency (regression to the mean). Thus, the reported reduction of the incident rate may have occurred even without the start of clozapine treatment. Despite these problems, Group 1 studies have the advantage of measuring real aggressive incidents rather than a proxy variable such as the hostility item on standard rating scales. Retrospective chart review studies usually do not require subjects' consent.

Group 2 studies had double-blind design and random assignment of subjects to treatments (see Tables 11–1 and 11–3) (Cantillon et al. 1997). The principal outcome measure was the hostility item of a standard rating scale, or a combination of items including the hostility item such as the hostility/excitement factor. High levels of verbally expressed hostility predict physical assault (P. D. Werner et al. 1983). Furthermore, high severity levels of this item do imply overt physical aggression, but this information is usually difficult to extract from studies reporting aggregate values. Therefore, these rating scales provide valuable insights (see Chapter 1 for a discussion of hostility) but yield only indirect information about incidents of overt physical aggression. All studies in Group 2 required subjects' consent.

Consent selection bias. Patients' likelihood of consenting to participate in studies varies with demographic factors (Robinson et al. 1996) and other variables; thus the sample of patients entering the trial may not be representative of the population of eligible patients. The problem of selection bias is particularly troubling in the studies of antiaggressive drugs because patients who are hostile are less likely to consent (Edlund et al. 1985). This problem, inherent in research on violence, can be somewhat mitigated by estimating the effect of consent bias on the generalizability of findings; details can be found elsewhere (Volavka and Citrome 1999).

Specificity of antiaggressive effect. Specificity is considered in terms of relative independence of antiaggressive action from effects on sedation and from general antipsychotic effects. Antiaggressive effect can of course be accomplished by nonspecific sedation, but this method is practical only for short periods of time in emergencies. Ideally, a specific antiaggressive drug should not interfere with behaviors other than aggression. The antiaggressive effects of clozapine do not appear to be mediated by sedation (Chiles et al. 1994; Citrome et al. 2001b).

Independence from general antipsychotic effects represents another aspect of antiaggressive specificity. Nonspecific antiaggressive effect may, for example, be seen when the aggressive behavior that was driven by paranoid delusions diminishes as these delusions are reduced by antipsychotic treatment. Various statistical methods have been used to demonstrate that clozapine (Citrome et al. 2001b; Rabinowitz et al. 1996; Volavka et al. 1993) and risperidone (Czobor et al. 1995) have antiaggressive/antihostility effects that are relatively independent of the effects against other positive symptoms. Methodological aspects of antiaggressive drug studies are discussed more extensively elsewhere (Volavka and Citrome 1999).

Mood Stabilizers

Mood stabilizers are widely used in the management of mood disorders. Lithium has been used as a mood stabilizer, primarily in patients with bipolar disorder, since the 1960s; more recently, mood stabilizing properties have been ascribed to several medications that are generally used as anticonvulsants. Valproate, carbamazepine, and gabapentin are in this category. Although the antiaggressive effect of mood stabilizers in schizophrenic patients is generally not mentioned in textbooks of psychopharmacology, these compounds are apparently used quite widely for this indication (Citrome 1995). An expert consensus statement recommends mood stabilizers as adjunctive treatment for persistent aggression in schizophrenic patients receiving antipsychotics (McEvoy et al. 1999, pp. 43–44).

Lithium

Lithium affects multiple neurotransmitter systems. It stimulates serotonin synthesis (Perez-Cruet et al. 1971), downregulates β-adrenergic receptors, blocks dopamine receptors, enhances muscarinic-cholinergic action, and inhibits processes mediated by cyclic adenosine monophosphate (Bunney and Garland-Bunney 1987). Each mechanism may contribute to the anti-aggressive action of lithium observed under a variety of experimental conditions in laboratory animals. These antiaggressive effects occur at doses that are lower than those required to reduce nonaggressive motor activity (Miczek 1987, p. 229). The mechanism of antiaggressive activity in humans may depend on the basic disorder during which aggression develops. It is possible that some of the antiaggressive action of lithium involves serotoninergic stimulation (see Chapter 3).

Aggressivity is frequently observed during manic episodes (Yesavage 1983a). Reduction of aggressivity is an important part of the therapeutic effect of lithium in manic patients.

The antiaggressive properties of lithium in mentally retarded persons were first demonstrated in an open study (Dostal and Zvolsky 1970) showing that the effect of this treatment was not specifically limited to aggressive behavior; there were additional reductions in restlessness and hyperactivity. The antiaggressive effects of lithium in mentally retarded persons were confirmed in another open trial (Tyrer et al. 1984), a retrospective study (Spreat et al. 1989), and a double-blind, placebo-controlled trial (Craft et al. 1987). The recommended serum lithium concentration for antiaggressive effects was 0.7–1.0 mEq/L (Craft et al. 1987) or 0.5–0.8 mEq/L (Tyrer et al. 1984). Although the original report (Dostal and Zvolsky 1970) mentioned uncontrollable polydipsia and enuresis, these side effects of lithium treatment were not prominent in the placebo-controlled larger trial (Craft et al. 1987) or in the other open study with slightly lower serum lithium levels (Tyrer et al. 1984). A small, retrospective, uncontrolled study (Luchins and Dojka 1989) confirmed the antiaggressive effects of lithium in mentally retarded persons; self-injurious behavior exhibited by these aggressive individuals was also reduced by the treatment. Interestingly, the effect of propranolol on these two behaviors was similar to that of lithium, leading the authors to speculate about a common biochemical mechanism underlying both treatments (Luchins and Dojka 1989).

A belligerent patient recovering from a head injury failed to respond to propranolol or haloperidol, but disappeared when the patient was given lithium; the effective levels were 0.4–0.8 mEq/L (Haas and Cope 1985). Keeping the plasma levels relatively low may be important, because a severe closed head injury was reported to reduce tolerance to lithium neurocognitive side effects in a bipolar patient maintained on lithium (Hornstein and Seliger 1989).

Lithium reduced aggression in a large placebo-controlled study of children with *conduct disorder*. The other active drug used in that study, haloperidol, had a similar effect on aggression, but haloperidol was more often associated with adverse effects than lithium (Campbell et al. 1984). The beneficial effects of both treatments were not limited to the suppression of aggression: the patients improved in many other ways as well. Very importantly, the doses of medications in this trial did not seriously affect the cognitive performance of the patients (Platt et al. 1981). In a more recent study, 86 children with conduct disorder who were hospitalized because of severe and chronic aggression were randomly assigned to treatment with lithium or placebo (Malone et al. 2000). Lithium was statistically and clinically superior to placebo in antiaggressive effect, but more than half of the subjects in the lithium group experienced nausea, vomiting, and urinary frequency.

Lithium treatment of recurrently violent prisoners reduced the number of infractions involving violent behavior in open trials (Sheard 1971; Tupin et al. 1973), as well as in a double-blind, placebo-controlled study (Sheard et al. 1976). Plasma lithium levels in these trials were mostly below 1.0 mEq/L; such relatively low levels are not generally associated with lethargy or general suppression of motor activity in adult patients. Thus, the antiaggressive effect of lithium was "specific" in the sense that animal experimenters understand the concept of specificity. Of course, there might have been some subtle nonspecific effects; for example, lithium might have affected the prisoners' mood or perhaps their personality. Most prisoners in the open trial (Tupin et al. 1973) had various organic mental syndromes or schizophrenia, whereas the subjects in the controlled trial were described as having "nonpsychotic personality disorders" (Sheard et al. 1976, p. 1411). The authors (Sheard et al. 1976) appear to assume that the beneficial effects of lithium are specifically limited to *impulsive* aggression (presumably excluding premeditated assaults). However, no definition of impulsive or nonimpulsive aggression is given in their report (see Chapter 7). In general, such differentiation of types of aggression is not provided in published reports on the psychopharmacology of violence.

These encouraging results of the lithium trial in prisoners who had no organic brain disease or psychosis (Sheard et al. 1976) are important for the theory of lithium effects. These results imply that the antiaggressive effects of lithium in patient samples need not be mediated through effects on an underlying coarse brain disease or on bipolar disorder. The study (Sheard et al. 1976) used a double-blind, parallel group design. However, 80% of the subjects in the lithium group correctly guessed their treatment because of the side effects. Future studies should therefore use a different design (perhaps an active placebo or a concentration-controlled trial [Peck 1990]).

The effectiveness of lithium therapy in schizophrenia has not been established. Active affective symptoms, previous affective episodes, and a family history of affective disorder may predict a favorable response to lithium (Atre-Vaidya and Taylor 1989), but these features also provide clues that the diagnosis may be something other than schizophrenia (Citrome 1989). A double-blind, placebo-controlled, parallel-design clinical trial involving seriously ill state hospital patients with schizophrenia who had not responded to prior trials of typical neuroleptics demonstrated no advantage of lithium combined with haloperidol over haloperidol alone (W.H. Wilson 1993). When lithium was added to neuroleptics for the treatment of patients with treatment-resistant schizophrenia who were classified as "dangerous, violent or criminal," no benefits were seen after 4 weeks of adjunctive lithium (Collins et al. 1991). However, there are case reports of patients with paranoid schizophrenia with aggressive or disorderly behaviors who have responded to the addition of lithium to their neuroleptic treatment, then deteriorated after the lithium was discontinued but subsequently improved when it was reinstituted (Prakash 1985).

The authors quoted above do not report any instances of a paradoxical increase of aggressivity during lithium treatment. One such paradoxical case was described (Schiff et al. 1982). This patient had a temporal lobe electroencephalographic spike focus. His electroencephalographic abnormality and aggressivity increased simultaneously after the start of lithium treatment and then improved after the treatment was stopped. However, a study reporting beneficial effects of lithium included at least four epileptic patients, one of whom had temporal lobe epilepsy (Tupin et al. 1973). Another study (Tyrer et al. 1984) observed eight epileptic patients, only one of whom showed a slight increase in seizure frequency during the lithium treatment.

In summary, lithium has been reported to reduce aggressive behavior in patients with various psychoses as well as in nonpsychotic, persistently aggressive prisoners. The mechanism of its antiaggressive action is not well understood. Primarily because of its toxicity and low therapeutic index, lithium is being gradually replaced by other mood stabilizers such as valproate in the armamentarium of antiaggressive drugs.

Valproate

Valproate has become one of the most commonly prescribed mood stabilizers for patients with bipolar disorder, schizoaffective disorder, and schizophrenia. In the inpatient facilities of the New York State Office of Mental Health, valproate was prescribed for 61% of patients with bipolar disorder, 54% of patients with schizoaffective disorder, and as many as 35% of patients diagnosed with schizophrenia (Citrome et al. 2000). Using valproate as an adjunctive treatment for schizophrenia is apparently a widespread practice that is not limited to New York (Ramesh and Sandson 2000). Indeed, valproate is the only mood stabilizer that is clearly considered the first-line adjunctive treatment for schizophrenia patients who exhibit persistent aggressive behavior (McEvoy et al. 1999, pp. 43–44).

However, published evidence supporting this treatment of schizophrenia is surprisingly weak. I know of only four published short-term (up to 5 weeks) double-blind studies of adjunctive valproate treatment in schizophrenia patients. Three of these studies failed to find overall beneficial effects of valproate (Dose et al. 1998; Hesslinger et al. 1999; Ko et al. 1985), although a reduction of "hostile belligerence" was observed in one of these three studies (Dose et al. 1998). There is one positive study that compared five patients receiving valproate adjunctive treatment with seven control subjects; all patients were diagnosed with acute exacerbation of chronic schizophrenia (Wassef et al. 2000). In that study, the patients assigned to the valproate group received this adjunctive treatment for 15 days and then received adjunctive placebo instead of valproate for the next 7 days. There was a significantly greater improvement in the valproate group than in control subjects in the third week of the study, when the valproate patients were switched to placebo, suggesting perhaps a carryover effect.

An open study of adjunctive valproate treatment in acutely excited psychotic (schizophrenic and manic) patients found significant reductions of aggressive, impulsive, and agitated behavior (Altamura et al. 1986), and another open study found generally positive effects of valproate augmentation in acutely exacerbating schizophrenia (Wassef et al. 2001). A retrospective chart review of adjunctive valproate treatment suggested a good response in bipolar disorder (manic or mixed), a moderate response in schizoaffective disorder, and no response in schizophrenia (McElroy et al. 1987). Additional evidence supporting adjunctive valproate treatment of schizophrenia relies on small uncontrolled studies (Bourguignon et al. 1984; Nagao et al. 1979; Wassef et al. 1996) and case reports (Chong et al. 1998) that are reviewed elsewhere (Wassef et al. 1999). One study using valproate as monotherapy reported a deterioration in six of eight schizophrenic patients (Lautin et al. 1980).

The antiaggressive effects of valproate in patients with dementia, mental retardation, and brain injuries were described in uncontrolled studies and case reports (Donovan et al. 1997; Geracioti 1994; Giakas et al. 1990; Hollander et al. 1996; Horne and Lindley 1995; Lott et al. 1995;

Mattes 1992; Mazure et al. 1992; Mellow et al. 1993; Wilcox 1994; Wroblewski et al. 1997).

Open-label valproate was used in 21 incarcerated male patients with a primary diagnosis of borderline personality disorder, referred for hospitalization because of aggressive behavior. After discharge, patients were followed up within the correctional system for 6 months. Eighteen of the 21 patients demonstrated a reduction in the frequency and severity of aggression. All patients demonstrated a reduction in subjective irritability (Hegarty 2000).

Thus, in summary, valproate is widely used to control aggressive behavior in many types of patients. Published evidence for its efficacy is relatively strong in mania, weaker in schizoaffective disorder, and weakest in schizophrenia. Nevertheless, many schizophrenia patients are treated with valproate; the principal intended target of this adjunctive treatment is impulsive aggressive behavior. More research is urgently needed to determine the effectiveness and safety of this treatment. Future studies of adjunctive valproate treatment should include measurements of plasma levels of valproate and the coadministered neuroleptic, because pharmacokinetic interactions are possible (Facciola et al. 1999).

Carbamazepine

The antiaggressive effects of carbamazepine as an adjunctive treatment in schizophrenia and schizoaffective disorder were suggested by two placebo-controlled studies (Neppe 1983; Okuma et al. 1989). The first study was small and included patients with other diagnoses. The second study (Okuma et al. 1989) involved 162 schizophrenic or schizoaffective patients receiving various antipsychotics (open-label) who were randomized to one of two adjunctive treatments: carbamazepine or placebo (double-blind). The study demonstrated a significantly better effect of carbamazepine on agitation and aggression; unfortunately, these two behaviors were commingled in data analysis. Thus, the report does not permit an assessment of antiaggressive effects per se. In addition to these placebo-controlled studies, other observations suggest antiaggressive effects of carbamazepine in schizophrenic and schizoaffective patients (Hakola and Laulumaa 1982; Luchins 1984; Yassa and Dupont 1983). A brief letter (Mattes 1984) reported that carbamazepine was administered to 34 adult inpatients with rage outbursts of various etiologies. Most patients ($n=19$) had intermittent explosive disorder. This was apparently an open, uncontrolled trial. Several descriptors were employed to assess the effect of carbamazepine on violent behavior. Significant improvement was noted in one of them (severity of physical assaults). Ten patients who developed agitated and aggressive behavior after closed head injury were treated with open-label carbamazepine; 8 of these patients improved (Azouvi et al. 1999). Thus, adjunctive carbamazepine may indeed have antiaggressive effects in patients with various brain disorders.

Similar to the studies of valproate, adjunctive carbamazepine treatment studies included plasma carbamazepine levels, but not the plasma levels of concomitant neuroleptic medication. This leaves open the possibility of pharmacokinetic interactions. Such an interaction has been reported for haloperidol (R.H. Levy and Kerr 1988) and may exist for other neuroleptics. However, definitive studies demonstrating such effects are lacking.

Gabapentin

Gabapentin has been proposed as a treatment for bipolar disorder (Schaffer and Schaffer 1997) and for behavior dyscontrol (Bozikas et al. 2001; Ryback and Ryback 1995). Similar to valproate, gabapentin has also been used as an adjunctive agent in the treatment of schizophrenia. In 1998, the prescription rate of gabapentin in New York State psychiatric hospital patients diagnosed with schizophrenia exceeded that for carbamazepine (Citrome et al. 2000).

Benzodiazepines

Benzodiazepines showed antiaggressive or "taming" effects in initial animal studies. However, more detailed studies of the dose-response relationship revealed bidirectional effects; low doses of benzodiazepines increased the frequency of attacks, whereas higher doses decreased the frequency of attacks by rodents in many experimental conditions (Miczek 1987). Increased levels of aggression were also reported in animals during withdrawal from long-term benzodiazepine treatment (Herman et al. 1976).

The use of benzodiazepines for short-term control of aggressive behavior is mentioned under "Emergency Treatment" above. The clinical reports reviewed below were largely concerned with ongoing or repeated administration of benzodiazepines.

Early tests of benzodiazepines as treatment for human aggression were inspired by the effects of these compounds in animals. Clinical observations of psychiatric inpatients with diverse diagnoses suggested that chlordiazepoxide reduced hostility and overt aggression "regardless of the underlying pathology" (Boyle and Tobin 1961). Similar results were noted with diazepam treatment of variously diagnosed forensic patients

(Kalina 1964) and with chlordiazepoxide in patients with "episodic behavior disorders" (Monroe 1975). Benzodiazepines were also used with success to control aggression in elderly patients with dementia (Yudofsky et al. 1990) and in mentally retarded persons (W.S. Bond et al. 1989). Patients with personality disorders and a history of temper outbursts were treated with chlordiazepoxide, oxazepam, or placebo in a double-blind experiment; oxazepam reduced hostility (as measured by the Buss-Durkee hostility scale [Buss and Durkee 1957]), but no effect on overt aggression was mentioned (Lion 1979).

Benzodiazepines are sometimes used as a long-term adjunctive treatment (coadministered with antipsychotics) to control persistent aggressive behavior in patients with schizophrenia. Expert consensus guidelines suggest this combination as a first- or second-line treatment for aggressive schizophrenic patients who have no history of substance abuse (McEvoy et al. 1999, p. 44). However, the efficacy of such treatment has not been established. In fact, a double-blind, placebo-controlled trial of adjunctive clonazepam treatment in 13 schizophrenia patients showed no beneficial effects. Four of the patients behaved aggressively during the study; three of these four had not been previously violent (Karson et al. 1982). Long-term use of benzodiazepines may result in tolerance and dependence. However, these problems have not been reported in schizophrenic patients receiving adjunctive benzodiazepines. It is possible that the tolerance develops primarily to the sedative effects, whereas other effects (e.g., anxiolytic) are relatively unaffected.

Paradoxical Reactions

In several patients, hostility or violence worsened after administration of benzodiazepines (Feldman 1962; Ingram and Timbury 1960; Murray 1961). Three of 79 psychiatric patients treated with chlordiazepoxide developed "acute rage reactions"; these three patients had had similar episodes in the past (Tobin et al. 1960), as did one of the two patients described elsewhere (Lion et al. 1975). These reactions (termed *paradoxical* because they were opposite to the expected effect) were later explored in a series of studies in nonpatient (psychologically healthy) subjects. Various paper-and-pencil tests assessing hostility provided dependent variables in these studies. The Buss-Durkee Hostility Inventory was the most widely used test. Hostility after a single dose of diazepam was more pronounced in subjects who had high predrug (baseline) levels of anxiety and depression (McDonald 1967). Similarly, chlordiazepoxide increased hostility in subjects with higher levels of baseline anxiety;

however, oxazepam had no marked effect on hostility scores (Gardos et al. 1968). Chlordiazepoxide increased hostility among psychologically healthy volunteers (Salzman et al. 1974); these increases were more frequent and intense than those associated with oxazepam or placebo (Kochansky et al. 1975). On the basis of these and other observations, it has been suggested that oxazepam may be the benzodiazepine specifically suited to reduce hostility (Salzman et al. 1975).

A similar conclusion regarding oxazepam was reached by experimenters who examined the effects of placebo, 10 mg diazepam, 15 mg chlorazepate, or 50 mg oxazepam on human aggressive behavior under laboratory conditions in 44 medically healthy men (Weisman et al. 1998). Participants were given the opportunity to administer electric shocks to an increasingly provocative fictitious opponent during a competitive reaction-time task. Aggression was defined as the level of shock the participant was willing to administer to the opponent. All three benzodiazepines elicited more aggressive behavior than placebo, but only the effect of diazepam reached statistical significance.

The robust, replicable nature of the benzodiazepine-increased hostility and aggression in normal volunteers makes the label "paradoxical reaction" inappropriate because there is nothing unexpected about them anymore. Similar to many other substances (e.g., alcohol), benzodiazepines have a wide, bidirectional spectrum of effects in animals and humans. The dose-response relationships governing this spectrum are understood much better in animals than in humans.

The relationship between hostility (determined by paper-and-pencil tests) in normal volunteers and overt aggression in psychiatric patients (rage reaction) is unclear. At least some of the persons who showed such reactions had a history of temper outbursts preceding their exposure to the drug (Lion et al. 1975; Tobin et al. 1960). However, forensic patients with a clear history of violence, destructiveness, and assaultiveness improved with diazepam therapy; no paradoxical reactions were noted (Kalina 1964). It has been suggested that paradoxical rage reactions in patients occur with higher doses of benzodiazepines (A. Bond and Lader 1979), but the evidence is not convincing. Most paradoxical reactions occurred after multiple doses, sometimes after weeks of continuous benzodiazepine treatment. However, most of the current use of benzodiazepines to control violence is limited to one or two injections at a time as needed; this practice should therefore reduce the likelihood of paradoxical reactions. The mechanism of the paradoxical reactions to benzodiazepines in psychiatric patients remains unclear. The frequency of occurrence of these reactions is low, and their effect on clinical practice is limited.

Antidepressants

In animals, short-term experiments with tricyclics demonstrated relatively modest antiaggressive effects; however, the effects of long-term treatment (e.g., 10 days) were in the opposite direction (Miczek 1987, p. 227). Increased hostility or aggressiveness after administration of tricyclics was reported in several adult, mostly depressed patients (Gottschalk et al. 1965; Rampling 1978); similar results were obtained in a double-blind, placebo-controlled study of amitriptyline in borderline patients (Soloff et al. 1986, 1987). Case reports of similar observations in children exist (Pallmeyer and Petti 1979; Tec 1963). A patient developed agitated, physically threatening behavior after a closed head injury; amitriptyline, started several months after the injury, reduced the threatening behavior (Jackson et al. 1985). The value of amitriptyline for the treatment of post-traumatic agitation (including some threatening behavior) was confirmed in additional patients (Mysiw et al. 1988).

The current interest in the role of certain antidepressants in treating aggression is based on the confluence of two developments. First, the crucial role of serotoninergic regulation of impulsive aggression against self and others has been recognized (see Chapter 3). Second, antidepressants with specific effects on 5-hydroxytryptamine (5-HT) receptors have become available. Trazodone, a selective 5-HT$_2$ antagonist, reduced violent outbursts in an open trial of four dementia patients who showed no clinical signs of depression (Simpson and Foster 1986); these observations were partially replicated in another sample of seven aggressive patients with dementia, three of whom improved (Pinner and Rich 1988). A combination of trazodone and tryptophan (a serotonin precursor) was used successfully to reduce aggressive behavior and temper tantrums in a mentally retarded patient (O'Neil et al. 1986) and in several elderly patients with dementia (Greenwald et al. 1986; Wilcock et al. 1987). A similar effect was reported in a retarded adult patient with Down syndrome when trazodone was given in combination with a "serotonin-enhancing" diet (Gedye 1991b).

Fluoxetine, a selective serotonin reuptake inhibitor, decreased impulsive aggression (including assaultiveness) in a double-blind, placebo-controlled trial conducted in 40 individuals with personality disorders and current histories of impulsive aggressive behavior and irritability (Coccaro and Kavoussi 1997). Fluoxetine treatment resulted in sustained reductions of irritability and aggression that were first apparent during months 2 and 3 of treatment, respectively. These results were not influenced by secondary measures of depression, anxiety, or alcohol use.

Patients with chronic schizophrenia who remained symptomatic while receiving maintenance antipsychotic treatment were given adjunctive fluoxetine; violent incidents decreased in four cases and increased in one case in this retrospective, uncontrolled study (Goldman and Janecek 1990). Fluoxetine was effective against anger attacks in irritable and hostile patients with unipolar depression (Fava et al. 1993). Interestingly, these patients showed a blunted prolactin response to thyrotropin-releasing hormone (TRH) before fluoxetine treatment; the response to TRH increased after the treatment. Thus, the results of this neuroendocrine challenge provided indirect evidence suggesting a central serotoninergic dysregulation in these patients with anger attacks (J.F. Rosenbaum et al. 1993).

Fluoxetine was reported to paradoxically increase suicidal ideation in six depressed patients (Teicher et al. 1990). Although four of these patients were also taking other medications than fluoxetine, that report received wide publicity, and some other patients subsequently claimed to have increased feelings of hostility while taking fluoxetine. Furthermore, adjunctive treatment with fluoxetine was associated with increased levels of aggressive behavior in 9 of 19 adult inpatients with mental retardation and epilepsy (Troisi et al. 1995). The mechanism of this effect was unclear; all patients were being coadministered multiple other medications, and the authors could not exclude the possibility of adverse interactions. It is also possible that patients with mental retardation and epilepsy belong to a small, vulnerable subpopulation (hypothesized by Mann and Kapur) that shows paradoxical responses to antidepressant treatment. These authors postulated that "in a subset of patients, the introduction of a serotonin reuptake inhibitor or an increase in dose may result in an exaggerated initial decrease of serotonergic transmission" and thus enhance suicidal or aggressive behavior early in treatment (Mann and Kapur 1991, p. 1032).

There has been considerable controversy regarding these paradoxical effects of fluoxetine, and the drug was blamed for inducing murder or suicide in several court cases. Responding to the controversy, Eli Lilly and Company researchers reanalyzed data from several fluoxetine trials comprising a total of 3,992 subjects. Statistically significantly, fewer fluoxetine-treated patients (0.15%) than placebo-treated patients (0.65%) experienced events suggestive of aggression. Another reanalysis of the pooled data from some of these trials showed that fluoxetine was not associated with suicidality (Tollefson et al. 1994). These reanalyses of large data sets may have missed some rare phenomena occurring in a small subset of patients. Nevertheless, they are reassuring.

Citalopram, another selective serotonin reuptake inhibitor, was used as adjunctive treatment in 15 persistently violent schizophrenia inpatients hospitalized at a forensic facility (Vartiainen et al. 1995). This was a crossover study in which the subjects were treated with adjunctive citalopram for 24 weeks and with adjunctive placebo for another 24 weeks (in addition to their antipsychotic medication). The study was double-blind. During citalopram treatment, the frequency of aggressive incidents was significantly lower than during placebo treatment. The design and execution of this study are outstanding.

Buspirone, an anxiolytic with antidepressant properties, is a 5-HT$_{1A}$ receptor agonist with demonstrated antiaggressive effects in the monkey (Tompkins et al. 1980). It was reported to improve aggressive and self-injurious behavior in 9 of 14 mentally retarded patients (Ratey et al. 1989); this effect was confirmed in a controlled study by the same group (Ratey et al. 1991). Several case studies reporting similar results were published (Gedye 1991a; Quiason et al. 1991). A case of posttraumatic belligerence (the patient was described as "extremely hostile, argumentative, impulsive, and threatening") was successfully managed with buspirone, which was started several months after the head injury (Levine 1988).

Serotonin Precursor Treatment

Disturbances of central serotoninergic function may lead to aggressive behavior (see Chapter 3). A decrease of serotonin availability has been inferred from decreased cerebrospinal fluid levels of 5-hydroxyindoleacetic acid (5-HIAA). Tryptophan is hydroxylated to 5-hydroxytryptophan, which is then decarboxylated to 5-HT (serotonin). Increased availability of tryptophan may lead to increased synthesis of serotonin. Raising the levels of tryptophan by increasing its dietary intake may therefore reduce aggressive behavior.

Tryptophan deficiency in the diet increased fighting in animals (see Chapter 2). However, altering tryptophan blood levels in psychiatrically healthy humans had no effect on aggressiveness that was measured by a test (Young et al. 1988).

Tryptophan was used in combination with trazodone in several studies (Gedye 1991b; Greenwald et al. 1986; O'Neil et al. 1986; Wilcock et al. 1987). Aggressive patients with XYY syndrome who had low cerebrospinal fluid levels of 5-HIAA were treated with tryptophan for 5 months, and the investigators claimed beneficial clinical effects (Bioulac et al. 1980). In another study, a group of 12 violent schizophrenic patients received tryptophan (4 or 8 mg/day) for 4 weeks, and a reduction in violent incidents was noted in this placebo-controlled experiment (Morand et al. 1983). An attempt to replicate that study was not completely successful: tryptophan did not affect the number of violent incidents but did reduce the need for injections of antipsychotics and sedatives (Volavka et al. 1990). This finding provided indirect support for a beneficial effect of tryptophan in aggressive psychiatric patients.

β-Adrenergic Blockers

Propranolol was briefly noted to reduce aggressive behavior in isolated mice in an early report (Valzelli et al. 1967). However, it appears that β-blockers were not systematically tested as a treatment for animal aggression before the first observations of the antiaggressive effects of propranolol in humans were published. The first report of propranolol use in humans for the control of "belligerent behavior following acute brain damage" did not include any theoretical rationale for this successful open trial (Elliott 1977).

Animal data indicate that the doses of propranolol required to reduce aggression are considerably smaller than those that decrease other motor activity (Miczek 1987; Vassout and Delini-Stula 1977). It is not clear whether the antiaggressive effects of β-blockers are in fact mediated by β-adrenergic receptors. It is possible that these effects are mediated through blockade of serotoninergic (Hjorth and Carlsson 1986; Weinstock and Weiss 1980) or other receptors.

Propranolol

Propranolol has been used to control aggression primarily in patients with organic brain disease. The diagnoses included mental retardation (Ratey et al. 1983, 1986); posttraumatic organic brain syndromes (Elliott 1977; Mansheim 1981; Yudofsky et al. 1981); various types of dementia (Greendyke et al. 1986; Petrie and Ban 1981; Yudofsky et al. 1984); Huntington's disease (Stewart et al. 1987); one case of Wilson's disease (Yudofsky et al. 1981); one case of postencephalitic psychosis (Schreier 1979); and "apparent or presumed chronic central nervous system dysfunction" inferred from soft neurological signs, abnormal electroencephalograms, or clinical seizures (Williams et al. 1982).

The time of onset of the antiaggressive effect of propranolol is difficult to glean from the reports; it appeared to range between 12 hours (Elliott 1977) and 2 months (Yudofsky et al. 1981). The reasons for this variability are not clear. Perhaps some descriptions of early effects reflected nonspecific sedation elicited by propranolol. Current literature suggests that onset of the antiaggressive effects can be seen 4–8 weeks after the effective dose is reached (Yudofsky et al. 1990). The effective dose can only be reached after a gradual buildup.

The dose of propranolol perceived as effective by the researchers was remarkably variable, ranging between 30 and 1,600 mg/day; this variability may reflect genuine differences among patients and perhaps among several mechanisms whereby propranolol exerts its antiaggressive effects. The dose-response relationship has not been systematically studied. Such a study would be complicated by the wide variation in the time of onset of action of propranolol.

Except for one small study (Greendyke et al. 1986), the propranolol studies were not controlled for placebo effects. Most were retrospective. These propranolol studies in patients with organic brain disease show a high success rate, which should be viewed with caution in view of the limitations just mentioned and also because negative results tend to remain unpublished (Easterbrook et al. 1991). Nevertheless, I believe that propranolol exhibits antiaggressive activity in patients with a wide spectrum of organic brain disorders.

Propranolol has been added to antipsychotic regimens as an adjunctive treatment for schizophrenia in patients who were not specifically selected for aggressivity (Sheppard 1979; Yorkston et al. 1977); it reduced symptoms, including aggression. Isolated cases of successful treatment of aggression with propranolol in particularly assaultive schizophrenic patients have been reported (Sorgi et al. 1986; J.R. Whitman et al. 1987). Propranolol was used as adjunctive treatment in a diagnostically heterogeneous sample of 20 psychiatric inpatients (5 diagnosed with schizophrenia, 1 with schizoaffective disorder, 7 with atypical psychosis, and other—sometimes multiple—diagnoses) (Silver et al. 1999). The patients were enrolled if they exhibited repeated verbal or physical aggression in the prior 6 months. The duration of the open-label trial varied among patients. Seven patients showed definite reduction of aggressive behavior, and an additional 5 showed equivocal response to propranolol augmentation. After the open-label trial, several patients were entered into a double-blind discontinuation phase, and some of the improvers got worse when propranolol was discontinued. This study showed that some aggressive patients do respond to propranolol. It also demonstrated the tremendous difficulties involved in implementing long-term pharmacologic studies of aggressive patients.

The mechanism of the antiaggressive effects of propranolol is not clear. When used as an antihypertensive drug, propranolol may cause drowsiness, fatigue, or lethargy. Thus, it is possible that some of the antiaggressive effect was due to nonspecific sedation. Unfortunately, none of the studies mentioned above employed specific measures of drowsiness, sedation, or fatigue. Williams et al. (1982) mention that somnolence occurred in 6 of 30 patients during the course of dose adjustment of propranolol; dose reductions alleviated this problem. Case descriptions published by other authors do not mention sedation. Therefore, it appears that the antiaggressive effects of propranolol may not be mediated through sedation; however, this issue has not been adequately addressed in human studies and requires more research. Animal work suggests separate mechanisms for antiaggressive and sedative effects.

In most studies, propranolol was added to other medications that the patients were receiving. There is therefore a possibility of drug interactions. Pharmacokinetic interactions have been identified: propranolol increases plasma levels of chlorpromazine (Peet et al. 1981) and thioridazine (Greendyke and Kanter 1987; Silver et al. 1986) and perhaps of other antipsychotic medications.

Pharmacodynamic interactions are also possible. Propranolol reduces akathisia, which in turn may be linked to violence; thus, propranolol may indirectly reduce violence in patients treated with antipsychotics by treating an antipsychotic side effect (Lipinski et al. 1988) rather than by exerting a direct antiaggressive effect of its own.

Propranolol is a lipophilic, nonselective (β_1 and β_2) adrenergic blocker that easily penetrates the brain. It has multiple peripheral and central effects. It is not clear whether β_1- or β_2-adrenergic receptors (or both) are involved in the antiaggressive effects. Furthermore, it is not clear whether the effect is central or peripheral. Studies using selective or lipophobic blockers (see below) address these questions.

At the high doses employed in some of the studies of aggression, propranolol may have effects on receptors other than the adrenergic ones. Animal literature suggesting that serotoninergic receptors may be affected by β-blocking agents is mentioned above. These receptors perhaps mediate the sedative effects of propranolol observed in humans. Furthermore, it has been suggested that antipsychotic and antiakathisic effects of propranolol may be mediated through an enhanced firing rate of tegmental dopamine neurons (Lipinski et al. 1988).

Other β-Adrenergic Blockers

Nadolol is a nonselective β-adrenergic blocker that is relatively lipophobic and accordingly is believed not to cross the blood-brain barrier to any great extent (although this belief is not universal; see J.R. Whitman et al. 1987). A retrospective chart review demonstrated antiaggressive effects of nadolol (40–160 mg/day) in six patients with chronic schizophrenia (Sorgi et al. 1986). Furthermore, it was as effective as propranolol in suppressing aggressive behavior in a mentally retarded patient who received a separate trial of each of these two agents (Polakoff et al. 1986). A double-blind, placebo-controlled, parallel-group trial of nadolol in aggressive, mostly schizophrenic patients (N=41) demonstrated the superiority of nadolol in reducing incidents of overt aggression (Ratey et al. 1992). Unfortunately, there appeared to be a considerable difference in the level of aggression between the two treatment groups at the baseline; it is not clear whether this difference affected the outcome. These encouraging results with a lipophobic drug suggest that at least some of the antiaggressive action of β-blocking agents may be peripheral. Peripheral components of akathisia, tension, or anxiety might be improved by nadolol, and the antiaggressive effect may be mediated by these improvements.

Metoprolol, a selective β_1-adrenergic receptor blocker, was effective in two cases of intermittent explosive disorder (Mattes 1985) and two cases of mental retardation (Kastner et al. 1990). Thus, some or all of the antiaggressive effects of nonselective β-blockers may be mediated through the β_1 receptor.

Similar to propranolol, the main practical problem with the administration of metoprolol for aggression is the high frequency of cardiovascular side effects (reduction of pulse rate and blood pressure).

Pindolol, besides its nonselective β-adrenergic blocking activity, has a partial agonist effect (intrinsic sympathomimetic activity). As a result, pindolol has fewer cardiovascular side effects than propranolol in normotensive populations, making it a safer and more attractive compound for psychiatric indications. Pindolol also blocks the 5-HT_{1A} receptors; this property may be at least partly responsible for antiaggressive effects. Pindolol was tested in a double-blind, placebo-controlled, crossover study with 11 patients with dementias of varying origin. It reduced assaultiveness and hostility without producing lethargy (Greendyke and Kanter 1986). Another double-blind, placebo-controlled, crossover study enrolled 30 male schizophrenia patients involved in four or more aggressive incidents in the two previous months. In addition to their antipsychotic treatment, patients were randomly and blindly assigned to either pindolol (15 mg/day) or placebo augmentation for 6 weeks, then switched for another 6 weeks to the other treatment (placebo or pindolol) (Caspi et al. 2001). No significant differences were found in the PANSS scores between the placebo and pindolol treatments. Significant reductions of the number and severity of aggressive incidents were obtained with pindolol. This sophisticated study clearly demonstrates the antiaggressive effects of pindolol.

In summary, adjunctive β-adrenergic blocking agents may have antiaggressive effects. The recent expert consensus guidelines list adjunctive β-blockers as a second-line treatment for persistently aggressive schizophrenia patients (McEvoy et al. 1999, p. 44), but the treatment is not much used in clinical practice.

Patients vary considerably in the degree to which they respond to β blockers. It is possible that that variability is influenced by genetic factors The gene for catechol-*O*-methyltransferase (COMT) shows a functional polymorphism, and the allele that codes for the low activity of this enzyme was associated with aggressive behavior in several studies (see Chapter 3). Blocking β-adrenergic transmission would partially correct for the relatively inadequate biotransformation of catecholamines. Therefore, we are now testing the hypothesis that the COMT allele coding for the low-activity form of the enzyme will be associated with a greater antiaggressive effect of a β-adrenergic blocking agent.

Antiandrogen Treatment

Antiandrogen treatment has been used successfully in sex offenders such as transvestites and exhibitionists (McConaghy et al. 1988; Money 1991) and rapists (Barry and Ciccone 1975). Medroxyprogesterone acetate (MPA) has marked antiandrogen properties. It lowers testosterone levels and sexual drive in male patients; the effects at higher doses are equivalent to a functional and reversible castration, but sexual activity can be maintained at lower doses (McConaghy et al. 1988). MPA decreases sexual drive, but it does not change the object of the drive (e.g., pedophiles remain interested in children) (Kiersch 1990).

Somewhat surprisingly, MPA also reduced aggressive outbursts in patients with temporal lobe epilepsy ($n=11$) and in four XYY subjects (Blumer and Migeon 1975). These effects were tentatively attributed by the authors to sedation and sleepiness elicited by MPA. As far as I know, the results in epileptic patients and XYY subjects have not been replicated.

The use of MPA in sex offenders raises complicated medical, ethical, and legal issues (Berlin 1989; Dyer 1988; Melella et al. 1989). The treatment should not (and probably cannot) be forced on an unwilling patient, but the extent to which a convicted sex offender can exercise a truly noncoerced choice is a matter of dispute. Furthermore, it is not clear whether sex offenders have a right to MPA treatment on request. MPA treatment can perhaps be a viable alternative to imprisonment in consenting offenders. As far as I know, clear ethical guidelines for the MPA treatment of sex offenders are not available.

Electroconvulsive Treatment

The effect of electroconvulsive treatment (ECT) in combination with risperidone was examined in an open trial in 10 male schizophrenic patients with significant aggressive behaviors (Hirose et al. 2001).

Patients were given bilateral ECT five times a week in combination with risperidone. The mean total number of administrations of ECT was 6.6 (range, 5–9). In 5 of the 6 patients who showed positive symptoms, the aggressive behavior was rapidly ameliorated within 12 days. The ECT/risperidone regimen also eliminated aggressive behavior in 4 patients who showed no positive symptoms within 10 days. These treatment effects lasted for at least 6 months in 9 of the 10 patients. The results suggest that the combination of ECT and risperidone produces a rapid and effective elimination of aggressive behaviors in schizophrenic patients. In addition, there was a resolution of aggression in 4 patients with no positive symptoms. This suggests that aggression in some schizophrenic patients develops as a primary symptom of schizophrenia and is not related to other positive symptoms of the disease or the patient's personality traits.

In a retrospective review of the medical records of 5 patients who received at least 12 sessions of ECT for treatment-resistant psychosis with severe episodic aggression at a forensic facility, the patients showed overall behavioral improvement and a decreased number of violent episodes during the year following treatment. (Parikh et al. 2000). In summary, ECT may be useful in reducing the frequency of violent incidents in patients with treatment-resistant aggression and psychosis.

SUMMARY AND CONCLUSIONS

Research on the psychopharmacological treatment of violence is beset by methodological, political, and ethical problems. Antipsychotics have been used widely to reduce aggression in patients with many clinical conditions. High doses of antipsychotics have probably been overused. Clozapine, an atypical antipsychotic, reduces hostility and aggression even in patients who do not respond to typical antipsychotics. Other atypical drugs are being tested for their potential antiaggressive effects. The data available to date suggest that clozapine will maintain its superiority as an antiaggressive drug in comparison with other atypical antipsychotics.

Mood stabilizers, particularly valproate, have been widely used as antiaggressive agents, although the evidence of their effectiveness for this indication is not strong. β-Adrenergic blockers were reported to be particularly effective antiaggressive agents in patients with organic conditions; more recent evidence suggests that aggressive schizophrenic patients may also benefit from this treatment. Benzodiazepines are useful for short-term control of acute aggressive episodes. ECT may emerge as an effective treatment for persistently aggressive psychotic patients who do not respond to medications.

12 | Summary and Conclusions

SUMMARY AND INTERPRETATION

There is no simple one-to-one relationship between biological factors and violence. Animal research reveals the importance of the interaction of biological and social factors that act jointly to generate aggressive behavior. Research on nonhuman primates documents that these interactions become increasingly more important and complex as we ascend the phylogenic scale. The direction of causation is not simply from biological factors to behaviors; rather, there are multiple bidirectional transactions between the organism and its environment, each influencing the other. For example, in monkeys the results of aggressive encounters affect levels of neurotransmitters and hormones; these levels in turn exert regulatory effects on aggressive behavior.

Both the organism and its environment are modified and evolve over time as a direct result of these mutual influences. Study of the developmental aspects of such transactional processes yielded important results in nonhuman primates; it was found, for example, that manipulation of the rearing environment resulted in changes in neurotransmitter functions that persisted into adulthood. One of the possible mechanisms for such transactions is the effect of environment on gene expression.

In the past 20 years, work with neurotransmitters has been a mainstay of biological research into aggression. It is an area in which there has been a productive integration between animal and human research. This work has also led to new hypotheses regarding the ways in which early experiences, alcohol intake, and other variables may exert their influence over aggression.

In many populations, a disturbance in central serotoninergic transmission is related to impulsive aggression. The serotoninergic system inhibits quick motor responses; disturbances of the system may result in disinhibition of such responses. The serotoninergic hypothesis of aggres-

299

sion opens possibilities for antiaggressive pharmacologic treatments.

When interpreting this literature, one should keep in mind that serotonin is not the only neurotransmitter involved in aggression. The underlying neurobiological dysfunction is more extensive, involving other neurotransmitters interacting with serotonin. Several lines of evidence point to the role of catecholamines in the modulation of irritability and aggression. Furthermore, impulsive aggression in humans often appears in a context of multiple abnormal behaviors and traits that are sufficiently pervasive and chronic to warrant a diagnosis of personality disorder (or intermittent explosive disorder). Serotoninergic or catecholaminergic effects were demonstrated in populations with these disorders. It is not clear how these results will generalize to other populations.

Alcohol plays a central role in violence and violent crime. Short-term effects of alcohol include increases in aggressiveness in laboratory experiments with psychiatrically healthy subjects. Alcohol ingestion by perpetrators precedes a large proportion of violent crimes. Alcohol ingestion by victims is also important, underscoring the dyadic dimension of the violent incident.

Drugs of abuse also play an important role. Short-term effects of cocaine, amphetamine, phencyclidine, and related substances may include aggressiveness. Withdrawal syndromes from various drugs of abuse (particularly opioids) include irritability and occasionally aggressiveness.

Alcohol abuse is, in part, genetically transmitted. As a result, there are further interactions among genetic predisposition, neurotransmitter dysfunction, alcohol abuse, and violence. Patients with major psychiatric disorders such as schizophrenia and mania show higher levels of alcohol and drug abuse, and substance abuse increases the risk of violent behavior among such patients.

Although central serotoninergic disturbance and aggressive behavior can be elicited by brain lesions in animals, almost no data exist to support an analogous linkage in humans. There is a very large body of literature on structural brain damage and violence in humans, but this literature has essentially no connection to neurotransmitters or receptors. Much of this neurological and neurosurgical literature predates the current flowering of neurotransmitter work. Although no brain "center for aggression" exists, evidence converging from clinical observations, electroencephalograms, and more recent imaging methods suggests that lesions or dysfunctions of anterior parts of the temporal lobes and the orbitomedial part of the frontal lobes may elicit violent behavior. Recent work suggests that impulsive violent behavior may be associated with dysfunctional connections between the orbitomedial frontal cortex and other parts of the brain; such dysfunction is suggested by disturbed microanatomy of the white matter revealed by diffusion tensor imaging. Subtle, diffuse neurological dysfunctions are associated with recidivistic violence among patients with major mental disorders. Similarly to serotoninergic dysfunction, neurological impairments may result in disinhibition of violent behaviors.

Genetic effects on criminal and violent behavior are supported by twin and adoption studies. Some of these genetic effects may be attributable to polymorphisms of various genes that are involved in the regulation of serotonin and catecholamine activity; several of these candidate genes are being intensively studied. Joint effects of genetic, prenatal, and perinatal factors contribute to the propensity for violent criminal behavior. These joint effects may be mediated by influences on neurotransmitters, by subtle neurodevelopmental abnormalities, by brain injuries sustained in the prenatal and perinatal periods, or by some other mechanisms. Subtle neurological dysfunctions reported in adult violent subjects might have developed as a result of these early events.

Studies of postnatal development have detected behavioral precursors of future aggressive behavior in early childhood, and they underscore the importance of learning and environmental influences in the control of violent behavior. Inhibition of aggressive responses to environmental influences has to be learned in childhood. Parents or other caregivers teach this inhibition by imposing limits of acceptable behavior and by setting an example with their own conduct. Environmental and constitutional obstacles to learning inhibition exist and interact with each other over time. Children will not learn to inhibit their aggressive responses in environments that are not conducive to such learning (e.g., in an abusive family). Furthermore, the child's capability to learn is important. That capability may be limited by various brain dysfunctions. These dysfunctions, then, cause violence only indirectly, by restricting the capability to learn. Besides various neurological abnormalities, several physiologic traits have been proposed to account for difficulties in learning to inhibit aggressive responses. A mini-theory involving one such trait (slow recovery of skin response) was presented. Another mini-theory, involving child abuse and biological factors, was developed to explain intergenerational transmission of violence.

Major mental disorders such as schizophrenia, severe mood disorders, and various other Axis I disorders are associated with increased arrest rates for violent crime and with increased levels of violent behavior in the community. Some of that behavior is related to psychotic symptoms, indicating that the relationship between psychosis and violence may be direct. Comorbid substance abuse, noncompliance with outpatient treatment, and homelessness are risk factors for violent behavior of patients with major mental disorders in the community. Although psychiatrists are familiar with these and other risk factors, risk assessment for violent behavior in the community has not been particularly accurate. Short-term prediction of violent behavior of such patients in the hospital has yielded more accurate results.

It appears that there are at least two subtypes of violent behavior in schizophrenic patients. Type 1, which is more frequent, occurs in acutely decompensated patients. These patients usually decompensate because they stop taking antipsychotic medications and/or start using alcohol and drugs. Once their medication regimen has been resumed and the substance abuse is stopped (which may require hospitalization), these patients improve, and their violent behavior disappears.

Type 2, which is less frequent, occurs in patients whose behavior is resistant to treatment with typical neuroleptics, have multiple violent incidents (recidivistic violence), and frequently show signs of subtle neurological dysfunction.

No specific antiaggressive drug is available for clinical use. Clozapine, an atypical neuroleptic, reduces hostile and aggressive behavior among patients with treatment-resistant schizophrenia. Preliminary evidence suggests that other atypical neuroleptics may have similar, albeit perhaps somewhat weaker, effects.

β-Adrenergic blocking agents reduce violent behavior in patients with organic mental syndromes and perhaps also in patients with schizophrenia. Anticonvulsants, lithium, and various serotoninergic agents may also be effective.

At the end of this book, then, we are still very far from a unified theory of aggression. First steps toward integration take the form of several mini-theories: the relationship between genes, neurotransmitters, and violence; intergenerational transmission of violence; learning of inhibitory behavior; and subtypes of violence in schizophrenia.

Expanding these mini-theories and connecting them with each other is a challenge for future research.

CRITIQUE OF THE RESEARCH

When reviewing research approaches to violence, one is struck by their mutual isolation. The work remains fragmented, and attempts at integration are rare. The literature is difficult to interpret because much of the research has been atheoretical, sometimes even lacking explicit hypotheses. This has been conducive to various problems in study design, which I now discuss.

Violence or Aggression as the Dependent Variable

Some authors used scores on a personality questionnaire—whereas others used conviction of murder—to define their dependent variable. Other definitions include official report of arrest, self-report of arrest or of fights, or hospital incident report. Some measures address trait aggressiveness; others, state aggressiveness.

These issues are discussed in Chapter 1. In general, the divergent measures of violence or aggression used in various studies make those studies difficult to compare. These measures address different aspects of violence or aggression. In many cases, the measures were selected not because they were theoretically important or particularly valid and reliable but because they were relatively easy to obtain (e.g., arrest records or hospital incident reports).

The Independent Variables

Violence is a complex and heterogeneous phenomenon unlikely to be explained by a small set of variables. Nevertheless, most studies consisted of relating very few (one or two) variables to a measure of violent behavior. The selection of these variables was sometimes based more on expediency than on a theory.

Subject Selection

The selection of subjects was typically biased. For example, many electroencephalographic studies reported on subjects who were incarcerated and who were sent for the electroencephalographic test because a prison medical officer suspected a neurological problem. Such samples of opportunity are, of course, not representative of any population of interest. Some of the bias is due to the necessity of obtaining informed consent from the subjects who participate in research. Paranoid and hostile people do not readily volunteer as research subjects; this results in a biased selection of the samples used for research. Because many of the studies had no explicit hypothesis to test, there was no power analysis and the samples were quite small.

Retrospective or Cross-Sectional Design

With some recent exceptions, most research into violence was retrospective or cross-sectional. The inherent weakness of these designs is the inability to distinguish between the antecedents and the consequences of violence.

Data Analyses

Researchers who studied more variables at a time only rarely attempted to develop an explanatory model using multivariate statistics. Instead, they performed large numbers of univariate tests, usually without correcting for the effect of chance in obtaining "statistically significant" results with multiple tests.

Furthermore, the difference between correlation and causality was not always fully appreciated.

FUTURE RESEARCH

In general, the most comprehensive explanation of violence could be obtained by joining the fragmented theories and pieces of evidence available today, developing a more inclusive theory, formulating hypotheses based on that theory, and finding a way of testing them. This more inclusive theory would incorporate genetic influences, prenatal and perinatal events, studies of rearing environment performed jointly with studies of biological variables such as neurotransmitters and subtle neurological and neuropsychological dysfunctions, and concurrent studies of aggressive and violent behavior. This project would use a longitudinal prospective design, and it would involve studying a large number of subjects, including those at high risk for violent behavior. Violent behavior would be studied in its environmental context, including the roles of the victims. Longitudinal prospective research in progress has already acquired some of the characteristics of this approach (Arseneault et al. 2000; Brennan et al. 2000; Raine et al. 1998b; Rasanen et al. 1998).

Protective factors should receive attention in future research. Most studies discussed in this book found that certain factors (e.g., male gender, mental illness, head injury, alcohol intoxication) increase the risk of violent behavior. However, most persons at risk fortunately are not violent. Why? What factors protect them from developing violent behavior? Intelligence is probably one of the protective factors (see Chapter 4). Moral sense, it seems, is another protective factor.

I suspect that moral sense has a powerful regulatory effect on violent behavior. This sounds obvious; however, I am not aware of any formal research in this area. The training of psychiatrists and behavioral scientists does not usually include much ethics. Discussing the moral values of a patient is unusual; most health professionals think that they should be nonjudgmental. Moral relativism is an implicit stance. These attitudes may perhaps be useful in some therapeutic situations, but they inhibit open discussion of moral sense and its regulatory role. Therefore, this area has been neglected; we lack definitions, rating instruments, norms, and—most important—the realization that it needs to be addressed. I expect that explorations of moral sense and its manifestations (such as empathy, altruism, and remorse for past violent acts) in the context of neuropsychiatry and neuroscience will yield exciting results.

Attention has been focused on risk assessment and management in research on violence and mental illness. This attention is understandable; daily practice of psychiatry and decisions on long-term policy depend on these issues. Still, we should understand that risk-assessment research is not designed primarily to uncover causes of violent behavior. One can, in principle, make predictions about phenomena that are incompletely understood. However, the accuracy of the predictions can be greatly improved if one knows the causes of the phenomena. The upper limit of the accuracy of risk assessment is determined by the extent of our knowledge of the underlying causative mechanisms. I think that we may have reached that limit. If this is true, only marginal improvements in accuracy can now be achieved without expansion of our knowledge of the underlying causes. In my opinion, such expansion cannot be accomplished by studying solely social or solely biological factors that cause violent behavior. One has to study both. If the reader is now persuaded that this statement is true, the book has accomplished one of its main goals.

Appendix | Statistical Explanation of the Actuarial Method

Bayes Decision

Actuarial prediction of violence can be seen as a statistical classification task. The true future status or class of an individual is considered as a random variable C taking values in the set $[1, 2,...M]$, where $C=i$ represents the outcome of classifying an individual in class i. Based on a set of measured features of the individual at time zero (t_0), we want to classify that individual at a future time point (t_f). Most of the literature considers the future status as a binary variable (violent or nonviolent); therefore, my discussion of the mathematical methods focuses on this case (i.e., $M=2$).

At t_0, the individual is represented by a set of features (variables) hypothesized to contain sufficient information to distinguish among the possible classes of C; this set (or vector) of N features is denoted as $x=(x_1, x_2,...x_N)$. For example, x_1 may be age, x_2 prior arrests, and so forth. In many cases, the set of potential features is quite large, and in the initial step of the prediction process, the researcher is faced with a feature selection or feature extraction problem.

In each special case, on the basis of prior knowledge, the investigator adopts a feature extraction strategy assumed to be most compatible with the particular problem of prediction. In many cases, the researcher has a specific model that reflects his or her hypothesis. The model specifies which informative features of an individual should be measured to achieve a high prediction accuracy (e.g., prior arrests). In other cases, however, there is no specific hypothesis about the features informative for the classification, and generally a large number of potentially informative features are collected. Statistical methods (e.g., principal component or factor analysis) are then applied to extract characteristic (derived) features based on this large set of predictors.

A principal problem with the latter approach is that the derived features, which may explain a high percentage of variation in the data, are not necessarily good predictors. Although the approach based on a specific model is clearly preferable to this statistical approach, the researcher may still want to use this approach when not enough is known to formulate a hypothesis. At this initial stage, the researcher frequently changes the set of possible predictor features and experiments with different strategies of feature extraction.

For the problem of classification, in addition to the random variable C and the set of potential features x, we should consider a loss matrix $W = (w_i)$. The elements of this matrix, w_i, represent the loss or cost occurring when an individual is predicted to belong to class i, and in reality he or she belongs to class j. Thus, the elements of this matrix indicate the cost or "loss" (e.g., possible hazard for society, financial loss) associated with each possible outcome of the prediction; when individuals are classified as violent or nonviolent, this loss matrix takes the general form depicted in Table A–1.

Table A–1. Loss matrix

		Actual group membership (j)	
		Violent ($j=1$)	Nonviolent ($j=2$)
Predicted group membership (i)	Violent ($i=1$)	w_{11}	w_{12}
	Nonviolent ($i=2$)	w_{21}	w_{22}

In practice, the losses associated with the correct positive (w_{11}) and negative (w_{22}) decisions are considered as zero ($w_{11}=w_{22}=0$). On the other hand, the losses attributable to the false-positive or false-negative decisions are given a nonzero value (i.e., $w_i>0$, where i does not equal j). The w_i values of the loss matrix depend on the special problem of prediction being dealt with. In most cases, w_{12} and w_{21} are given the same values; however, there are important areas of application where w_{12} and w_{21} are considered to be genuinely different.

Policy considerations influence the values of w_i. For the prediction of violence, a civil libertarian policy would attribute a higher value of loss to w_{12} than to w_{21} ($w_{21}<w_{12}$). In contrast, public protectionists think that

the cost (the danger for society) associated with false-negative decisions is greater compared with that of false-positive decisions (i.e., $w_{12} < w_{21}$).

In a mathematical-statistical approach to the prediction problem, we attempt to find a $d(x)$ decision function or "rule" that minimizes the expected loss of prediction. The decision function providing the minimal expected loss among all possible decision functions is called the *Bayes decision function*.

This function (and the underlying Bayes theorem) are frequently used and quoted by researchers developing actuarial predictions; however, these terms are almost never explained. This is regrettable, because the Bayes theorem is "one of the medical literature's greatest communicative terrors" (Feinstein 1985, p. 437). Unfortunately, real understanding of actuarial prediction is difficult without it. I would therefore like to appeal to the reader to plow through the following paragraphs of dense text; several figures were created to help the reader understand this section.

The Bayes decision function is determined by three fundamental factors: 1) the losses associated with the possible different decisions, 2) the prior probabilities of being violent or nonviolent, and 3) the conditional distribution of the feature vector x within class i.

Assuming that the correct prediction is not associated with any cost (i.e., $w_{11} = w_{22} = 0$), in our special case (i.e., when there are only two classes; $M=2$), the optimal or Bayes decision has the following form:

$$d(x) = 1, \text{ if } w_{21} \bullet p_2 \bullet f_2(x) \leq w_{12} \bullet p_1 \bullet f_1(x), \text{ and}$$
$$d(x) = 2, \text{ if } w_{21} \bullet p_2 \bullet f_2(x) \geq w_{12} \bullet p_1 \bullet f_1(x),$$

where w_{12} and w_{21} are losses associated with false-positive and false-negative decisions, p_1 and p_2 are the prior probabilities or base rates of being violent or nonviolent, and $f_1(x)$ and $f_2(x)$ are the known conditional probability density functions ("frequency distributions") of the feature vector x in class 1 (violent) or class 2 (nonviolent). Simply put, the Bayes decision rule forms the product of the loss, the prior probability, and the conditional probability density function.

To understand the Bayes decision function, let us examine the situation when both types of false decisions are associated with the same loss; for the sake of simplicity, suppose here that $w_{12} = w_{21} = 1$. In this case, the Bayes decision function minimizes the probability of false decisions (i.e., the false decision per se is considered as a loss), and the decision rule is reduced to the examination of the $p_1 \bullet f_1(x)$ and the $p_2 \bullet f_2(x)$ terms in the above equation. These two terms at each observed x_i value are proportional to the posterior probabilities of being violent or nonviolent. Thus, the Bayes decision rule under the above condition (i.e., $w_{12}=w_{21}$) is to observe an x_i and classify the individual in the class that yields the largest posterior probability (i.e., yields the largest value for the $p \bullet f(x)$ term in the above equation).

Figures A–1 through A–3 illustrate the Bayes decision function when the costs of the false-positive and false-negative decisions are equal, and the predictor set contains only one variable. In these figures the conditional $f_i(x)$ densities for the violent and nonviolent class are considered as normal densities.

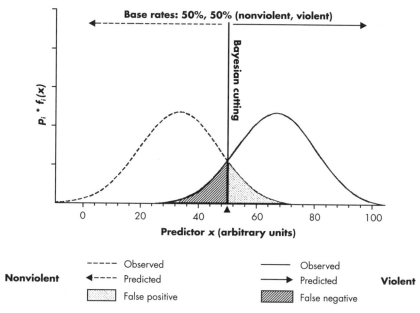

Figure A–1. Bayes decision with equal base rates. Prior probabilities (p) for occurrence of nonviolent and violent individuals are equal in examined sample. Vertical axis displays the product of the prior probability and the $f(x)$ probability density function for each of the two groups. These $x \bullet f(x)$ products, at each x_i value of the predictor variable, are proportional to posterior probabilities of belonging to a particular class (violent or nonviolent). Thus, an observation (x_i) is classified into the class that yields the highest probability [i.e., the largest value for $x_i \bullet f(x_i)$] for that observation. In this example, the cutting point for the Bayes decision is 50. *Hatched* and *shaded areas* show the probabilities of false-negative and false-positive findings in the given sample.

Figure A–1 illustrates the (special) case when the prior probabilities or base rates of violent and nonviolent individuals in the examined population are equal (i.e., $p_1=p_2=0.5$). In this case, for normal densities, the cutting point for classifying an individual into the violent or the nonviolent class is determined by the point of intersection of the two probability density functions.

In Figure A–1, for each of the two groups, the vertical axis displays the product of the prior probability (p) and the $f(x)$ probability density function. As mentioned above, at each x_i value of the predictor variable, these $x \bullet f(x)$ products are proportional to the posterior probabilities of belonging to a particular class (violent or nonviolent). The figure displays the cutting point (Bayes cutting) that minimizes the overall rate of false predictions; at this value ($x=50$), the probability of membership in each of the two groups is equal. At any value of the predictor variable greater than the Bayes cutting point, the probability of membership in the violent group is higher than that of membership in the nonviolent group; thus, individuals with these values are classified as violent. Similarly, individuals with an x value smaller than the cutting point are classified as nonviolent. Referring to Figure A–1, the resulting Bayes decision function may be given as follows: if $x \leq 50$, then the prediction is nonviolence; otherwise, the prediction is violence.

Figure A–2 demonstrates how the cutting point for the Bayes decision function is influenced by unequal base rates; in the special case I used for illustration, the base rates of violent and nonviolent individuals in the examined sample were 80% and 20%, respectively.

Please note that the Bayes cutting point ($x=58$), compared with the cutting point ($x=50$) of Figure A–1, shifted to the right because the prior probability of being violent ($p=0.2$) is smaller than that of being nonviolent ($p=0.8$). Figure A–2 illustrates the problem of predicting events that have low base rates: at the optimal cutting point, there is a relatively higher misclassification rate for the violent group compared with the nonviolent one.

Figure A–3 shows the consequence of a non-Bayesian decision. Here the Bayesian cutting point for equal base rates (i.e., the value of 50; see Figure A–1) is applied in a population in which the base rates are in fact unequal. This cutting point does not minimize the probability of misclassification under these conditions. Furthermore, the use of this cutting point results in a disproportional increase of false-positive predictions (i.e., overprediction of violence).

As mentioned above, for the Bayes decision we need to have *prior* knowledge about the conditional $f(x)$ probability density function of x in the two classes of C (violence and nonviolence). Most authors use linear

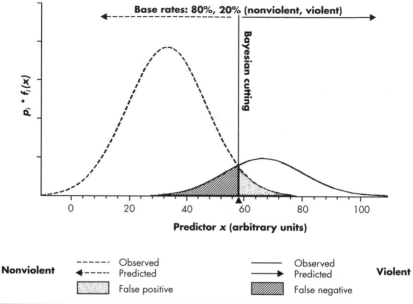

Figure A–2. Bayes decision with unequal base rates. Displayed is the cutting point (Bayesian cutting) that minimizes the overall rate of false predictions. Individuals with *x* values greater or smaller than the Bayesian cutting point are classified as violent or nonviolent, respectively. See Figure A–1 legend for more details.

discriminant analysis for prediction; this analysis is based on numerous assumptions about the data (Fukunaga 1972; Giri 1977; Shumway 1982). Under these generally unrealistic assumptions, the Bayes decision yields the linear discriminant equations that are used by most authors who attempt actuarial predictions.

In practical applications, the prior determinations of the conditional $f_i(x)$ and the derivation of the linear discriminant equation(s) or prediction rule are accomplished in the initial phase of the research by using a sample of individuals thought to be representative for the total population ("learning" or "calibration" sample). Then, in the next (cross-validation) phase of the research, the performance of the prediction rule derived at the previous step is evaluated by using a validation sample. This cross-validation step is indispensable because, for each of the three principal input parameters (i.e., costs, base rates, prior knowledge of the probability density functions) of the decision, there is a great deal of uncertainty. For example, the estimation of base rates can vary greatly from study to study or from one target population to the other.

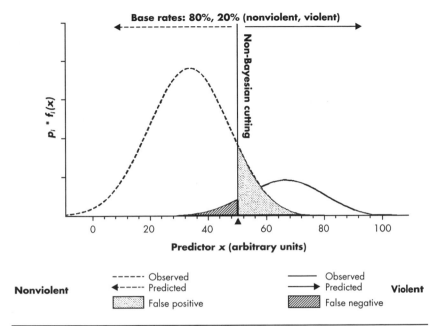

Figure A–3. Non-Bayesian decision with unequal base rates. Displayed is the cutting point that minimizes the overall rate of false predictions at *equal* base rates. *Hatched* and *shaded areas* indicate probabilities of false-negative and false-positive findings in the given sample when the non-Bayesian cutting point is used. See Figure A–1 legend for more details.

Although in many cases there is insufficient information to apply the Bayes decision function—for example, the prior probabilities or the $f_i(x)$ probability densities are not known—the Bayes approach is routinely used in practice. Because the adequacy of the Bayes decision function is questionable in such cases, I think that alternative statistical approaches that require less prior knowledge about data should also be explored in practice.

References

Abel EL: The relationship between cannabis and violence: a review. Psychol Bull 84:193–211, 1977

Abram K: The effect of co-occurring disorders on criminal careers: interaction of antisocial personality, alcoholism, and drug disorders. Int J Law Psychiatry 12:133–148, 1989

Abram KM, Teplin LA: Drug disorder, mental illness, and violence. NIDA Res Monogr 103:222–238, 1990

Abram KM, Teplin LA: Co-occurring disorders among mentally ill jail detainees. Implications for public policy. Am Psychol 46:1036–1045, 1991

Abramson MF: The criminalization of mentally disordered behavior: possible side-effect of a new mental health law. Hosp Community Psychiatry 23:101–105, 1972

Ackerman PT, Dykman RA, Peters JE: Teenage status of hyperactive and nonhyperactive learning disabled boys. Am J Orthopsychiatry 47:577–596, 1977

Adams JJ, Meloy JR, Moritz MS: Neuropsychological deficits and violent behavior in incarcerated schizophrenics. J Nerv Ment Dis 178:253–256, 1990

Ahn H, Prichep L, John ER, et al: Developmental equations reflect brain dysfunctions. Science 210:1259–1262, 1980

Albanese MJ, Khantzian EJ, Murphy SL, et al: Decreased substance use in chronically psychotic patients treated with clozapine (letter). Am J Psychiatry 151:780–781, 1994

Albert DJ, Walsh ML: The inhibitory modulation of agonistic behavior in the rat brain: a review. Neurosci Biobehav Rev 6:125–143, 1982

Altamura AC, Basile R, Mauri M, et al: Valpromide (Depamide) in the treatment of acute psychotic states: an open clinical study [in French]. Acta Psychiatr Belg 86:297–304, 1986

Alterman AI: Methodological issues and prevalence estimates of substance abuse in schizophrenia. J Nerv Ment Dis 180:593–594, 1992

Aman MG, Marks RE, Turbott SH, et al: Methylphenidate and thioridazine in the treatment of intellectually subaverage children: effects on cognitive-motor performance. J Am Acad Child Adolesc Psychiatry 30:816–824, 1991

American Psychiatric Association: Diagnostic and Statistical Manual: Mental Disorders. Washington, DC, American Psychiatric Association, 1952

American Psychiatric Association: Diagnostic and Statistical Manual of Mental Disorders, 2nd Edition. Washington, DC, American Psychiatric Association, 1968

American Psychiatric Association: Diagnostic and Statistical Manual of Mental Disorders, 3rd Edition. Washington, DC, American Psychiatric Association, 1980

American Psychiatric Association: Diagnostic and Statistical Manual of Mental Disorders, 3rd Edition, Revised. Washington, DC, American Psychiatric Association, 1987

American Psychiatric Association: Diagnostic and Statistical Manual of Mental Disorders, 4th Edition. Washington, DC, American Psychiatric Association, 1994

American Psychiatric Association: Diagnostic and Statistical Manual of Mental Disorders, 4th Edition, Text Revision. Washington, DC, American Psychiatric Association, 2000

Anderson SW, Bechara A, Damasio H, et al: Impairment of social and moral behavior related to early damage in human prefrontal cortex. Nat Neurosci 2:1032–1037, 1999

Anglin D, Spears KL, Hutson HR: Flunitrazepam and its involvement in date or acquaintance rape. Acad Emerg Med 4:323–326, 1997

Angrist BM, Gershon S: Amphetamine abuse in New York City—1966 to 1968. Semin Psychiatry 1:195–207, 1969

Anonymous: After bodybuilder is accused of murder, many point finger at steroid use. The New York Times, July 3, 1993, p 45

Appelbaum PS, Robbins PC, Monahan J: Violence and delusions: data from the MacArthur Violence Risk Assessment Study. Am J Psychiatry 157:566–572, 2000

Applegate CD: 5,7-Dihydroxytryptamine-induced mouse killing and behavioral reversal with ventricular administration of serotonin in rats. Behav Neural Biol 30:178–190, 1980

Arango C, Barba CA, Gonzalez-Salvador T, et al: Violence in inpatients with schizophrenia: a prospective study. Schizophr Bull 25:493–503, 1999

Archer J: The influence of testosterone on human aggression. Br J Psychol 82:1–28, 1991

Armond AD: Violence in the semi-secure ward of a psychiatric hospital. Med Sci Law 22:203–209, 1982

Arseneault L, Moffitt TE, Caspi A, et al: Mental disorders and violence in a total birth cohort: results from the Dunedin Study. Arch Gen Psychiatry 57:979–986, 2000

Arvanitis LA, Miller BG, and the Seroquel Trial 13 Study Group: Multiple fixed doses of "Seroquel" (quetiapine) in patients with acute exacerbation of schizophrenia: a comparison with haloperidol and placebo. Biol Psychiatry 42:233–246, 1997

Asberg M, Traskman L, Thoren P: 5-HIAA in the cerebrospinal fluid: a biochemical suicide predictor? Arch Gen Psychiatry 33:1193–1197, 1976

Ashford JB: Offense comparisons between mentally disordered and non-mentally disordered inmates. Canadian Journal of Criminology 31:35–48, 1989

Atre-Vaidya N, Taylor MA: Effectiveness of lithium in schizophrenia: do we really have an answer? J Clin Psychiatry 50:170–173, 1989

Axelrod J, Tomchick R: Enzymatic O-methylation of epinephrine and other catechols. J Biol Chem 233:702–705, 1958

Azouvi P, Jokic C, Attal N, et al: Carbamazepine in agitation and aggressive behaviour following severe closed-head injury: results of an open trial. Brain Inj 13:797–804, 1999

Babigian HM: Schizophrenia: epidemiology, in Comprehensive Textbook of Psychiatry/IV, 4th Edition, Vol 1. Edited by Kaplan HI, Sadock BJ. Baltimore, MD, Williams & Wilkins, 1985, pp 643–650

Bach-y-Rita G, Veno A: Habitual violence: a profile of 62 men. Am J Psychiatry 131:1015–1017, 1974

Bach-y-Rita G, Lion JR, Ervin FR: Pathological intoxication: clinical and electroencephalographic studies. Am J Psychiatry 127:698–703, 1970

Bach-y-Rita G, Lion JR, Climent CE, et al: Episodic dyscontrol: a study of 130 violent patients. Am J Psychiatry 127:1473–1478, 1971

Bain J, Langevin R, Dickey R, et al: Sex hormones in murderers and assaulters. Behav Sci Law 5:95–101, 1987

Bain J, Langevin R, Dickey R, et al: Hormones in sexually aggressive men. I. Baseline values for eight hormones. II. The ACTH test. Annals of Sex Research 1:63–78, 1988

Baldwin JD: Determinants of aggression in squirrel monkeys (Saimiri), in Aggression and Peacefulness in Humans and Other Primates. Edited by Silverberg J, Gray PJ. New York, Oxford University Press, 1992, pp 72–99

Barkley MS, Goldman BD: The effects of castration and silastic implants of testosterone on intermale aggression in the mouse. Horm Behav 9:32–48, 1977

Barratt ES: Impulsiveness defined within a system model of personality, in Advances in Personality Assessment, Vol 5. Edited by Butcher JN, Spielberger CD. Hillsdale, NJ, Erlbaum, 1985a, pp 113–132

Barratt ES: Impulsiveness subtraits: arousal and information processing, in Motivation, Emotion and Personality. Edited by Spence JT, Izard CE. Amsterdam, Elsevier, 1985b, pp 137–146

Barratt ES, Patton JH: Impulsivity: cognitive, behavioral, and psychophysiological correlates, in Biological Bases of Sensation Seeking, Impulsivity, and Anxiety. Edited by Zuckerman M. Hillsdale, NJ, Erlbaum, 1983, pp 77–116

Barry DJ, Ciccone JR: Use of Depo-Provera in the treatment of aggressive sexual offenders: preliminary report of three cases. Bull Am Acad Psychiatry Law 3:179–184, 1975

Basser PJ, Mattiello J, LeBihan D: MR diffusion tensor spectroscopy and imaging. Biophys J 66:259–267, 1994

Bear D, Levin K, Blumer D, et al: Interictal behaviour in hospitalised temporal lobe epileptics: relationship to idiopathic psychiatric syndromes. J Neurol Neurosurg Psychiatry 45:481–488, 1982

Beck NC, Greenfield SR, Gotham H, et al: Risperidone in the management of violent, treatment-resistant schizophrenics hospitalized in a maximum security forensic facility. J Am Acad Psychiatry Law 25:461–468, 1997

Begleiter H, Porjesz B, Bihari B, et al: Event-related brain potentials in boys at risk for alcoholism. Science 225:1493–1496, 1984

Bender L: The concept of pseudopsychopathic schizophrenia in adolescents. Am J Orthopsychiatry 29:491–512, 1959

Beresford HR: Legal implications of epilepsy. Epilepsia 29 (suppl 2):S114–S121, 1988

Bergeman CS, Seroczynski AD: Genetic and environmental influences on aggression and impulsivity, in Neurobiology and Clinical Views on Aggression and Impulsivity. Edited by Maes M, Coccaro EF. Chichester, Wiley, 1998, pp 63–80

Berken GH, Stone MM, Stone SK: Methadone in schizophrenic rage: a case study. Am J Psychiatry 135:248–249, 1978

Berlin FS: The paraphilias and Depo-Provera: some medical, ethical and legal considerations. Bull Am Acad Psychiatry Law 17:233–239, 1989

Bick PA, Hannah AL: Intramuscular lorazepam to restrain violent patients (letter). Lancet 1:206, 1986

Binder RL, McNiel DE: Effects of diagnosis and context on dangerousness. Am J Psychiatry 145:728–732, 1988

Binder RL, McNiel DE: The relationship of gender to violent behavior in acutely disturbed psychiatric patients. J Clin Psychiatry 51:110–114, 1990

Bioulac B, Benezech M, Renaud B, et al: Serotoninergic dysfunction in the 47,XYY syndrome. Biol Psychiatry 15:917–923, 1980

Blumer D, Benson DF: Personality changes with frontal and temporal lobe lesions, in Psychiatric Aspects of Neurologic Disease. Edited by Benson DF, Blumer D. New York, Grune & Stratton, 1975, pp 151–170

Blumer D, Migeon C: Hormone and hormonal agents in the treatment of aggression. J Nerv Ment Dis 160:127–137, 1975

Bohman M, Cloninger CR, Sigvardsson S, et al: Predisposition to petty criminality in Swedish adoptees. I. Genetic and environmental heterogeneity. Arch Gen Psychiatry 39:1233–1241, 1982

Bolton R: Hostility in fantasy: a further test of the hypoglycemia-aggression hypothesis. Aggressive Behavior 2:257–274, 1976

Bond A, Lader M: Benzodiazepines and aggression, in Psychopharmacology of Aggression. Edited by Sandler M. New York, Raven, 1979, pp 173–182

Bond WS, Mandos LA, Kurtz MB: Midazolam for aggressivity and violence in three mentally retarded patients. Am J Psychiatry 146:925–926, 1989

Bourguignon A, Monfort J-C, de Medeiros P, et al: Treatment of several psychotic states with the combination of valproic acid with diazepam [in French]. Ann Med Psychol (Paris) 142:1214–1218, 1984

Bouwknecht JA, Hijzen TH, van der Gugten J, et al: Absence of 5-HT(1B) receptors is associated with impaired impulse control in male 5-HT(1B) knockout mice. Biol Psychiatry 49:557–568, 2001

Boyle D, Tobin JM: Pharmaceutical management of behavior disorders. Journal of the Medical Society of New Jersey 58:427–429, 1961

Bozikas V, Bascialla F, Yulis P, et al: Gabapentin for behavioral dyscontrol with mental retardation. Am J Psychiatry 158:965–966, 2001

Brahams D: Premenstrual syndrome: a disease of the mind? Lancet 2:1238–1240, 1981

Brahams D: Hypoglycaemia and intent. Lancet 337:1030, 1991

Branchey L, Branchey M, Shaw S, et al: Depression, suicide, and aggression in alcoholics and their relationship to plasma amino acids. Psychiatry Res 12:219–226, 1984

Branchey MH, Buydens-Branchey L, Lieber CS: P3 in alcoholics with disordered regulation of aggression. Psychiatry Res 25:49–58, 1988

Brase DA, Loh HH: Possible role of 5-hydroxytryptamine in minimal brain dysfunction. Life Sci 16:1005–1015, 1975

Breier A, Meehan K, Birkett M, et al: A double-blind, placebo-controlled dose-response comparison of intramuscular olanzapine and haloperidol in the treatment of acute agitation in schizophrenia. Arch Gen Psychiatry 59:441–448, 2002

Brennan PA, Mednick BR, Mednick SA: Parental psychopathology, congenital factors, and violence, in Mental Disorder and Crime. Edited by Hodgins S. Newbury Park, CA, Sage, 1993, pp 244–261

Brennan PA, Grekin ER, Mednick SA: Maternal smoking during pregnancy and adult male criminal outcomes. Arch Gen Psychiatry 56:215–219, 1999

Brennan PA, Mednick SA, Hodgins S: Major mental disorders and criminal violence in a Danish birth cohort. Arch Gen Psychiatry 57:494–500, 2000

Breslau N, Klein N, Allen L: Very low birthweight: behavioral sequelae at nine years of age. J Am Acad Child Adolesc Psychiatry 27:605–612, 1988

Brizer DA, Convit A, Krakowski M, et al: A rating scale for reporting violence on psychiatric wards. Hosp Community Psychiatry 38:769–770, 1987

Brizer DA, Crowner ML, Convit A, et al: Videotape recording of inpatient assaults: a pilot study. Am J Psychiatry 145:751–752, 1988

Brody SL: Violence associated with acute cocaine use in patients admitted to a medical emergency department. NIDA Res Monogr 103:44–59, 1990

Brook S, Lucey JV, Gunn KP: Intramuscular ziprasidone compared with intramuscular haloperidol in the treatment of acute psychosis. Ziprasidone I.M. Study Group. J Clin Psychiatry 61:933–941, 2000

Brooks N, Campsie L, Symington C, et al: The five year outcome of severe blunt head injury: a relative's view. J Neurol Neurosurg Psychiatry 49:764–770, 1986

Brower KJ, Hierholzer R, Maddahian E: Recent trends in cocaine abuse in a VA psychiatric population. Hosp Community Psychiatry 37:1229–1234, 1986

Brower KJ, Blow FC, Beresford TP: Forms of cocaine and psychiatric symptoms (letter). Lancet 1:50, 1988

Brown CS, Kent TA, Bryant SG, et al: Blood platelet uptake of serotonin in episodic aggression. Psychiatry Res 27:5–12, 1989

Brown GI, Linnoila M, Goodwin FK: Clinical assessment of human aggression and impulsivity in relationship to biochemical measures, in Violence and Suicidality: Perspectives in Clinical and Psychobiological Research. Edited by Van Praag HM, Plutchik R, Apter A. New York, Brunner/Mazel, 1990, pp 184–217

Brown GL, Goodwin FK, Ballenger JC, et al: Aggression in humans correlates with cerebrospinal fluid amine metabolites. Psychiatry Res 1:131–139, 1979

Brown GL, Ebert MH, Goyer PF, et al: Aggression, suicide, and serotonin: relationship to CSF amine metabolites. Am J Psychiatry 139:741–746, 1982

Brunner HG, Nelen M, Breakefield XO, et al: Abnormal behavior associated with a point mutation in the structural gene for monoamine oxidase A. Science 262:578–580, 1993a

Brunner HG, Nelen MR, van Zandvoort P, et al: X-linked borderline mental retardation with prominent behavioral disturbance: phenotype, genetic localization, and evidence for disturbed monoamine metabolism. Am J Hum Genet 52:1032–1039, 1993b

Bryan JW, Freed FW: Corporal punishment: normative data and sociological and psychological correlates in a community college population. J Youth Adolesc 11:77–87, 1982

Buchanan A: Criminal conviction after discharge from special (high security) hospital. Incidence in the first 10 years. Br J Psychiatry 172:472–476, 1998

Buchsbaum MS, Coursey RD, Murphy DL: The biochemical high-risk paradigm: behavioral and familial correlates of low platelet monoamine oxidase activity. Science 194:339–341, 1976

Buckley P, Thompson P, Way L, et al: Substance abuse among patients with treatment-resistant schizophrenia: characteristics and implications for clozapine therapy. Am J Psychiatry 151:385–389, 1994

Buckley P, Bartell J, Donenwirth K, et al: Violence and schizophrenia: clozapine as a specific antiaggressive agent. Bull Am Acad Psychiatry Law 23:607–611, 1995

Buckley P, Ibrahim Z, Singer B, et al: Aggression and schizophrenia: efficacy of risperidone. J Am Acad Psychiatry Law 25:173–181, 1997

Buckley P, McCarthy M, Chapman P, et al: Clozapine treatment of comorbid substance abuse and schizophrenia (abstract). Biol Psychiatry 45:14S, 1999

Buckley P, McCarthy M, Chapman P, et al: Craving reduction and clozapine response in patients with comorbid substance abuse and schizophrenia (abstract). Biol Psychiatry 47:18S–19S, 2000

Bunney WE Jr, Garland-Bunney BL: Mechanisms of action of lithium in affective illness: basic and clinical implications, in Psychopharmacology: The Third Generation of Progress. Edited by Meltzer HY. New York, Raven, 1987, pp 553–565

Bushman BJ, Cooper HM: Effects of alcohol on human aggression: an integrative research review. Psychol Bull 107:341–354, 1990

Buss AH, Durkee A: An inventory for assessing different kinds of hostility. J Consult Psychol 21:343–349, 1957

Cadoret RJ, Troughton E, Bagford J, et al: Genetic and environmental factors in adoptee antisocial personality. Eur Arch Psychiatry Neurol Sci 239:231–240, 1990

Cadoret RJ, Yates WR, Troughton E, et al: Genetic-environmental interaction in the genesis of aggressivity and conduct disorders. Arch Gen Psychiatry 52:916–924, 1995

Campbell M, Small AM, Green WH, et al: Behavioral efficacy of haloperidol and lithium carbonate. A comparison in hospitalized aggressive children with conduct disorder. Arch Gen Psychiatry 41:650–656, 1984

Cantillon M, Arvanitis LA, Miller BG, et al: 'Seroquel' (quetiapine fumarate) reduces hostility and aggression in patients with acute schizophrenia (abstract). Paper presented at the 36th Annual Meeting of the American College of Neuropsychopharmacology, Waikoloa, Hawaii, December 8–12, 1997, p 171

Carey G: Twin imitation for antisocial behavior: implications for genetic and family environment research. J Abnorm Psychol 101:18–25, 1992

Carlier M, Roubertoux PL, Kottler ML, et al: Y-chromosome and aggression in strains of laboratory mice. Behav Genet 20:137–156, 1990

Carmel H, Tanke ED, Yesavage JA: Physician Staffing and Patient Violence. Bull Am Acad Psychiatry Law 19:49–51, 1991

Cases O, Seif I, Grimsby J, et al: Aggressive behavior and altered amounts of brain serotonin and norepinephrine in mice lacking MAOA. Science 268:1763–1766, 1995

Caspi N, Modai I, Barak P, et al: Pindolol augmentation in aggressive schizophrenic patients: a double-blind crossover randomized study. Int Clin Psychopharmacol 16:111–115, 2001

Centerwall BS: Race, socioeconomic status, and domestic homicide, Atlanta, 1971–72. Am J Public Health 74:813–815, 1984

Centerwall BS: Race, socioeconomic status, and domestic homicide. JAMA 273:1755–1758, 1995

Chamberlain B, Ervin FR, Pihl RO, et al: The effect of raising or lowering tryptophan levels on aggression in vervet monkeys. Pharmacol Biochem Behav 28:503–510, 1987

Chen C-H, Lee Y-R, Chung M-Y, et al: Systematic mutation analysis of the catechol O-methyltransferase gene as a candidate gene for schizophrenia. Am J Psychiatry 156:1273–1275, 1999

Cherek DR, Lane SD: Effects of d,l-fenfluramine on aggressive and impulsive responding in adult males with a history of conduct disorder. Psychopharmacology 146:473–481, 1999

Chiles JA, Davidson P, McBride D: Effects of clozapine on use of seclusion and restraint at a state hospital. Hosp Community Psychiatry 45:269–271, 1994

Choi PYL, Parrott AC, Cowan D: High dose anabolic steroids in strength athletes: effects upon hostility and aggression (abstract). J Psychopharmacol 3:102, 1989

Chong S-A, Tan C-H, Lee E-L, et al: Augmentation of risperidone with valproic acid (letter). J Clin Psychiatry 59:430, 1998

Chow EW, Bassett AS, Weksberg R: Velo-cardio-facial syndrome and psychotic disorders: implications for psychiatric genetics. Am J Med Genet 54:107–112, 1994

Christiansen KO: A review of studies of criminality among twins, in Biosocial Bases of Criminal Behavior. Edited by Mednick SA, Christiansen KO. New York, Gardner, 1977, pp 45–88

Christiansen K, Knussmann R: Androgen levels and components of aggressive behavior in men. Horm Behav 21:170–180, 1987

Christmas AJ, Maxwell DR: A comparison of the effects of some benzodiazepines and other drugs on aggressive and exploratory behaviour in mice and rats. Neuropharmacology 9:17–29, 1970

Cirincione C, Steadman HJ, Robbins PC, et al: Schizophrenia as a contingent risk factor for criminal violence. Int J Law Psychiatry 15:347–358, 1992

Citrome L: Differential diagnosis of psychosis. A brief guide for the primary care physician. Postgrad Med 85:273–274, 1989

Citrome L: Use of lithium, carbamazepine, and valproic acid in a state-operated psychiatric hospital. J Pharm Technol 11:55–59, 1995

Citrome L, Levine J, Allingham B: Changes in use of valproate and other mood stabilizers for patients with schizophrenia from 1994 to 1998. Psychiatr Serv 51:634–638, 2000

Citrome L, Krakowski M, Greenberg WM, et al: Antiaggressive effect of quetiapine in a patient with schizoaffective disorder (letter). J Clin Psychiatry 62:901, 2001a

Citrome L, Volavka J, Czobor P, et al: Effects of clozapine, olanzapine, risperidone, and haloperidol on hostility among patients with schizophrenia. Psychiatr Serv 52:1510–1514, 2001b

Cleckley H: The Mask of Sanity. Saint Louis, MO, Mosby, 1976

Climent CE, Rollins A, Ervin FR, et al: Epidemiological studies of women prisoners. I. Medical and psychiatric variables related to violent behavior. Am J Psychiatry 130:985–990, 1973

Cloninger CR: A systematic method for clinical description and classification of personality variants. A proposal. Arch Gen Psychiatry 44:573–588, 1987

Cloninger CR, Bohman M, Sigvardsson S: Inheritance of alcohol abuse. Cross-fostering analysis of adopted men. Arch Gen Psychiatry 38:861–868, 1981

Coccaro EF: Central serotonin and impulsive aggression. Br J Psychiatry Suppl 155:52–62, 1989

Coccaro EF, Kavoussi RJ: Fluoxetine and impulsive aggressive behavior in personality-disordered subjects. Arch Gen Psychiatry 54:1081–1088, 1997

Coccaro EF, Siever LJ, Klar HM, et al: Serotonergic studies in patients with affective and personality disorders. Arch Gen Psychiatry 46:587–599, 1989

Coccaro EF, Gabriel S, Siever LJ: Buspirone challenge: preliminary evidence for a role for central 5-HT1a receptor function in impulsive aggressive behavior in humans. Psychopharmacol Bull 26:393–405, 1990

Coccaro EF, Harvey PD, Kupsaw-Lawrence E, et al: Development of neuropharmacologically based behavioral assessments of impulsive aggressive behavior. J Neuropsychiatry Clin Neurosci 3:S44–S51, 1991

Coccaro EF, Bergeman CS, McClearn GE: Heritability of irritable impulsiveness: a study of twins reared together and apart. Psychiatry Res 48:229–242, 1993

Coccaro EF, Bergeman CS, Kavoussi RJ, et al: Heritability of aggression and irritability: a twin study of the Buss-Durkee aggression scales in adult male subjects. Biol Psychiatry 41:273–284, 1997a

Coccaro EF, Berman ME, Kavoussi RJ: Assessment of life history of aggression: development and psychometric characteristics. Psychiatry Res 73:147–157, 1997b

Cocozza JJ, Steadman HJ: The failure of psychiatric predictions of dangerousness: clear and convincing evidence. Rutgers Law Review 29:1084–1101, 1976

Coid J: The epidemiology of abnormal homicide and murder followed by suicide. Psychol Med 13:855–860, 1983

Coleman FH, Christensen HD, Gonzalez CL, et al: Behavioral changes in developing mice after prenatal exposure to paroxetine (Paxil). Am J Obstet Gynecol 181:1166–1171, 1999

Collins JJ, Schlenger WE: Acute and chronic effects of alcohol use on violence. J Stud Alcohol 49:516–521, 1988

Collins PJ, Larkin EP, Shubsachs APW: Lithium carbonate in chronic schizophrenia—a brief trial of lithium carbonate added to neuroleptics for treatment of resistant schizophrenic patients. Acta Psychiatr Scand 84:150–154, 1991

Conacher GN, Workman DG: Violent crime possibly associated with anabolic steroid use (letter). Am J Psychiatry 146:679, 1989

Conn LM, Lion JR: Assaults in a university hospital, in Assaults Within Psychiatric Facilities. Edited by Lion JR, Reid WH. New York, Grune & Stratton, 1983, pp 61–69

Constantino JN, Morris JA, Murphy DL: CSF 5-HIAA and family history of antisocial personality disorder in newborns. Am J Psychiatry 154:1771–1773, 1997

Convit A, Jaeger J, Lin SP, et al: Predicting assaultiveness in psychiatric inpatients: a pilot study. Hosp Community Psychiatry 39:429–434, 1988a

Convit A, Jaeger J, Lin SP, et al: Prediction of violence in psychiatric inpatients, in Biological Contributions to Crime Causation. Edited by Moffitt T, Mednick S. Amsterdam, Martinus Nijhoff, 1988b, pp 223–245

Convit A, Nemes ZC, Volavka J: History of phencyclidine use and repeated assaults in newly admitted young schizophrenic men (letter). Am J Psychiatry 145:1176, 1988c

Convit A, Jaeger J, Lin SP, et al: Prediction of assaultive behavior in psychiatric inpatients: is it possible? in Current Approaches to the Prediction of Violence. Edited by Brizer DA, Crowner ML. Washington, DC, American Psychiatric Press, 1989, pp 37–62

Convit A, Isay D, Otis D, et al: Characteristics of repeatedly assaultive psychiatric inpatients. Hosp Community Psychiatry 41:1112–1115, 1990a

Convit A, O'Donnell J, Volavka J: Validity of self-reports of criminal activity in psychiatric inpatients. J Nerv Ment Dis 178:48–51, 1990b

Convit A, Czobor P, Volavka J: Lateralized abnormality in the EEG of persistently violent psychiatric inpatients. Biol Psychiatry 30:363–370, 1991

Cooke W: Presidential address: differential psychology of American women. Am J Obstet Gynecol 65:457, 1945

Corder BF, Ball BC, Haizlip TM, et al: Adolescent parricide: a comparison with other adolescent murder. Am J Psychiatry 133:957–961, 1976

Cordilia A: Alcohol and property crime: exploring the causal nexus. J Stud Alcohol 46(2):161–171, 1985

Corrigan B: Anabolic steroids and the mind (review, 51 refs). Med J Aust 165:222–226, 1996

Cote G, Hodgins S: Co-occurring mental disorders among criminal offenders. Bull Am Acad Psychiatry Law 18:271–281, 1990

Craft M, Ismail IA, Krishnamurti D, et al: Lithium in the treatment of aggression in mentally handicapped patients. A double-blind trial. Br J Psychiatry 150:685–689, 1987

Craig TJ: An epidemiologic study of problems associated with violence among psychiatric inpatients. Am J Psychiatry 139:1262–1266, 1982

Critchley HD, Simmons A, Daly EM, et al: Prefrontal and medial temporal correlates of repetitive violence to self and others. Biol Psychiatry 47:928–934, 2000

Crowe R: The adopted offspring of woman criminal offenders. Arch Gen Psychiatry 27:600–603, 1972

Crowner M: Environmental concomitants of psychiatric inpatient violence, in Current Approaches to the Prediction of Violence. Edited by Brizer DA, Crowner ML. Washington, DC, American Psychiatric Press, 1989, pp 101–120

Crowner ML, Douyon R, Convit A, et al: Akathisia and violence. Psychopharmacol Bull 26:115–117, 1990

Crowner ML, Douyon R, Convit A, et al: Videotape recording of assaults on a state hospital inpatient ward. J Neuropsychiatry Clin Neurosci 3:S9–S14, 1991

Crowner ML, Stepcic F, Peric G, et al: Typology of patient-patient assaults detected by videocameras. Am J Psychiatry 151:1669–1672, 1994

Crowner M, Peric G, Stepcic F, et al: Psychiatric patients' explanations for assaults. Psychiatr Serv 46:614–615, 1995

Cuffel BJ: Prevalence estimates of substance abuse in schizophrenia and their correlates. J Nerv Ment Dis 180:589–592, 1992

Currie S, Heathfield KWG, Henson RA, et al: Clinical course and prognosis of temporal lobe epilepsy. A survey of 666 patients. Brain 94:173–190, 1971

Curtis GC: Violence breeds violence—perhaps? Am J Psychiatry 120:386–387, 1963

Czobor P, Volavka J: Violence in mentally ill: questions remain (letter). Arch Gen Psychiatry 56:193, 1999

Czobor P, Volavka J, Meibach RC: Effect of risperidone on hostility in schizophrenia. J Clin Psychopharmacol 15:243–249, 1995

Dabbs JM Jr, Hargrove MF: Age, testosterone, and behavior among female prison inmates. Psychosom Med 59:477–480, 1997

Dabbs JM Jr, Frady R, Carr TS, et al: Saliva testosterone and criminal violence in young adult prison inmates. Psychosom Med 49:174–182, 1987

Dabbs JM Jr, Ruback RB, Frady RL, et al: Saliva testosterone and criminal violence among women. Pers Individ Dif 9:269–275, 1988

Dabbs JM Jr, Carr TS, Frady RL, et al: Testosterone, crime, and misbehavior among 692 male prison inmates. Pers Individ Dif 18:627–633, 1995

Daderman AM, Lidberg L: Flunitrazepam (Rohypnol) abuse in combination with alcohol causes premeditated, grievous violence in male juvenile offenders. J Am Acad Psychiatry Law 27:83–99, 1999

Dalby JT: Brief anabolic steroid use and sustained behavioral reaction (letter). Am J Psychiatry 149:271–272, 1992

Dalton K: Menstruation and crime. Br Med J 2:1752–1753, 1961

Dalton K: The Premenstrual Syndrome. Springfield, IL, Charles C Thomas, 1964

Dalton K: Paramenstrual baby battering (letter). Br Med J 2:279, 1975

Dalton K: Cyclical criminal acts in premenstrual syndrome. Lancet 2:1070–1071, 1980

Damasio H, Grabowski T, Frank R, et al: The return of Phineas Gage: clues about the brain from the skull of a famous patient. Science 264:1102–1105, 1994

Davidson RJ, Putnam KM, Larson CL: Dysfunction in the neural circuitry of emotion regulation—a possible prelude to violence. Science 289:591–594, 2000

Dawson M, Greville GD: Biochemistry, in Electroencephalography. Edited by Hill JDN, Parr G. London, MacDonald, 1963, pp 158–161

De Baudouin, Haumonte A, Bessing M, et al: Study of a population of 97 incarcerated murderers [in French]. Ann Med Psychol (Paris) 1:625–686, 1961

DeJong J, Virkkunen M, Linnoila M: Factors associated with recidivism in a criminal population. J Nerv Ment Dis 180:543–550, 1992

Delgado JMR: Cerebral heterostimulation in a monkey colony. Science 141:161–163, 1963

Delgado JMR: Neuronal constellations in aggressive behavior, in Aggression and Violence: A Psycho/Biological and Clinical Approach. Proceedings of the First Saint Vincent Special Conference, October 14–15, 1980. Edited by Valzelli L, Morgese L. Rome, Edizioni Saint Vincent, 1981, pp 82–98

Delgado-Escueta AV, Mattson RH, King L, et al: The nature of aggression during epileptic seizures. N Engl J Med 305:711–716, 1981

Delini-Stula A, Vassout A: The effects of antidepressants on aggressiveness induced by social deprivation in mice. Pharmacol Biochem Behav 14:33–41, 1981

Denicoff KD, Hoban C, Grover GN, et al: Glucose tolerance testing in women with premenstrual syndrome. Am J Psychiatry 147:477–480, 1990

Denno DW: Biology and violence: from birth to adulthood. Cambridge, England, Cambridge University Press, 1990

Depp FC: Violent behavior patterns on psychiatric wards. Aggress Behav 2:295–306, 1976

Depp FC: Assaults in a public mental hospital, in Assaults Within Psychiatric Facilities. Edited by Lion JR, Reid WH. New York, Grune & Stratton, 1983, pp 21–45

Devinsky O, Bear D: Varieties of aggressive behavior in temporal lobe epilepsy. Am J Psychiatry 141:651–656, 1984

Dicks D, Myers RE, Kling A: Uncus and amygdala lesions: effects on social behavior in the free-ranging rhesus monkey. Science 165:69–71, 1969

Dietz PE, Rada RT: Battery incidents and batterers in a maximum security hospital. Arch Gen Psychiatry 39:31–34, 1982

DiLalla LF, Gottesman II: Biological and genetic contributors to violence—Widom's untold tale. Psychol Bull 109:125–129, 1991

Dolan RJ: On the neurology of morals. Nat Neurosci 2:927–929, 1999

Dole VP, Joseph H: Long-term outcome of patients treated with methadone maintenance. Ann N Y Acad Sci 311:181–189, 1978

Donohue J, Levitt S: The impact of legalized abortion on crime. Working Paper 10. Berkeley Olin Program in Law & Economics, Working Paper Series. Berkeley, CA, University of California, 2000

Donovan SJ, Susser ES, Nunes EV, et al: Divalproex treatment of disruptive adolescents: a report of 10 cases. J Clin Psychiatry 58:12–15, 1997

d'Orban PT, Dalton J: Violent crime and the menstrual cycle. Psychol Med 10:353–359, 1980

Dorevitch A, Katz N, Zemishlany Z, et al: Intramuscular flunitrazepam versus intramuscular haloperidol in the emergency treatment of aggressive psychotic behavior. Am J Psychiatry 156:142–144, 1998

Dose M, Hellweg R, Yassouridis A, et al: Combined treatment of schizophrenic psychoses with haloperidol and valproate. Pharmacopsychiatry 31:122–125, 1998

Dostal T, Zvolsky P: Antiaggressive effect of lithium salts in severe mentally retarded adolescents. Int Pharmacopsychiatry 5:203–207, 1970

Dotson LE, Robertson LS, Tuchfeld B: Plasma alcohol, smoking, hormone concentrations and self-reported aggression: a study in a social-drinking situation. J Stud Alcohol 36:578–586, 1975

Douglas KS, Ogloff JRP, Nicholls TL, et al: Assessing risk for violence among psychiatric patients: the HCR-20 violence risk assessment scheme and the Psychopathy Checklist: Screening Version. J Consult Clin Psychol 67:917–930, 1999

Drake ME, Pakalnis A, Brown ME, et al: Auditory event related potentials in violent and nonviolent prisoners. Eur Arch Psychiatry Neurol Sci 238:7–10, 1988

Driver MV, West LR, Faulk M: Clinical and EEG studies of prisoners charged with murder. Br J Psychiatry 125:583–587, 1974

Dufek M: Forensic Psychiatry for Lawyers and Physicians [in Czech]. Praha, Orbis, 1975

Dugger CW: Subway killing suspect escaped 4 times in 1994. The New York Times, January 5, 1995, p B3

Dwivedi KN, Beaumont G, Brandon S: Electrophysiological responses in high and low aggressive young adolescent boys. Acta Paedopsychiatr 50:179–190, 1984

Dyer C: Mental Health Commission defeated over paedophile. Br Med J 296: 1660–1661, 1988

Easterbrook PJ, Berlin JA, Gopalan R, et al: Publication bias in clinical research (see comments). Lancet 337:867–872, 1991

Ebrahim GM, Gibler B, Gacono CB, et al: Patient response to clozapine in a forensic psychiatric hospital. Hosp Community Psychiatry 45:271–273, 1994

Edlund MJ, Craig TJ, Richardson MA: Informed consent as a form of volunteer bias. Am J Psychiatry 142:624–627, 1985

Egan MF, Goldberg TE, Kolachana BS, et al: Effect of COMT Val108/158 Met genotype on frontal lobe function and risk for schizophrenia. Proc Natl Acad Sci U S A 98:6917–6922, 2001

Ehlers CL, Rickler KC, Hovey JE: A possible relationship between plasma testosterone and aggressive behavior in a female outpatient population, in Limbic Epilepsy and the Dyscontrol Syndrome. Edited by Girgis M, Kiloh LG. New York, Elsevier, 1980, pp 183–194

Ehrenberg BL, Hardy PM, Zifkin BG: Psychomotor epilepsy and violence (letter). Am J Psychiatry 140:647, 1983

Ehrenkranz J, Bliss E, Sheard MH: Plasma testosterone: correlation with aggressive behavior and social dominance in man. Psychosom Med 36:469–475, 1974

Ehrhardt AA, Baker SW: Fetal androgens, human central nervous system differentiation, and behavior sex differences, in Sex Differences in Behavior. Edited by Friedman RC, Richart RM, Vande Wiele RL. New York, Wiley, 1974, pp 33–51

Ehrhardt AA, Epstein R, Money J: Fetal androgens and female gender identity in the early treated adrenogenital syndrome. Johns Hopkins Med J 122:160–167, 1968

Ehrhardt AA, Meyer-Bahlburg HFL, Rosen LR, et al: The development of gender-related behavior in females following prenatal exposure to diethylstilbestrol (DES). Horm Behav 23:526–541, 1989

Eichelman B: The limbic system and aggression in humans. Neurosci Biobehav Rev 7:391–394, 1983

Eichelman B, Hartwig A: The Carolina Nosology of Destructive Behavior (CNDB). J Neuropsychiatry Clin Neurosci 2:288–296, 1990

Ellinwood EH: Assault and homicide associated with amphetamine abuse. Am J Psychiatry 127:1170–1175, 1971

Elliott FA: Propranolol for the control of belligerent behavior following acute brain damage. Ann Neurol 1:489–491, 1977

Elliott FA: The episodic dyscontrol syndrome and aggression. Neurol Clin 2:113–125, 1984

Ellis DP, Austin P: Menstruation and aggressive behavior in a correctional center for women. J Crim Law Criminol Police Sci 62:388–395, 1971

Else LT, Wonderlich SA, Beatty WW, et al: Personality characteristics of men who physically abuse women. Hosp Community Psychiatry 44:54–58, 1993

Engel J Jr, Caldecott-Hazard S, Bandler R: Neurobiology of behavior: anatomic and physiological implications related to epilepsy. Epilepsia 27 (suppl 2):3–13, 1986

Eppright TD, Kashani JH, Robinson BD, et al: Comorbidity of conduct disorder and personality disorders in an incarcerated juvenile population. Am J Psychiatry 150:1233–1236, 1993

Eriksson T, Lidberg L: Increased plasma concentrations of the 5-HT precursor amino acid tryptophan and other large neutral amino acids in violent criminals. Psychol Med 27:477–481, 1997

Eron LD, Huesmann LR: The genesis of gender differences in aggression, in Psychological Development: Perspectives Across the Life-Span. Edited by Luszcz MA, Nettelbeck T. Amsterdam, Elsevier, 1989, pp 55–67

Eronen M: Mental disorders and homicidal behavior in female subjects. Am J Psychiatry 152:1216–1218, 1995

Eronen M, Hakola P, Tiihonen J: Factors associated with homicide recidivism in a 13-year sample of homicide offenders in Finland. Psychiatr Serv 47:403–406, 1996a

Eronen M, Hakola P, Tiihonen J: Mental disorders and homicidal behavior in Finland. Arch Gen Psychiatry 53:497–501, 1996b

Eronen M, Tiihonen J, Hakola P: Schizophrenia and homicidal behavior. Schizophr Bull 22:83–89, 1996c

Estroff SE, Zimmer C: Social networks, social support, and violence among persons with severe, persistent mental illness, in Violence and Mental Disorder: Developments in Risk Assessment. Edited by Monahan J, Steadman HJ. Chicago, IL, University of Chicago Press, 1994, pp 259–295

Estroff SE, Zimmer C, Lachicotte WS, et al: The influence of social networks and social support on violence by persons with serious mental illness. Hosp Community Psychiatry 45:669–679, 1994

Evans J, Platts H, Lightman S, et al: Impulsiveness and the prolactin response to d-fenfluramine. Psychopharmacology (Berl) 149:147–152, 2000

Evenson RC, Sletten IW, Altman H, et al: Disturbing behavior: a study of incident reports. Psychiatr Q 48:266–275, 1974

Eysenck HJ: Crime and Personality. Boston, MA, Houghton Mifflin, 1964

Eysenck HJ, Gudjonsson GH: The Causes and Cures of Criminality. New York, Plenum, 1989

Eysenck SBG, Eysenck HJ: The place of impulsiveness in a dimensional system of personality description. Br J Soc Clin Psychol 16:57–68, 1977

Eysenck SBG, Eysenck HJ: Impulsiveness and venturesomeness: their position in a dimensional system of personality description. Psychol Rep 43:1247–1255, 1978

Facciola G, Avenoso A, Scordo MG, et al: Small effects of valproic acid on the plasma concentrations of clozapine and its major metabolites in patients with schizophrenic or affective disorders. Ther Drug Monit 21:341–345, 1999

Falconer DS, Mackay TFC: Introduction to Quantitative Genetics, 4th Edition. Essex, England, Longman, 1996

Farrington DP: Age and crime, in An Annual Review of Research (Crime and Justice Series, Vol 7). Edited by Tonry M, Morris N. Chicago, IL, University of Chicago Press, 1986, pp 189–250

Farrington DP: Early predictors of adolescent aggression and adult violence. Violence Vict 4:79–100, 1989

Fauman MA, Fauman BJ: Violence associated with phencyclidine abuse. Am J Psychiatry 136:1584–1586, 1979

Fauman MA, Fauman BJ: Chronic phencyclidine (PCP) abuse: a psychiatric perspective, part I: general aspects and violence (proceedings). Psychopharmacol Bull 16:70–72, 1980

Fava M, Rosenbaum JF, Pava JA, et al: Anger attacks in unipolar depression, part 1: clinical correlates and response to fluoxetine treatment. Am J Psychiatry 150:1158–1163, 1993

Fava M, Vuolo RD, Wright EC, et al: Fenfluramine challenge in unipolar depression with and without anger attacks. Psychiatry Res 94:9–18, 2000

Federal Bureau of Investigation: Crime in the United States. Washington, DC, U.S. Department of Justice, 1987

Feinstein AR: Clinical Epidemiology: The Architecture of Clinical Research. Philadelphia, PA, Saunders, 1985

Feldman PE: An analysis of the efficacy of diazepam. J Neuropsychiatry 3 (suppl):S62–S67, 1962

Felthous AR: Childhood antecedents of aggressive behaviors in male psychiatric patients. Bull Am Acad Psychiatry Law 8:104–110, 1980

Fenton GW, Tennent TG, Fenwick PB, et al: The EEG in antisocial behaviour: a study of posterior temporal slow activity in special hospital patients. Psychol Med 4:181–186, 1974

Fernstrom JD, Wurtman RJ: Brain serotonin content: physiological regulation by plasma neutral amino acids. Science 178:414–416, 1972

Finger S, Stein DG: Brain Damage and Recovery. New York, Academic Press, 1982

Fink M: Study of long-term hashish users in Greece: summary and discussion, in Hashish: Studies of Long-Term Use. Edited by Stefanis C, Dornbush R, Fink M. New York, Raven, 1977, pp 151–158

Fishbein DH, Herning R, Pickworth WB, et al: EEG and brainstem auditory evoked response potentials in adult male drug abusers with self-reported histories of aggressive behavior. Biol Psychiatry 26:595–611, 1989a

Fishbein DH, Lozovsky D, Jaffe JH: Impulsivity, aggression, and neuroendocrine responses to serotonergic stimulation in substance abusers. Biol Psychiatry 25:1049–1066, 1989b

Fishbein DH, Dax E, Lozovsky DB, et al: Neuroendocrine responses to a glucose challenge in substance users with high and low levels of aggression, impulsivity, and antisocial personality. Neuropsychobiology 25:106–114, 1992

Floody OR: Hormones and aggression in female mammals, in Hormones and Aggressive Behavior. Edited by Svare BB. New York, Plenum, 1983, pp 39–90

Flor-Henry P: Psychosis, neurosis and epilepsy. Developmental and gender-related effects and their aetiological contribution. Br J Psychiatry 124:144–150, 1974

Flor-Henry P: Lateralized temporal-limbic dysfunction and psychopathology. Ann N Y Acad Sci 280:777–797, 1976

Flor-Henry P: Commentary and synthesis, in Laterality and Psychopathology. Edited by Flor-Henry P, Gruzelier J. Amsterdam, Elsevier, 1983, pp 1–18

Ford FR: Diseases of the Nervous System in Infancy, Childhood and Adolescence. Springfield, IL, Charles C Thomas, 1960

Forssman H, Frey TS: Electroencephalograms of boys with behavior disorders. Acta Psychiatr Neurol Scand 28:61–73, 1953

Fottrell E: A study of violent behavior among patients in psychiatric hospitals. Br J Psychiatry 136:216–221, 1980

Fox KA, Tockosh JR, Wilcox AH: Increased aggression among grouped male mice fed chlordiazepoxide. Eur J Pharmacol 11:119–121, 1970

Frank LG, Glickman SE, Licht P: Fatal sibling aggression, precocial development, and androgens in neonatal spotted hyenas. Science 252:702–704, 1991

Frank RT: The hormonal causes of premenstrual tension. Arch Neurol Psychiatr 26:1053–1057, 1931

Frankel FH: Adult reconstruction of childhood events in the multiple personality literature. Am J Psychiatry 150:954–958, 1993

Fukunaga K: Introduction to Statistical Pattern Recognition. New York, Academic Press, 1972

Gabrielli WF, Mednick SA: Sinistrality and delinquency. J Abnorm Psychol 89:654–661, 1980

Garattini S, Valzelli L: Is the isolated animal a possible model for phobia and anxiety? Prog Neuropsychopharmacol 5:159–165, 1981

Gardos G, DiMascio A, Salzman C, et al: Differential actions of chlordiazepoxide and oxazepam on hostility. Arch Gen Psychiatry 18:757–760, 1968

Gearing FR, Schweitzer MD: An epidemiologic evaluation of long-term methadone maintenance treatment for heroin addiction. Am J Epidemiol 100:101–112, 1974

Gedye A: Buspirone alone or with serotonergic diet reduced aggression in a developmentally disabled adult. Biol Psychiatry 30:88–91, 1991a

Gedye A: Serotonergic treatment for aggression in a Down's syndrome adult showing signs of Alzheimer's disease. J Ment Defic Res 35:247–258, 1991b

Gelernter J, Kranzler H, Coccaro EF, et al: Serotonin transporter protein gene polymorphism and personality measures in African American and European American subjects. Am J Psychiatry 155:1332–1338, 1998

Geracioti TD Jr: Valproic acid treatment of episodic explosiveness related to brain injury (letter). J Clin Psychiatry 55:416–417, 1994

Gercenzon AA: Introduction to Soviet Criminology [in Czech]. Moscow, Publishing House for Legal Literature, 1965

Geyer MA, Segal DS: Shock-induced aggression: Opposite effects of intraventricularly infused dopamine and norepinephrine. Behav Biol 10:99–104, 1974

Giakas WJ, Seibyl JP, Mazure CM: Valproate in the treatment of temper outbursts (letter). J Clin Psychiatry 51:525, 1990

Gianoulakis C: Rats exposed prenatally to alcohol exhibit impairment in spatial navigation test. Behav Brain Res 36:217–228, 1990

Gibbons JL, Barr GA, Bridger WH, et al: Effects of para-chlorophenylalanine and 5-hydroxytryptophan on mouse killing behavior in killer rats. Pharmacol Biochem Behav 9:91–98, 1978

Gibbons JL, Barr GA, Bridger WH, et al: Manipulations of dietary tryptophan: effects on mouse killing and brain serotonin in the rat. Brain Res 169:139–153, 1979

Giri NC: Multivariate Statistical Inference. New York, Academic Press, 1977

Gitlin MJ, Pasnau RO: Psychiatric syndromes linked to reproductive function in women: a review of current knowledge. Am J Psychiatry 146:1413–1422, 1989

Glueck S, Glueck E: Unraveling Juvenile Delinquency. New York, The Commonwealth Fund, 1950

Goff DC, Brotman AW, Kindlon D, et al: Self-reports of childhood abuse in chronically psychotic patients. Psychiatry Res 37:73–80, 1991

Gogos JA, Morgan M, Luine V, et al: Catechol-O-methyltransferase-deficient mice exhibit sexually dimorphic changes in catecholamine levels and behavior. Proc Natl Acad Sci U S A 95:9991–9996, 1998

Goldberg R, Motzkin B, Marion R, et al: Velo-cardio-facial syndrome: a review of 120 patients. Am J Med Genet 45:313–319, 1993

Goldman MB, Janecek HM: Adjunctive fluoxetine improves global function in chronic schizophrenia. J Neuropsychiatry Clin Neurosci 2:429–431, 1990

Goldstein PJ: The drugs/violence nexus: a tripartite conceptual framework. J Drug Issues 493–506, 1985

Gondolf EW, Mulvey EP, Lidz CW: Psychiatric admission of family violent versus nonfamily violent patients. Int J Law Psychiatry 14:245–254, 1991

Gorenstein EE, Newman JP: Disinhibitory psychopathology: a new perspective and a model for research. Psychol Rev 87:301–315, 1980

Gottfredson MR, Hirschi TA: A General Theory of Crime. Stanford, CA, Stanford University Press, 1990

Gottschalk LA, Gleser GC, Wylie HW Jr, et al: Effect of imipramine on anxiety and hostility levels. Psychopharmacologia 7:303–310, 1965

Grafman J, Schwab K, Warden D, et al: Frontal lobe injuries, violence, and aggression: a report of the Vietnam head injury study. Neurology 46:1231–1238, 1996

Graham LR: Science in Russia and the Soviet Union. A Short History. Cambridge, England, Cambridge University Press, 1993

Greendyke RM, Kanter DR: Therapeutic effects of pindolol on behavioral disturbances associated with organic brain disease: a double-blind study. J Clin Psychiatry 47:423–426, 1986

Greendyke RM, Kanter DR: Plasma propranolol levels and their effect on plasma thioridazine and haloperidol concentrations. J Clin Psychopharmacol 7:178–182, 1987

Greendyke RM, Kanter DR, Schuster DB, et al: Propranolol treatment of assaultive patients with organic brain disease. J Nerv Ment Dis 174:290–294, 1986

Greenebaum JV, Lurie LA: Encephalitis as a causative factor in behavior disorders of children. JAMA 136:923–930, 1948

Greenfield TK, McNiel DE, Binder RL: Violent behavior and length of psychiatric hospitalization. Hosp Community Psychiatry 40:809–814, 1989

Greenwald BS, Marin DB, Silverman SM: Serotoninergic treatment of screaming and banging in dementia (letter). Lancet 2:1464–1465, 1986

Grinfeld MJ: Task force to report on jailed mentally ill. Psychiatric Times 9:28–30, 1992

Grossman LS, Haywood TW, Cavanaugh JL, et al: State psychiatric hospital patients with past arrests for violent crimes. Psychiatr Serv 46:790–795, 1995

Gudmundsson G: Epilepsy in Iceland. A clinical and epidemiological investigation. Acta Neurol Scand 43 (suppl 25):1–124, 1966

Guillemin R, Vargo T, Rossier J, et al: Beta-endorphin and adrenocorticotropin are secreted concomitantly by the pituitary gland. Science 197:1367–1369, 1977

Guilleminault C, Moscovitch A, Leger D: Forensic sleep medicine: nocturnal wandering and violence. Sleep 18:740–748, 1995

Gunn J: Epileptic homicide: a case report. Br J Psychiatry 132:510–513, 1978

Gunn J, Bonn J: Criminality and violence in epileptic prisoners. Br J Psychiatry 118:337–343, 1971

Gunn J, Fenton G: Epilepsy in prisons: a diagnostic survey. Br Med J 4:326–329, 1969

Gunn JC, Fenton GW: Epilepsy, automatism and crime. Lancet 1:1173–1176, 1971

Guy W: ECDEU Assessment Manual for Psychopharmacology. Rockville, MD, National Institute of Mental Health, 1976

Guy W: ECDEU Assessment Manual for Psychopharmacology. Rockville, MD, National Institute of Mental Health, 1986

Haas JF, Cope DN: Neuropharmacologic management of behavior sequelae in head injury: a case report. Arch Phys Med Rehabil 66:472–474, 1985

Hafner H, Boker W: Crimes of Violence by Mentally Abnormal Offenders. A Psychiatric and Epidemiological Study in the Federal German Republic. Cambridge, England, Cambridge University Press, 1982

Hahn RA, Hynes MD, Fuller RW: Apomorphine-induced aggression in rats chronically treated with oral clonidine: Modulation by central serotonergic mechanisms. J Pharmacol Exp Ther 220:389–393, 1982

Hakola HPA, Laulumaa VA: Carbamazepine in treatment of violent schizophrenics (letter). Lancet 1:1358, 1982

Haller RM, Deluty RH: Assaults on staff by psychiatric in-patients. A critical review. Br J Psychiatry 152:174–179, 1988

Hallikainen T, Saito T, Lachman HM, et al: Association between low activity serotonin transporter promoter genotype and early onset alcoholism with habitual impulsive violent behavior. Mol Psychiatry 4:385–388, 1999

Hallsteinsen A, Kristensen M, Dahl AA, et al: The Extended Staff Observation Aggression Scale (SOAS-E): development, presentation and evaluation. Acta Psychiatr Scand 97:423–426, 1998

Halperin JM, Newcorn JH, Schwartz ST, et al: Age-related changes in the association between serotonergic function and aggression in boys with ADHD. Biol Psychiatry 41:682–689, 1997

Hamilton JA, Gallant SJ: Debate on late luteal phase dysphoric disorder. Am J Psychiatry 147:1106–1107, 1990

Hands J, Herbert V, Tennent G: Menstruation and behaviour in a special hospital. Med Sci Law 14:32–35, 1974

Hanlon TE, Nurco DN, Kinlock TW, et al: Trends in criminal activity and drug use over an addiction career. Am J Drug Alcohol Abuse 16:223–238, 1990

Hare RD: Twenty years of experience with the Cleckley psychopath, in Unmasking the Psychopath. Antisocial Personality and Related Syndromes. Edited by Reid WH, Dorr D, Walker JI, et al. New York, WW Norton, 1986, pp 3–27

Hare RD: Psychopathy and antisocial personality disorder: a case of diagnostic confusion. Psychiatric Times, February 1996, pp 39–40

Hare RD, McPherson LM: Violent and aggressive behavior by criminal psychopaths. Int J Law Psychiatry 7:35–50, 1984

Hare RD, McPherson LM, Forth AE: Male psychopaths and their criminal careers. J Consult Clin Psychol 56:710–714, 1988

Harlow H, Harlow M: The young monkeys. Psychology Today 1:40–47, 1967

Harris GT, Rice ME: Risk appraisal and management of violent behavior. Psychiatr Serv 48:1168–1176, 1997

Harris GT, Varney GW: A ten-year study of assaults and assaulters on a maximum security psychiatric unit. Journal of Interpersonal Violence 1:173–191, 1986

Harry B, Steadman HJ: Arrest rates of patients treated at a community mental health center [published erratum appears in Hosp Community Psychiatry 40(12):1303, 1989]. Hosp Community Psychiatry 39:862–866, 1988

Hart SD, Hare RD: Discriminant validity of the psychopathy checklist in a forensic psychiatric population. Psychol Assess 1:211–218, 1989

Hart SD, Hare RD, Forth AE: Psychopathy as a risk marker for violence: development and validation of a screening version of the revised psychopathy checklist, in Violence and Mental Disorder: Developments in Risk Assessment. Edited by Monahan J, Steadman HJ. Chicago, IL, University of Chicago Press, 1994, pp 81–98

Haug M, Simler S, Kim L, et al: Studies on the involvement of GABA in the aggression directed by groups of intact or gonadectomized male and female mice towards lactating intruders. Pharmacol Biochem Behav 12:189–193, 1980

Hausfater G, Skoblick B: Perimenstrual behavior changes among female yellow baboons: some similarities to premenstrual syndrome (PMS) in women. Am J Primatol 9:165–172, 1985

Hechtman L, Weiss G, Perlman T: Hyperactives as young adults: past and current substance abuse and antisocial behavior. Am J Orthopsychiatry 54:415–425, 1984

Hedlund JL, Sletten IW, Altman H, et al: Prediction of patients who are dangerous to others. J Clin Psychol 29:443–447, 1973

Hegarty AM: Treatment of impulsive aggression with divalproex (abstract no NR518), in 2000 New Research Program and Abstracts, American Psychiatric Association 153rd Annual Meeting, Chicago, IL, May 13–18, 2000. Washington, DC, American Psychiatric Association, 2000, p 198

Hegstrand LR, Eichelman B: Increased shock-induced fighting with supersensitive beta- adrenergic receptors. Pharmacol Biochem Behav 19:313–320, 1983

Heilbrun AB: Psychopathy and violent crime. J Consult Clin Psychol 47:509–516, 1979

Heilbrun AB: Cognitive models of criminal violence based upon intelligence and psychopathy levels. J Consult Clin Psychol 50:546–557, 1982

Heilbrun AB, Knopf IJ, Bruner P: Criminal impulsivity and violence and subsequent parole outcome. Br J Criminol 16:367–377, 1976

Heinrichs DW, Buchanan RW: Significance and meaning of neurological signs in schizophrenia. Am J Psychiatry 145:11–18, 1988

Heinrichs RW: Frontal cerebral lesions and violent incidents in chronic neuropsychiatric patients. Biol Psychiatry 25:174–178, 1989

Heinz A, Higley JD, Gorey JG, et al: In vivo association between alcohol association, aggression, and serotonin transporter availability in nonhuman primates. Am J Psychiatry 155:1023–1028, 1998

Hellman DS, Blackman N: Enuresis, firesetting and cruelty to animals: a triad predictive of adult crime. Am J Psychiatry 122:1431–1435, 1966

Herman ZS, Drybanski A, Trzeciak HI: Increased aggression in rats after withdrawal of long term used oxazepam. Experientia 32:1305–1306, 1976

Herrera JN, Sramek JJ, Costa JF, et al: High potency neuroleptics and violence in schizophrenics. J Nerv Ment Dis 176:558–561, 1988

Herrmann N, Lanctot KL, Eryavec GM, et al: Serotonergic function and aggression in Alzheimer's disease (abstract no NR439), in 1998 New Research Program and Abstracts, American Psychiatric Association 151st Annual Meeting, Toronto, Canada, May 30–June 4, 1998. Washington, DC, American Psychiatric Association, 1998, p 186

Herzberg JL, Fenwick PB: The aetiology of aggression in temporal-lobe epilepsy. Br J Psychiatry 153:50–55, 1988

Hess WR, Brugger M: Das subkortikale zentrum der affektiven abwehrreaktion. Helvetica Physiologica Acta 1:33–52, 1943

Hesslinger B, Normann C, Langosch JM, et al: Effects of carbamazepine and valproate on haloperidol plasma levels and on psychopathologic outcome in schizophrenic patients. J Clin Psychopharmacol 19:310–315, 1999

Hiday VA, Swartz MS, Swanson JW, et al: Male-female differences in the setting and construction of violence among people with severe mental illness. Soc Psychiatry Psychiatr Epidemiol 33 (suppl 1):S68–S74, 1998

Higley JD, Suomi SJ, Linnoila M: CSF monoamine metabolite concentrations vary according to age, rearing, and sex, and are influenced by the stressor of social separation in rhesus monkeys. Psychopharmacology 103:551–556, 1991

Higley JD, Mehlman PT, Taub DM, et al: Cerebrospinal fluid monoamine and adrenal correlates of aggression in free-ranging rhesus monkeys. Arch Gen Psychiatry 49:436–441, 1992

Higley JD, Thompson WW, Champoux M, et al: Paternal and maternal genetic and environmental contributions to cerebrospinal fluid monoamine metabolites in rhesus monkeys (Macaca mulatta). Arch Gen Psychiatry 50:615–623, 1993

Higley JD, Mehlman PT, Higley SB, et al: Excessive mortality in young free-ranging male nonhuman primates with low cerebrospinal fluid 5-hydroxyindoleacetic acid concentrations. Arch Gen Psychiatry 53:537–543, 1996

Higley JD, Bennett AJ, Heils A, et al: Early rearing and genotypic influences on CNS serotonin and behavior in nonhuman primates (abstract). Biol Psychiatry 47 (suppl):10S–11S, 2000

Hill D: Cerebral dysrhythmia: its significance in aggressive behaviour. Proc R Soc Med 37:317–328, 1944

Hill D: EEG in episodic and psychopathic behaviour. Electroencephalogr Clin Neurophysiol 4:419–442, 1952

Hill D, Pond DA: Reflections on one hundred capital cases submitted to electroencephalography. Journal of Mental Science 98:23–43, 1952

Hill D, Sargant W: A case of matricide. Lancet 244(1):526–527, 1943

Hill D, Watterson D: Electro-encephalographic studies of psychopathic personalities. Journal of Neurology and Psychiatry 5:47–65, 1942

Hindelang MJ, Hirschi T, Weis JG: Measuring Delinquency. Beverly Hills, CA, Sage, 1981

Hinsie LE, Campbell RJ: Psychiatric Dictionary. New York, Oxford University Press, 1960

Hirose S, Ashby CR Jr, Mills MJ: Effectiveness of ECT combined with risperidone against aggression in schizophrenia. J ECT 17:22–26, 2001

Hirschi T, Hindelang MJ: Intelligence and delinquency: a revisionist review. Am Sociol Rev 42:571–587, 1977

Hitchcock E, Cairns V: Amygdalotomy. Postgrad Med J 49:894–904, 1973

Hjorth S, Carlsson A: Is pindolol a mixed agonist-antagonist at central serotonin (5-HT) receptors? Eur J Pharmacol 129:131–138, 1986

Hodgins S: Mental disorder, intellectual deficiency, and crime. Evidence from a birth cohort. Arch Gen Psychiatry 49:476–483, 1992

Hodgins S, Mednick SA, Brennan PA, et al: Mental disorder and crime. Evidence from a Danish birth cohort. Arch Gen Psychiatry 53:489–496, 1996

Holcomb WR, Ahr PR: Arrest rates among young adult psychiatric patients treated in inpatient and outpatient settings. Hosp Community Psychiatry 39:52–57, 1988

Hollander E: Managing aggressive behavior in patients with obsessive-compulsive disorder and borderline personality disorder. J Clin Psychiatry 60 (suppl 15):38–44, 1999

Hollander E, Rosen J: Impulsivity. J Psychopharmacol 14 (suppl 1):S39–S44, 2000

Hollander E, Grossman R, Stein DJ, et al: Borderline personality disorder and impulsive-aggression: the role for divalproex sodium treatment. Psychiatr Ann 26 (suppl):S464–S469, 1996

Hollander E, Cohen L, Simon L: Impulse-control disorder measures, in Handbook of Psychiatric Measures. Edited by Rush AJ Jr, Pincus HA, First MB, et al. Washington, DC, American Psychiatric Association, 2000, pp 687–712

Honer WG, Gewirtz G, Turey M: Psychosis and violence in cocaine smokers (letter). Lancet 2:451, 1987

Honigfeld G, Gillis RD, Klett CJ: NOSIE-30: a treatment-sensitive ward behavior scale. Psychol Rep 19:180–182, 1966

Hoptman MJ, Volavka J, Johnson G, et al: Decreased fractional anisotropy in frontal white matter is associated with impulsivity in men with schizophrenia (abstract). Schizophr Res 49 (suppl):157, 2001

Horne M, Lindley SE: Divalproex sodium in the treatment of aggressive behavior and dysphoria in patients with organic brain syndromes (letter). J Clin Psychiatry 56:430–431, 1995

Hornstein A, Seliger G: Cognitive side effects of lithium in closed head injury (letter). J Neuropsychiatry Clin Neurosci 1:446–447, 1989

Huber G: Psychiatrie: systematischer Lehrtext für Studenten und Ärzte. Stuttgart, Schattauer, 1987

Huesmann LR, Eron LD, Lefkowitz MM, et al: Stability of aggression over time and generations. Devel Psychol 20:1120–1134, 1984

Hunter ME, Love CC: Total quality management and the reduction of inpatient violence and costs in a forensic psychiatric hospital. Psychiatr Serv 47:751–754, 1996

Huntingford FA, Turner AK: Animal Conflict. London, Chapman & Hall, 1987

Hutchinson RR, Azrin NH, Hunt GM: Attack produced by intermittent reinforcement of a concurrent operant response. J Exp Anal Behav 11:489–495, 1968

Ingram IM, Timbury GC: Side-effects of Librium. Lancet 2:766, 1960

Ito TA, Miller N, Pollock VE: Alcohol and aggression: a meta-analysis on the moderating effects of inhibitory cues, triggering events, and self-focused attention. Psychol Bull 120:60–82, 1996

Jablensky A, Sartorius N, Ernberg G, et al: Schizophrenia: manifestations, incidence and course in different cultures. A World Health Organization ten-country study. Psychol Med Monogr Suppl 20:1–97, 1992

Jackson RD, Corrigan JD, Arnett JA: Amitriptyline for agitation in head injury. Arch Phys Med Rehabil 66:180–181, 1985

Jenkins RL, Pacella BL: Electroencephalographic studies of delinquent boys. Am J Orthopsychiatry 13:107–120, 1943

Johanson CE, Fischman MW: The pharmacology of cocaine related to its abuse. Pharmacol Rev 41:3–52, 1989

John ER, Karmel BZ, Corning WC, et al: Neurometrics. Science 196:1393–1410, 1977

John ER, Ahn H, Prichep L, et al: Developmental equations for the electroencephalogram. Science 210:1255–1258, 1980

John V, Rapp M, Pies R: Aggression, agitation, and mania with olanzapine (letter). Can J Psychiatry 43:1054, 1998

Johnson DAW, Pasterski G, Ludlow JM, et al: The discontinuance of maintenance neuroleptic therapy in chronic schizophrenic patients: drug and social consequences. Acta Psychiatr Scand 67:339–352, 1983

Jolly A: The Evolution of Primate Behavior. New York, Macmillan, 1985

Jones G, Zammit S, Norton N, et al: Aggressive behaviour in patients with schizophrenia is associated with catechol-O-methyltransferase genotype. Br J Psychiatry 179:351–355, 2001

Jones KL, Smith DW, Ulleland CN, et al: Pattern of malformation in offspring of chronic alcoholic mothers. Lancet 1:1267–1271, 1973

Junginger J: Command hallucinations and the prediction of dangerousness. Psychiatr Serv 46:911–914, 1995

Junginger J, McGuire L: The paradox of command hallucinations (letter). Psychiatr Serv 52:385, 2001

Junginger J, Parks-Levy J, McGuire L: Delusions and symptom-consistent violence. Psychiatr Serv 49:218–220, 1998

Jurik NC, Winn R: Gender and homicide: a comparison of men and women who kill. Violence Vict 5:227–242, 1990

Kahn MW: A comparison of personality, intelligence, and social history of two criminal groups. J Soc Psychol 49:33–40, 1959

Kalina RK: Diazepam: its role in a prison setting. Dis Nerv Syst 25:101–107, 1964

Kamin LJ: Criminality and adoption (letter). Science 227:983, 1985

Kandel ER: A new intellectual framework for psychiatry. Am J Psychiatry 155:457–469, 1998

Kandel E, Mednick SA, Kirkegaard-Sorensen L, et al: IQ as a protective factor for subjects at high risk for antisocial behavior. J Consult Clin Psychol 56:224–226, 1988

Kandel ER, Schwartz JH, Jessell TM: Principles of Neural Science. New York, McGraw-Hill, 2000

Kantak KM, Miczek KA: Social, motor, and autonomic signs of morphine withdrawal: differential sensitivities to catecholaminergic drugs in mice. Psychopharmacology 96:468–476, 1988

Karayiorgou M, Sobin C, Blundell ML, et al: Family based association studies support a sexually dimorphic effect of COMT and MAOA on genetic susceptibility to obsessive-compulsive disorder. Biol Psychiatry 45:1178–1189, 1999

Karli P: The Norway rat's killing response to the white mouse: an experimental analysis. Behaviour 10:81–103, 1956

Karson C, Bigelow LB: Violent behavior in schizophrenic inpatients. J Nerv Ment Dis 175:161–164, 1987

Karson CN, Weinberger DR, Bigelow L, et al: Clonazepam treatment of chronic schizophrenia: negative results in a double-blind, placebo-controlled trial. Am J Psychiatry 139:1627–1628, 1982

Kastner T, Burlingham K, Friedman DL: Metoprolol for aggressive behavior in persons with mental retardation. Am Fam Physician 42:1585–1588, 1990

Kauhanen J, Hallikainen T, Tuomainen T-P, et al: Association between the functional polymorphism of catechol-O-methyltransferase gene and alcohol consumption among social drinkers. Alcohol Clin Exp Res 24:135–139, 2000

Kay SR, Wolkenfeld F, Murrill LM: Profiles of aggression among psychiatric patients. I. Nature and prevalence. J Nerv Ment Dis 176:539–546, 1988

Kay SR, Opler LA, Lindenmayer JP: The Positive and Negative Syndrome Scale (PANSS): rationale and standardisation. Br J Psychiatry Suppl 155:59–65, 1989

Kaye AL, Shea MT: Personality disorders, personality traits, and defense mechanism measures, in Handbook of Psychiatric Measures. Edited by Rush AJ Jr, Pincus HA, First MB, et al. Washington, DC, American Psychiatric Association, 2000, pp 713–749

Keckich WA: Neuroleptics. Violence as a manifestation of akathisia. JAMA 240: 2185–2185, 1978

Kemppainen L, Jokelainen J, Jarvelin MR, et al: The one-child family and violent criminality: a 31-year follow-up study of the Northern Finland 1966 birth cohort. Am J Psychiatry 158:960–962, 2001

Kennard MA, Rabinovich MS, Schwartzman AE, et al: Factor of aggression as related to the electroencephalogram. Dis Nerv Syst 17:127–131, 1956

Khajawall AM, Erickson TB, Simpson GM: Chronic phencyclidine abuse and physical assault. Am J Psychiatry 139:1604–1606, 1982

Kiersch TA: Treatment of sex offenders with Depo-Provera. Bull Am Acad Psychiatry Law 18:179–187, 1990

King CH: The ego and the integration of violence in homicidal youth. Am J Orthopsychiatry 45:134–145, 1975

King DW, Ajmone Marsan C: Clinical features and ictal patterns in epileptic patients with EEG temporal lobe foci. Ann Neurol 2:138–147, 1977

King RJ, Jones J, Scheuer JW, et al: Plasma cortisol correlates of impulsivity and substance abuse. Pers Individ Dif 11:287–291, 1990

Klassen D, O'Connor WA: Crime, inpatient admissions, and violence among male mental patients. Int J Law Psychiatry 11:305–312, 1988a

Klassen D, O'Connor WA: A prospective study of predictors of violence in adult male mental health admissions. Law Hum Behav 12:143–158, 1988b

Kluver H, Bucy PC: Preliminary analysis of functions of the temporal lobes in monkeys. Archives of Neurology and Psychiatry 42:979–1000, 1939

Knoedler DW: The Modified Overt Aggression Scale (letter; comment). Am J Psychiatry 146:1081–1082, 1989

Ko GN, Korpi ER, Freed WJ, et al: Effect of valproic acid on behavior and plasma amino acid concentrations in chronic schizophrenic patients. Biol Psychiatry 20:209–215, 1985

Kochansky GE, Salzman C, Shader RI, et al: The differential effects of chlordiazepoxide and oxazepam on hostility in a small group setting. Am J Psychiatry 132:861–863, 1975

Kotler M, Barak P, Cohen H, et al: Homicidal behavior in schizophrenia associated with a genetic polymorphism determining low catechol O-methyltransferase (COMT) activity. Am J Med Genet 88:628–633, 1999

Kozol HL, Boucher RJ, Garofalo RF: The diagnosis and treatment of dangerousness. Crime Delinq 18:371–392, 1972

Krakowski MI, Convit A, Volavka J: Patterns of inpatient assaultiveness: effect of neurological impairment and deviant family environment on response to treatment. Neuropsychiatry Neuropsychol Behav Neurol 1:21–29, 1988a

Krakowski M, Jaeger J, Volavka J: Violence and psychopathology: a longitudinal study. Compr Psychiatry 29:174–181, 1988b

Krakowski MI, Convit A, Jaeger J, et al: Neurological impairment in violent schizophrenic inpatients. Am J Psychiatry 146:849–853, 1989

Krakowski MI, Kunz M, Czobor P, et al: Long-term high-dose neuroleptic treatment: who gets it and why? Hosp Community Psychiatry 44:640–644, 1993

Krakowski M, Czobor P, Chou JCY: Course of violence in patients with schizophrenia: relationship to clinical symptoms. Schizophr Bull 25:505–517, 1999

Kreuz LE, Rose RM: Assessment of aggressive behavior and plasma testosterone in a young criminal population. Psychosom Med 34:321–332, 1972

Kristianson P: The personality in psychomotor epilepsy compared with the explosive and aggressive personality. Br J Psychiatry 125:221–229, 1974

Krsiak M: Timid singly housed mice: Their value in prediction of psychotropic activity of drugs. Br J Pharmacol 55:141–150, 1975

Krsiak M: Effects of drugs on behaviour of aggressive mice. Br J Pharmacol 65:525–533, 1979

Krsiak M, Elis J, Poschlova N, et al: Increased aggressiveness and lower brain serotonin levels in offspring of mice given alcohol during gestation. J Stud Alcohol 38:1696–1704, 1977

Krueger RF, Moffitt TE, Caspi A, et al: Assortative mating for antisocial behavior: developmental and methodological implications. Behav Genet 28:173–186, 1998

Kruesi MJP, Rapoport JL, Hamburger S, et al: Cerebrospinal fluid monoamine metabolites, aggression, and impulsivity in disruptive behavior disorders of children and adolescents. Arch Gen Psychiatry 47:419–426, 1990

Krynicki VE: Cerebral dysfunction in repetitively assaultive adolescents. J Nerv Ment Dis 166:59–67, 1978

Kunugi H, Vallada HP, Sham PC, et al: Catechol-O-methyltransferase polymorphisms and schizophrenia: a transmission disequilibrium study in multiply affected families. Psychiatr Genet 7:97–101, 1997

Kunz M, Sikora J, Krakowski M, et al: Serotonin in violent patients with schizophrenia. Psychiatry Res 59:161–163, 1995

Kyriacou DN, Anglin D, Taliaferro E, et al: Risk factors for injury to women from domestic violence against women. N Engl J Med 341:1892–1898, 1999

Lacey JH, Evans CD: The impulsivist: a multi-impulsive personality disorder. Br J Addict 81:641–649, 1986

Lachman HM, Papolos DF, Saito T, et al: Human catechol-O-methyltransferase pharmacogenetics: description of a functional polymorphism and its potential application to neuropsychiatric disorders. Pharmacogenetics 6:243–250, 1996

Lachman HM, Nolan KA, Mohr P, et al: Association between catechol O-methyltransferase genotype and violence in schizophrenia and schizoaffective disorder. Am J Psychiatry 155:835–837, 1998

Lafave HG, Pinkney AA, Gerber GJ: Criminal activity by psychiatric clients after hospital discharge. Hosp Community Psychiatry 44:180–181, 1993

Lagos JM, Perlmutter K, Saexinger H: Fear of the mentally ill: empirical support for the common man's response. Am J Psychiatry 134:1134–1136, 1977

Lal H, O'Brien J, Puri SK: Morphine-withdrawal aggression: sensitization by amphetamines. Psychopharmacologia 22:217–223, 1971

Lammers AJ, van Rossum JM: Bizarre social behaviour in rats induced by a combination of a peripheral decarboxylase inhibitor and DOPA. Eur J Pharmacol 5:103–106, 1968

Lamprecht F, Eichelman B, Thoa NB, et al: Rat fighting behavior: serum dopamine-B-hydroxylase and hypothalamic tyrosine hydroxylase. Science 177:1214–1215, 1972

Langevin R, Paitich D, Orchard B, et al: Diagnosis of killers seen for psychiatric assessment. Acta Psychiatr Scand 66:216–228, 1982a

Langevin R, Paitich D, Orchard B, et al: The role of alcohol, drugs, suicide attempts and situational strains in homicide committed by offenders seen for psychiatric assessment. Acta Psychiatr Scand 66:229–242, 1982b

Langevin R, Ben-Aron M, Wortzman G, et al: Brain damage, diagnosis, and substance abuse among violent offenders. Behav Sci Law 5:77–94, 1987

Lapierre D, Braun CMJ, Hodgins S, et al: Neuropsychological correlates of violence in schizophrenia. Schizophr Bull 21:253–262, 1995a

Lapierre D, Braun CMJ, Hodgins S: Ventral frontal deficits in psychopathy: neuropsychological test findings. Neuropsychologia 33:139–151, 1995b

Lappalainen J, Long JC, Eggert M, et al: Linkage of antisocial alcoholism to the serotonin 5-HT1B receptor gene in 2 populations. Arch Gen Psychiatry 55:989–994, 1998

Lautin A, Angrist B, Stanley M, et al: Sodium valproate in schizophrenia: some biochemical correlates. Br J Psychiatry 137:240–244, 1980

Leckman JF, Goodman WK, Riddle MA, et al: Low CSF 5HIAA and obsessions of violence: report of two cases (letter). Psychiatry Res 33:95–99, 1990

Lenin VI: State and Revolution. New York, International Publishers, 1932

Leon DA: Failed or misleading adjustment for confounding. Lancet 342:479–481, 1993

Lesch K-P, Bengel D, Heils A, et al: Association of anxiety-related traits with a polymorphism in the serotonin transporter gene regulatory region. Science 274:1527–1531, 1996

Lesem MD, Zajecka JM, Swift RH, et al: Intramuscular ziprasidone, 2 mg versus 10 mg, in the short-term management of agitated psychotic patients. J Clin Psychiatry 62:12–18, 2001

Levine AM: Buspirone and agitation in head injury. Brain Inj 2:165–167, 1988

Levy RH, Kerr BM: Clinical pharmacokinetics of carbamazepine. J Clin Psychiatry 49 (suppl):58–61, 1988

Levy S: Post-encephalitic behavior disorder—a forgotten entity: a report of 100 cases. Am J Psychiatry 115:1062–1067, 1959

Lewis DO, Shanok SS: Medical histories of delinquent and nondelinquent children: an epidemiological study. Am J Psychiatry 134:1020–1025, 1977

Lewis DO, Pincus JH, Shanok SS, et al: Psychomotor epilepsy and violence in a group of incarcerated adolescent boys. Am J Psychiatry 139:882–887, 1982

Lewis DO, Moy E, Jackson LD, et al: Biopsychosocial characteristics of children who later murder: a prospective study. Am J Psychiatry 142:1161–1167, 1985

Lewis DO, Pincus JH, Bard B, et al: Neuropsychiatric, psychoeducational, and family characteristics of 14 juveniles condemned to death in the Unites States. Am J Psychiatry 145:584–589, 1988

Lewis DO, Lovely R, Yeager C, et al: Toward a theory of the genesis of violence: a follow-up study of delinquents. Am Acad Child Psychiatry 28:431–436, 1989

Lezak MD: Neuropsychological Assessment. New York, Oxford University Press, 1983

Li T, Sham PC, Vallada H, et al: Preferential transmission of the high activity allele of COMT in schizophrenia. Psychiatr Genet 6:131–133, 1996

Lidberg L, Asberg M, Sundqvist-Stensman UB: 5-Hydroxyindoleacetic acid levels in attempted suicides who have killed their children (letter). Lancet 2:928, 1984

Lidberg L, Modin I, Oreland L, et al: Platelet monoamine oxidase activity and psychopathy. Psychiatry Res 16:339–343, 1985a

Lidberg L, Tuck JR, Asberg M, et al: Homicide, suicide and CSF 5-HIAA. Acta Psychiatr Scand 71:230–236, 1985b

Lidz CW, Mulvey EP, Appelbaum PS, et al: Commitment: the consistency of clinicians and the use of legal standards. Am J Psychiatry 146:176–181, 1989

Lidz CW, Mulvey EP, Gardner W: The accuracy of predictions of violence to others. JAMA 269:1007–1011, 1993

Liebman J, Axler F, Kotranski L: Excess mortality in Harlem (letter). N Engl J Med 322:1606, 1990

Lindqvist P: Criminal homicide in northern Sweden 1970–1981: alcohol intoxication, alcohol abuse and mental disease. Int J Law Psychiatry 8:19–37, 1986

Lindqvist P, Allebeck P: Schizophrenia and assaultive behaviour: the role of alcohol and drug abuse. Acta Psychiatr Scand 82:191–195, 1990

Lindsley DA: A longitudinal study of the occipital alpha rhythm in normal children. J Genet Psychol 55:197–213, 1939

Link BG, Stueve A: Psychotic symptoms and the violent/illegal behavior of mental patients compared to community controls, in Violence and Mental Disorder: Developments in Risk Assessment. Edited by Monahan J, Steadman HJ. Chicago, IL, University of Chicago Press, 1994, pp 137–159

Link BG, Cullen FT, Andrews H: The violent and illegal behavior of mental patients reconsidered. Am Sociol Rev 57:275–292, 1992

Link BG, Stueve A, Phelan J: Psychotic symptoms and violent behaviors: probing the components of "threat/control-override" symptoms. Soc Psychiatry Psychiatr Epidemiol 33 (suppl 1):S55–S60, 1998

Linnoila M, Virkkunen M, Scheinin M, et al: Low cerebrospinal fluid 5-hydroxy-indole acetic acid concentration differentiates impulsive from non-impulsive violent behavior. Life Sci 33:2609–2614, 1983

Lion JR: Benzodiazepines in the treatment of aggressive patients. J Clin Psychiatry 40:70–71, 1979

Lion JR, Azcarate CL, Koepke HH: "Paradoxical rage reactions" during psychotropic medication. Dis Nerv Syst 36:557–558, 1975

Lion JR, Synder W, Merrill GL: Underreporting of assaults on staff in a state hospital. Hosp Community Psychiatry 32:497–498, 1981

Lipinski JF Jr, Keck PE Jr, McElroy SL: Beta-adrenergic antagonists in psychosis: is improvement due to treatment of neuroleptic-induced akathisia? J Clin Psychopharmacol 8:409–416, 1988

Litt SM: Perinatal complications and criminality. Unpublished doctoral dissertation, New School for Social Research, New York, 1972

Litwack TR, Kirschner SM, Wack RC: The assessment of dangerousness and predictions of violence: recent research and future prospects. Psychiatr Q 64:245–273, 1993

Lothstein LM, Jones P: Discriminating violent individuals by means of various psychological tests. J Pers Assess 42:237–243, 1978

Lott AD, McElroy SL, Keys MA: Valproate in the treatment of behavioral agitation in elderly patients with dementia. J Neuropsychiatry Clin Neurosci 7:314–319, 1995

Lowry PW, Hassig SE, Gunn RA, et al: Homicide victims in New Orleans: recent trends. Am J Epidemiol 128:1130–1136, 1988

Luchins DJ: Carbamazepine in violent non-epileptic schizophrenics. Psychopharmacol Bull 20:569–571, 1984

Luchins DJ, Dojka D: Lithium and propranolol in aggression and self-injurious behavior in the mentally retarded. Psychopharmacol Bull 25:372–375, 1989

Lykken DT: A study of anxiety in the sociopathic personality. Journal of Abnormal and Social Psychology 55:6–10, 1957

Maccoby EE, Jacklin CN: The Psychology of Sex Differences. Stanford, CA, Stanford University Press, 1974

Maguire K, Pastore AL (eds): Sourcebook of Criminal Justice Statistics, 1994. Washington, DC, U.S. Department of Justice, Bureau of Justice Statistics, 1995

Maguire K, Pastore AL (eds): Sourcebook of Criminal Justice Statistics, 2000. Washington, DC, U.S. Department of Justice, Bureau of Justice Statistics, 2001

Maguire K, Pastore AL, Flanagan TJ (eds): Sourcebook of Criminal Justice Statistics, 1992. Washington, DC, U.S. Department of Justice, Bureau of Justice Statistics, 1993

Maier GJ: The impact of clozapine on 25 forensic patients. Bull Am Acad Psychiatry Law 20:297–307, 1992

Malamud N: Psychiatric disorder with intracranial tumors of limbic system. Arch Neurol 17:113–123, 1967

Malaspina D, Goetz RR, Friedman JH, et al: Traumatic brain injury and schizophrenia in members of schizophrenia and bipolar disorder pedigrees. Am J Psychiatry 158:440–446, 2001

Maletzky BM: The diagnosis of pathological intoxication. J Stud Alcohol 37:1215–1228, 1976

Malina RM: Biological substrata, in Comparative Studies of Blacks and Whites in the United States. Edited by Miller KS, Dreger RM. New York, Seminar, 1973, pp 53–123

Mallya AR, Roos PD, Roebuck-Colgan K: Restraint, seclusion, and clozapine. J Clin Psychiatry 53:395–397, 1992

Malone RP, Biesecker KA, Luebbert JF, et al: Importance of placebo baseline in clinical drug trials involving aggressive children. Paper presented at the New Clinical Drug Evaluation Unit Program 35th Annual Meeting Orlando, FL, May 31–June 3, 1995

Malone RP, Delaney MA, Luebbert JF, et al: A double-blind placebo-controlled study of lithium in hospitalized aggressive children and adolescents with conduct disorder. Arch Gen Psychiatry 57:649–654, 2000

Mann JJ: The neurobiology of suicide. Nat Med 4:25–30, 1998

Mann JJ, Kapur S: The emergence of suicidal ideation and behavior during antidepressant pharmacotherapy. Arch Gen Psychiatry 48:1027–1033, 1991

Mann JJ, Waternaux C, Haas GL, et al: Toward a clinical model of suicidal behavior in psychiatric patients. Am J Psychiatry 156:181–189, 1999

Mannuzza S, Klein RG, Konig PH, et al: Hyperactive boys almost grown up. IV. Criminality and its relationship to psychiatric status. Arch Gen Psychiatry 46:1073–1079, 1989

Manschreck TC, Laughery JA, Weisstein CC, et al: Characteristics of freebase cocaine psychosis. Yale J Biol Med 61:115–122, 1988

Mansheim P: Treatment with propranolol of the behavioral sequelae of brain damage (letter). J Clin Psychiatry 42:132, 1981

Manuck SB, Flory JD, Ferrell RE, et al: Aggression and anger-related traits associated with a polymorphism of the tryptophan hydroxylase gene. Biol Psychiatry 45:603–614, 1999

Manuck SB, Flory JD, Ferrell RE, et al: A regulatory polymorphism of the monoamine oxidase-A gene may be associated with variability in aggression, impulsivity, and central nervous system serotonergic responsivity. Psychiatry Res 95:9–23, 2000

Marder SR, Meibach RC: Risperidone in the treatment of schizophrenia. Am J Psychiatry 151:825–835, 1994

Marder SR, Davis JM, Chouinard G: The effects of risperidone on the five dimensions of schizophrenia derived by factor analysis: combined results of the North American trials. J Clin Psychiatry 58:538–546, 1997

Marinacci AA, Von Hagen KO: Alcohol and temporal lobe dysfunction. Some of its psychomotor equivalents. Behav Neuropsychiatry 3:2–11, 1972

Mark VH: Epilepsy and episodic aggression (letter). Arch Neurol 39:384–386, 1982

Mark VH, Ervin FR: Violence and the Brain. New York, Harper & Row, 1970

Mark VH, Sweet W, Ervin FR: Deep temporal lobe stimulation and destructive lesions in episodically violent temporal lobe epileptics, in Neural Bases of Violence and Aggression. Edited by Fields WS, Sweet WH. St. Louis, MO, Warren H Green, 1975, pp 379–391

Marlowe M, Stellern J, Moon C, et al: Main and interaction effects of metallic toxins on aggressive classroom behavior. Aggress Behav 11:41–48, 1985

Martell DA: Homeless mentally disordered offenders and violent crimes. Preliminary research findings. Law Hum Behav 15:333–347, 1991

Martell DA: Estimating the prevalence of organic brain dysfunction in maximum-security forensic psychiatric patients. J Forensic Sci 37:878–893, 1992

Martell DA, Dietz PE: Mentally disordered offenders who push or attempt to push victims onto subway tracks in New York City. Arch Gen Psychiatry 49:472–475, 1992

Matousek M, Petersen I: Automatic evaluation of EEG background activity by means of age-dependent quotients. Electroencephalogr Clin Neurophysiol 35:603–612, 1973

Matousek M, Volavka J, Roubicek J, et al: EEG frequency analysis related to age in normal adults. Electroencephalogr Clin Neurophysiol 23:162–167, 1967

Matsui M, Gur RC, Turetsky BI, et al: The relation between tendency for psychopathology and reduced frontal brain volume in healthy people. Neuropsychiatry Neuropsychol Behav Neurol 13:155–162, 2000

Mattes JA: Carbamazepine for uncontrolled rage outbursts (letter). Lancet 2:1164–1165, 1984

Mattes JA: Metoprolol for intermittent explosive disorder. Am J Psychiatry 142:1108–1109, 1985

Mattes JA: Valproic acid for nonaffective aggression in the mentally retarded. J Nerv Ment Dis 180:601–602, 1992

Mattsson A, Schalling D, Olweus D, et al: Plasma testosterone, aggressive behavior, and personality dimensions in young male delinquents. J Am Acad Child Psychiatry 19:476–490, 1980

Mazur A: Hormones, aggression, and dominance in humans, in Hormones and Aggressive Behavior. Edited by Svare BB. New York, Plenum, 1983, pp 563–576

Mazur A, Lamb TA: Testosterone, status, and mood in human males. Horm Behav 14:236–246, 1980

Mazure CM, Druss BG, Cellar JS: Valproate treatment of older psychotic patients with organic mental syndromes and behavioral dyscontrol. J Am Geriatr Soc 40:914–916, 1992

Mazzanti CM, Lappalainen J, Long JC, et al: Role of the serotonin transporter promoter polymorphism in anxiety-related traits. Arch Gen Psychiatry 55:936–940, 1998

McCarthy M, Chapman P, Richman CG, et al: Clozapine treatment of comorbid substance abuse in patients with schizophrenia (abstract no NR273), in 1999 New Research Program and Abstracts, American Psychiatric Association 152nd Annual Meeting, May 15–20, 1999. Washington, DC, American Psychiatric Association, 1999, p 140

McConaghy N, Blaszczynski A, Kidson W: Treatment of sex offenders with imaginal desensitization and/or medroxyprogesterone. Acta Psychiatr Scand 77:199–206, 1988

McCord C, Freeman HP: Excess mortality in Harlem. N Engl J Med 322:173–177, 1990

McCord J: A longitudinal study of aggression and antisocial behavior, in Prospective Studies of Crime and Delinquency. Edited by Van Dusen KT, Mednick SA. Boston, MA, Kluwer-Nijhoff, 1983, pp 269–275

McCord J: Parental aggressiveness and physical punishment in long-term perspective, in Family Abuse and Its Consequences. New Directions in Research. Edited by Hotaling GT, Finkelhor D, Kirkpatrick JT, et al. Newbury Park, CA, Sage, 1988, pp 91–98

McDonald RL: The effects of personality type on drug response. Arch Gen Psychiatry 17:680–686, 1967

McElroy SL, Keck PEJ, Pope HGJ: Sodium valproate: its use in primary psychiatric disorders. J Clin Psychopharmacol 7:16–24, 1987

McEvoy JP, Scheifler PL, Frances A: The expert consensus guideline series. Treatment of schizophrenia 1999. J Clin Psychiatry 60 (suppl 11):1–80, 1999

McFarland BH, Faulkner LR, Bloom JD, et al: Chronic mental illness and the criminal justice system. Hosp Community Psychiatry 40:718–723, 1989

McGivern RF, Lobaugh NJ, Collier AC: Effect of naloxone and housing conditions on shock-elicited reflexive fighting: Influence of immediate prior stress. Physiological Psychology 9:251–256, 1981

McKinlay WW, Brooks DN, Bond MR, et al: The short-term outcome of severe blunt head injury as reported by relatives of the injured persons. J Neurol Neurosurg Psychiatry 44:527–533, 1981

McNiel DE, Binder RL: Predictive validity of judgments of dangerousness in emergency civil commitment. Am J Psychiatry 144:197–200, 1987

McNiel DE, Binder RL: Relationship between preadmission threats and later violent behavior by acute psychiatric inpatients. Hosp Community Psychiatry 40:605–608, 1989

McNiel DE, Binder RL: Clinical assessment of the risk of violence among psychiatric inpatients. Am J Psychiatry 148:1317–1321, 1991

McNiel DE, Binder RL: Correlates of accuracy in the assessment of psychiatric inpatients' risk of violence. Am J Psychiatry 152:901–906, 1995

McNiel DE, Binder RL, Greenfield TK: Predictors of violence in civilly committed acute psychiatric patients. Am J Psychiatry 145:965–970, 1988

McNiel DE, Eisner JP, Binder RL: The relationship between command hallucinations and violence. Psychiatr Serv 51:1288–1292, 2000

Mednick SA: Criminality and adoption. Science 227:984–989, 1985

Mednick SA, Volavka J: Biology of crime, in An Annual Review of Research (Crime and Justice Series, Vol 7). Edited by Tonry M, Morris N. Chicago, IL, University of Chicago Press, 1980, pp 85–158

Mednick SA, Volavka J, Gabrielli WF, et al: EEG as a predictor of antisocial behavior. Criminology 19:219–229, 1981

Mednick SA, Pollock VE, Volavka J, et al: Biology and violence, in Criminal Violence. Edited by Wolfgang ME, Weiner NA, Cook PJ, et al. Beverly Hills, CA, Sage, 1982, pp 21–80

Mednick SA, Gabrielli WF Jr, Hutchings B: Genetic influences in criminal convictions: evidence from an adoption cohort. Science 224:891–894, 1984

Megargee EI: Psychological determinants and correlates of criminal violence, in Criminal Violence. Edited by Wolfgang ME, Weiner NA, Cook PJ, et al. Beverly Hills, CA, Sage, 1982, pp 81–170

Megargee EI, Bohn MJ Jr: A new classification system for criminal offenders IV: empirically determined characteristics of the ten types. Crim Justice Behav 4:149–210, 1977

Melella JT, Travin S, Cullen K: Legal and ethical issues in the use of antiandrogens in treating sex offenders. Bull Am Acad Psychiatry Law 17:223–232, 1989

Mellow AM, Solano-Lopez C, Davis S: Sodium valproate in the treatment of behavioral disturbance in dementia. J Geriatr Psychiatry Neurol 6:205–209, 1993

Mendelson JH, Mello NK: Alcohol, aggression and androgens, in Aggression. Edited by Frazier SH. Baltimore, MD, Williams & Wilkins, 1974, pp 225–247

Mendelson JH, Mello NK, Ellingboe J: Effects of alcohol on pituitary-gonadal hormones, sexual function, and aggression in human males, in Psychopharmacology: A Generation of Progress. Edited by Lipton MA, DiMascio A, Killam KF. New York, Raven, 1978, pp 1677–1692

Mendelson W, Johnson N, Stewart MA: Hyperactive children as teenagers: a follow-up study. J Nerv Ment Dis 153:273–279, 1971

Mendez MF, Doss RC, Taylor JL: Interictal violence in epilepsy. Relationship to behavior and seizure variables. J Nerv Ment Dis 181:566–569, 1993

Menditto AA, Beck NC, Stuve P, et al: Effectiveness of clozapine and a social learning program for severely disabled psychiatric inpatients. Psychiatr Serv 47:46–51, 1996

Menzies RJ, Webster CD, Sepejak D: Hitting the forensic sound barrier: predictions of dangerousness in a pretrial psychiatric clinic, in Dangerousness. Edited by Webster CD, Ben Aron HM, Hucker SJ. New York, Cambridge University Press, 1985, pp 115–143

Meyer-Bahlburg HFL, Ehrhardt AA: Prenatal sex hormones and human aggression: a review, and new data on progestogen effects. Aggressive Behavior 8:39–62, 1982

Meyer-Bahlburg HFL, Nat R, Boon DA, et al: Aggressiveness and testosterone measures in man. Psychosom Med 36:269–274, 1974

Michals ML, Crismon ML, Roberts S, et al: Clozapine response and adverse effects in nine brain-injured patients. J Clin Psychopharmacol 13:198–203, 1993

Miczek KA: The Psychopharmacology of Aggression, in Handbook of Psychopharmacology, Vol 19. Edited by Iversen LL, Iversen SD, Snyder SH. New York, Plenum, 1987, pp 230–231

Miczek KA, Tidey JW: Amphetamines: aggressive and social behavior. NIDA Res Monogr 94:68–100, 1989

Miczek KA, Thompson ML, Shuster L: Opioid-like analgesia in defeated mice. Science 215:1520–1522, 1982

Miles DR, Carey G: Genetic and environmental architecture of human aggression. J Pers Soc Psychol 72:207–217, 1997

Milich R, Kramer J: Reflections on impulsivity: an empirical investigation of impulsivity as a construct. Advances in Learning and Behavioral Disabilities 3:57–94, 1984

Miller BL, Pachter JS, Valzelli L: Brain tryptophan in isolated aggressive mice. Neuropsychobiology 5:11–15, 1979

Miller MH: Dorsolateral frontal lobe lesions and behavior in the macaque: dissociation of threat and aggression. Physiology and Behavior 17:209–213, 1976

Millson RC, Delva NJ: Clozapine to olanzapine (letter). Am J Psychiatry 156:1121, 1999

Milton J, Amin S, Singh SP, et al: Aggressive incidents in first-episode psychosis. Br J Psychiatry 178:433–440, 2001

Mintzer J, Brawman-Mintzer O, Mirski DF, et al: Fenfluramine challenge test as a marker of serotonin activity in patients with Alzheimer's dementia and agitation. Biol Psychiatry 44:918–921, 1998

Mitchell C: Intoxication, criminality, and responsibility. Int J Law Psychiatry 13:1–7, 1990

Moffitt TE: Parental mental disorder and offspring criminal behavior: an adoption study. Psychiatry 50:346–360, 1987

Moffitt TE, Silva PA: Neuropsychological deficit and self-reported delinquency in an unselected birth cohort. J Am Acad Child Adolesc Psychiatry 27:233–240, 1988

Moffitt TE, Brammer GL, Caspi A, et al: Whole blood serotonin relates to violence in an epidemiological study. Biol Psychiatry 43:446–457, 1998

Monahan J: The psychiatrization of criminal behavior: a reply. Hosp Community Psychiatry 24:105–107, 1973

Monahan J: Predicting Violent Behavior. An Assessment of Clinical Techniques. Beverly Hills, CA, Sage, 1981

Monahan J: Mental disorder and violent behavior. Perceptions and evidence. Am Psychol 47:511–521, 1992

Monahan J: Limiting therapist exposure to Tarasoff liability. Guidelines for risk containment. Am Psychol 48:242–250, 1993

Monahan J, Steadman HJ: Crime and mental disorder: an epidemiological approach, in An Annual Review of Research (Crime and Justice Series, Vol 7). Edited by Tonry M, Morris N. Chicago, IL, University of Chicago Press, 1983, pp 145–189

Monahan J, Steadman HJ: Toward a rejuvenation of risk assessment research, in Violence and Mental Disorder: Developments in Risk Assessment. Edited by Monahan J, Steadman HJ. Chicago, IL, University of Chicago Press, 1994, pp 1–17

Monahan J, Steadman HJ, Appelbaum PS, et al: Developing a clinically useful actuarial tool for assessing violence risk. Br J Psychiatry 176:312–319, 2000

Money J: Use of an androgen-depleting hormone in the treatment of male sex offenders. J Sex Res 6(3):165–172, 1991

Money J, Ehrhardt AA: Gender dimorphic behavior and fetal sex hormones. Recent Prog Horm Res 28:735–763, 1972

Monroe RR: Episodic Behavioral Disorders. Cambridge, MA, Harvard University Press, 1970

Monroe RR: Anticonvulsants in the treatment of aggression. J Nerv Ment Dis 160:119–126, 1975

Monroe RR: Brain Dysfunction in Aggressive Criminals. Lexington, MA, Lexington Books, 1978

Monti PM, Brown WA, Corriveau DP: Testosterone and components of aggressive and sexual behavior in man. Am J Psychiatry 134:692–694, 1977

Morand C, Young SN, Ervin FR: Clinical response of aggressive schizophrenics to oral tryptophan. Biol Psychiatry 18:575–578, 1983

Morrow B, Goldberg R, Carlson C, et al: Molecular definition of the 22q11 deletions in velo-cardio-facial syndrome. Am J Hum Genet 56:1391–1403, 1995

Morton J, Additon H, Addison R, et al: A clinical study of premenstrual tension. Am J Obstet Gynecol 65:1182–1191, 1953

Moses LE: Criminality and adoption. Science 227:983–984, 1985

Moss HB, Panzak GL: Steroid use and aggression (letter). Am J Psychiatry 149:1616, 1992

Moss HB, Yao JK, Panzak GL: Serotonergic responsivity and behavioral dimensions in antisocial personality disorder with substance abuse. Biol Psychiatry 28:325–338, 1990

Moyer KE: The Psychobiology of Aggression. New York, Harper & Row, 1976

Mulvey EP, Blumstein A, Cohen J: Reframing the research question of mental patient criminality. Int J Law Psychiatry 9:57–65, 1986

Murdoch D, Pihl RO, Ross D: Alcohol and crimes of violence: present issues. Int J Addict 25:1065–1081, 1990

Murray N: Covert effects of chlordiazepoxide therapy. Journal of Neuropsychiatry 3:168–170, 1961

Muscat JE: Characteristics of childhood homicide in Ohio, 1974–84. Am J Public Health 78:822–824, 1988

Myers KM, Dunner DL: Self and other directed violence on a closed acute-care ward. Psychiatr Q 56:178–188, 1984

Mysiw WJ, Jackson RD, Corrigan JD: Amitriptyline for post-traumatic agitation. Am J Phys Med Rehabil 67:29–33, 1988

Nachshon I: Hemisphere dysfunction in psychopathy and behavior disorders, in Hemisyndromes: Psychobiology, Neurology, Psychiatry. Edited by Myslobodsky M. New York, Academic Press, 1983, pp 389–414

Nachshon I: Hemisphere function in violent offenders, in Biological Contributions to Crime Causation. Edited by Moffitt TE, Mednick SA. Dordrecht, Netherlands, Martinus Nijhoff, 1988, pp 55–67

Nagao T, Ohshimo T, Mitsunobu K, et al: Cerebrospinal fluid monoamine metabolites and cyclic nucleotides in chronic schizophrenic patients with tardive dyskinesia or drug-induced tremor. Biol Psychiatry 14:509–523, 1979

Neppe VM: Carbamazepine as adjunctive treatment in nonepileptic chronic inpatients with EEG temporal lobe abnormalities. J Clin Psychiatry 44:326–331, 1983

Ness JW, Franchina JJ: Effects of prenatal alcohol exposure on rat pups' ability to elicit retrieval behavior from dams. Dev Psychobiol 23:85–99, 1990

Nettler G: Explaining Crime. New York, McGraw-Hill, 1978

Neugebauer R, Hoek HW, Susser E: Prenatal exposure to wartime famine and development of antisocial personality disorder in early adulthood (see comments). JAMA 282:455–462, 1999

New AS, Gelernter J, Yovell Y, et al: Tryptophan hydroxylase genotype is associated with impulsive-aggression measures: a preliminary study. Am J Med Genet 81:13–17, 1998

New AS, Gelernter J, Mitropoulou V, et al: Impulsive aggression associated with HTR1B genotype in personality disorders (abstract no NR388), in New Research Program and Abstracts, American Psychiatric Association 152nd Annual Meeting, May 15–20, 1999. Washington, DC, American Psychiatric Association, 1999, p 172

New AS, Goodman M, Mitropoulou V, et al: Serotonin-related genes and impulsive aggression in personality disorders (abstract). Biol Psychiatry 47:118S, 2000

Ng B, Kumar S, Ranclaud M, et al: Ward crowding and incidents of violence on an acute psychiatric inpatient unit. Psychiatr Serv 52:521–525, 2001

Ng SK, Hauser WA, Brust JC, et al: Alcohol consumption and withdrawal in new-onset seizures. N Engl J Med 319:666–673, 1988

Niedermeyer E, Lopes da Silva F: Epileptic seizure disorders, in Electroencephalography: Basic Principles, Clinical Applications and Related Fields, 2nd Edition. Baltimore, MD, Urban & Schwarzenberg, 1987, pp 405–510

Nielsen DA, Virkkunen M, Lappalainen J, et al: A tryptophan hydroxylase gene marker for suicidality and alcoholism. Arch Gen Psychiatry 55:593–602, 1998

Nijman HLI, Muris P, Merckelbach HLGJ, et al: The Staff Observation Aggression Scale–Revised (SOAS-R). Aggressive Behavior 25:197–209, 1999

Niswander KR, Gordon M: The Women and Their Pregnancies. Washington, DC, National Institute of Health, 1972

Nolan KA, Citrome L, Volavka J: Violence in schizophrenia: the roles of psychosis and psychopathy. Journal of Practical Psychiatry and Behavioral Health 5:326–335, 1999a

Nolan KA, Volavka J, Mohr P, et al: Psychopathy and violent behavior among patients with schizophrenia or schizoaffective disorder. Psychiatr Serv 50:787–792, 1999b

Nolan KA, Volavka J, Lachman HM, et al: An association between a polymorphism of the tryptophan hydroxylase gene and aggression in schizophrenia and schizoaffective disorder. Psychiatr Genet 10:109–115, 2000

Oddy M, Coughlan T, Tyerman A, et al: Social adjustment after closed head injury: a further follow-up seven years after injury. J Neurol Neurosurg Psychiatry 48:564–568, 1985

O'Gorman JG, Lloyd JEM: Extraversion, impulsiveness, and EEG alpha activity. Pers Individ Dif 8:169–174, 1987

Okasha A, Sadek AO, Moneim SA: Psychosocial and electroencephalographic studies of Egyptian murderers. Br J Psychiatry 126:34–40, 1975

Okuma T, Yamashita I, Takahashi R, et al: A double-blind study of adjunctive carbamazepine versus placebo on excited states of schizophrenic and schizoaffective disorders. Acta Psychiatr Scand 80:250–259, 1989

Olivier B, Mos J, van Oorschot R: Maternal aggression in rats: effects of chlordiazepoxide and fluprazine. Psychopharmacology 86:68–76, 1985

Olivier B, Mos J, Rasmussen D: Behavioural pharmacology of the serenic, eltoprazine. Drug Metabol Drug Interact 8:31–83, 1990

Olweus D: Stability of aggressive reaction patterns in males: a review. Psychol Bull 86:852–875, 1979

Olweus D, Mattsson A, Schalling D, et al: Testosterone, aggression, physical, and personality dimensions in normal adolescent males. Psychosom Med 42:253–269, 1980

Olweus D, Mattsson A, Schalling D, et al: Circulating testosterone levels and aggression in adolescent males: a causal analysis. Psychosom Med 50:261–272, 1988

O'Neil M, Page N, Adkins WN, et al: Tryptophan-trazodone treatment of aggressive behaviour (letter). Lancet 2:859–860, 1986

Owen DR: The 47,XYY male: a review. Psychol Bull 78:209–233, 1972

Pallmeyer TP, Petti TA: Effects of imipramine on aggression and dejection in depressed children. Am J Psychiatry 136:1472–1473, 1979

Palmstierna T, Wistedt B: Staff Observation Aggression Scale, SOAS: presentation and evaluation. Acta Psychiatr Scand 76:657–663, 1987

Palmstierna T, Huitfeldt B, Wistedt B: The relationship of crowding and aggressive behavior on a psychiatric intensive care unit. Hosp Community Psychiatry 42:1237–1240, 1991

Palmstierna T, Nijman H, Wistedt B, et al: Revision of the Staff Observation Aggression Scale (SOAS): comment on Hallsteinsen et al. (letter). Acta Psychiatr Scand 100:80–81, 1999

Papolos DF, Faedda GL, Veit S, et al: Bipolar spectrum disorders in patients diagnosed with velo-cardio-facial-syndrome: does hemizygous deletion of chromosome 22q11 result in bipolar affective disorder? Am J Psychiatry 153:1541–1547, 1996

Papolos DF, Veit S, Faedda GL, et al: Ultra-ultra rapid cycling bipolar disorder is associated with the low activity catecholamine-O-methyltransferase allele. Mol Psychiatry 3:346–349, 1998

Parikh MK, Hegarty AM, Sancho EP: Use of ECT for severe episodic aggression in patients with treatment-refractory psychosis (abstract no NR76), in 2000 New Research Program and Abstracts, American Psychiatric Association 153rd Annual Meeting, Chicago, IL, May 13–18, 2000. Washington, DC, American Psychiatric Association, 2000, p 76

Pasamanick B, Knobloch H: Brain damage and reproductive casualty. Am J Orthopsychiatry 30:298–305, 1960

Pastore AL, Maguire K (eds): Sourcebook of Criminal Justice Statistics, 1999 (online). <http://www.albany.edu/sourcebook/> 2000

Patterson GR, Reid JB, Dishion TJ: A Social Interactional Approach. Vol 4: Antisocial Boys. Eugene, OR, Castalia, 1992

Peck C: The randomized concentration-controlled clinical trial (CCT): an information-rich alternative to the randomized placebo-controlled trial (PCT) (abstract). Clin Pharmacol Ther 47:148, 1990

Peet M, Middlemiss DN, Yates RA: Propranolol in schizophrenia. II. Clinical and biochemical aspects of combining propranolol with chlorpromazine. Br J Psychiatry 139:112–117, 1981

Perez-Cruet J, Tagliamonte A, Tagliamonte P, et al: Stimulation of serotonin synthesis by lithium. J Pharmacol Exp Ther 178:325–330, 1971

Perez-Pena R: Morgenthau says release was an error. The New York Times, July 23, 1993, p B3

Pernanen K: Alcohol in Human Violence. New York, Guilford, 1991

Persky H, Smith KD, Basu GK: Relation of psychologic measures of aggression and hostility to testosterone production in man. Psychosom Med 33:265–277, 1971

Petersen KGI, Matousek M, Mednick SA, et al: EEG antecedents of thievery. Acta Psychiatr Scand 65:331–338, 1982

Peterson BS, Vohr B, Staib LH, et al: Regional brain volume abnormalities and long-term cognitive outcome in preterm infants. JAMA 284:1939–1947, 2000

Petrich J: Psychiatric treatment in jail: an experiment in health-care delivery. Hosp Community Psychiatry 27:413–415, 1976

Petrie WM, Ban TA: Propranolol in organic agitation (letter). Lancet 1:324, 1981

Phillips MR, Wolf AS, Coons DJ: Psychiatry and the criminal justice system: testing the myths. Am J Psychiatry 145:605–610, 1988

Pietrini P, Guazzelli M, Basso G, et al: Neural correlates of imaginal aggressive behavior assessed by positron emission tomography in healthy subjects. Am J Psychiatry 157:1772–1781, 2000

Pihl RO, Ervin F: Lead and cadmium levels in violent criminals. Psychol Rep 66:839–844, 1990

Pihl RO, Peterson JB: Alcohol/drug use and aggressive behavior, in Mental Disorder and Crime. Newbury Park, CA, Sage, 1993, pp 263–283

Pillmann F, Rohde A, Ullrich S, et al: Violence, criminal behavior, and the EEG: significance of left hemispheric focal abnormalities. J Neuropsychiatry Clin Neurosci 11:454–457, 1999

Pine DS, Coplan JD, Wasserman GA, et al: Neuroendocrine response to fenfluramine challenge in boys. Associations with aggressive behavior and adverse rearing. Arch Gen Psychiatry 54:839–846, 1997

Pinner E, Rich CL: Effects of trazodone on aggressive behavior in seven patients with organic mental disorders. Am J Psychiatry 145:1295–1296, 1988

Platt JE, Campbell M, Green WH, et al: Effects of lithium carbonate and haloperidol on cognition in aggressive hospitalized school-age children. J Clin Psychopharmacol 1:8–13, 1981

Plomin R, Loehlin JC, DeFries JC: Genetic and environmental components of "environmental" influences. Dev Psychol 21:391–402, 1985

Plutchik R, Van Praag H: Psychosocial correlates of suicide and violence risk, in Violence and Suicidality: Perspectives in Clinical and Psychobiological Research. Edited by Van Praag HM, Plutchik R, Apter A. New York, Brunner/Mazel, 1990, pp 37–65

Plutchik R, Van Praag HM, Conte HR: Correlates of suicide and violence risk: III. A two-stage model of countervailing forces. Psychiatry Res 28:215–225, 1989

Polakoff SA, Sorgi PJ, Ratey JJ: The treatment of impulsive and aggressive behavior with nadolol (letter). J Clin Psychopharmacol 6:125–126, 1986

Pollak R: The epilepsy defense. Atlantic Monthly, May 1984, pp 20–28

Pollock VE, Volavka J, Goodwin DW, et al: The EEG after alcohol administration in men at risk for alcoholism. Arch Gen Psychiatry 40:857–861, 1983

Pollock VE, Briere J, Schneider L, et al: Childhood antecedents of antisocial behavior: parental alcoholism and physical abusiveness. Am J Psychiatry 147:1290–1293, 1990

Pontius AA: Specific stimulus-evoked violent action in psychotic trigger reaction: a seizure-like imbalance between frontal lobe and limbic systems? Percept Mot Skills 59:299–333, 1984

Pontius AA, Yudowitz BS: Frontal lobe dysfunction in some criminal actions shown in the narratives test. J Nerv Ment Dis 168:111–117, 1980

Pope HG Jr, Katz DL: Affective and psychotic symptoms associated with anabolic steroid use. Am J Psychiatry 145:487–490, 1988

Pope HG Jr, Katz DL: Homicide and near-homicide by anabolic steroid users. J Clin Psychiatry 51:28–31, 1990

Pope HG Jr, Katz DL: Psychiatric and medical effects of anabolic-androgenic steroid use. A controlled study of 160 athletes. Arch Gen Psychiatry 51:375–382, 1994

Pope HG Jr, Kouri EM, Powell KF, et al: Anabolic-androgenic steroid use among 133 prisoners. Compr Psychiatry 37:322–327, 1996

Pope HG Jr, Kouri EM, Hudson JI: Effects of supraphysiologic doses of testosterone on mood and aggression in normal men: a randomized controlled trial. Arch Gen Psychiatry 57:133–140, 2000

Poshivalov VP: Ethological analysis of neuropeptides and psychotropic drugs: effects on intraspecies aggression and sociability of isolated mice. Aggressive Behavior 8:355–369, 1982

Prakash R: Lithium-responsive schizophrenia: case reports. J Clin Psychiatry 46:141–142, 1985

Puglisi-Allegra S: Effects of sodium n-dipropylacetate, muscimol hydrobromide and (R,S) nipecotic acid amide on isolation-induced aggressive behavior. Psychopharmacology 70:287–290, 1980

Pulver AE, Nestadt G, Goldberg R, et al: Psychotic illness in patients diagnosed with velo-cardio-facial syndrome and their relatives. J Nerv Ment Dis 182:476–478, 1994

Quattrone A, Tedeschi G, Aguglia U, et al: Prolactin secretion in man: a useful tool to evaluate the activity of drugs on central 5-hydroxytryptaminergic neurones. Studies with fenfluramine. Br J Clin Pharmacol 16:471–475, 1983

Quiason N, Ward D, Kitchen T: Buspirone for aggression (letter). J Am Acad Child Adolesc Psychiatry 30:1026, 1991

Quinsey VL: The baserate problem and the prediction of dangerousness: a reappraisal. J Psychiatry Law 8:329–340, 1980

Quitkin F, Rifkin A, Klein DF: Neurologic soft signs in schizophrenia and character disorders. Organicity in schizophrenia with premorbid asociality and emotionally unstable character disorders. Arch Gen Psychiatry 33:845–853, 1976

Rabinowitz J, Avnon M, Rosenberg V: Effect of clozapine on physical and verbal aggression. Schizophr Res 22:249–255, 1996

Rabinowitz J, Mar M: Risk factors for violence among long-stay psychiatric patients: national study. Acta Psychiatr Scand 99:341–347, 1999

Rabkin JG: Criminal behavior of discharged mental patients: a critical appraisal of the research. Psychol Bull 86:1–27, 1979

Rada RT, Laws DR, Kellner R: Plasma testosterone levels in the rapist. Psychosom Med 38:257–268, 1976

Rada RT, Laws DR, Kellner R, et al: Plasma androgens in violent and nonviolent sex offenders. Bull Am Acad Psychiatry Law 11:149–158, 1983

Raine A: Evoked potentials and antisocial behavior, in Biological Contributions to Crime Causation. Edited by Moffitt TE, Mednick SA. Dordrecht, Netherlands, Martinus Nijhoff, 1988, pp 14–39

Raine A: The Psychopathology of Crime: Criminal Behavior as a Clinical Disorder. San Diego, CA, Academic Press, 1993

Raine A, Brennan P, Mednick SA: Birth complications combined with early maternal rejection at age 1 year predispose to violent crime at age 18 years. Arch Gen Psychiatry 51:984–988, 1994

Raine A, Brennan P, Mednick SA: Interaction between birth complications and early maternal rejection in predisposing individuals to adult violence: specificity to serious, early onset violence. Am J Psychiatry 154:1265–1271, 1997a

Raine A, Buchsbaum M, LaCasse L: Brain abnormalities in murderers indicated by positron emission tomography. Biol Psychiatry 42:495–508, 1997b

Raine A, Bihrle S, Buchsbaum M: Prefrontal glucose deficits in murderers lacking psychosocial deprivation. Neuropsychiatry Neuropsychol Behav Neurol 11:1–7, 1998a

Raine A, Reynolds C, Venables PH, et al: Fearlessness, stimulation-seeking, and large body size at age 3 years as early predispositions to childhood aggression at age 11 years. Arch Gen Psychiatry 55:745–751, 1998b

Raine A, Venables PH, Williams M: Autonomic orienting responses in 15-year-old male subjects and criminal behavior at age 24. Am J Psychiatry 147:933–937, 1990a

Raine A, Venables PH, Williams M: Relationships between central and autonomic measures of arousal at age 15 years and criminality at age 24 years. Arch Gen Psychiatry 47:1003–1007, 1990b

Raine A, Lencz T, Bihrle S, et al: Reduced prefrontal gray matter volume and reduced autonomic activity in antisocial personality disorder. Arch Gen Psychiatry 57:119–127, 2000

Raleigh MJ: Differential behavioral effects of tryptophan and 5-hydroxytryptophan in vervet monkeys: influence of catecholaminergic systems. Psychopharmacology 93:44–50, 1987

Raleigh MJ, Steklis HD, Ervin FR, et al: The effects of orbitofrontal lesions on the aggressive behavior of vervet monkeys (Cercopithecus aethiops sabaeus). Exp Neurol 66:158–168, 1979

Ralls K: Mammals in which females are larger than males. Q Rev Biol 51:245–276, 1976

Ramani V, Gumnit RJ: Intensive monitoring of epileptic patients with a history of episodic aggression. Arch Neurol 38:570–571, 1981

Ramesh N, Sandson NB: An analysis of recent valproate prescribing trends. (abstract no NR114), in 2000 New Research Program and Abstracts, American Psychiatric Association 153rd Annual Meeting, Chicago, IL, May 13–18, 2000. Washington, DC, American Psychiatric Association, 2000, p 87

Rampling D: Aggression: a paradoxical response to tricyclic antidepressants. Am J Psychiatry 135:117–118, 1978

Randall LO, Schallek W, Heise GA, et al: The psychosedative properties of methaminodiazepoxide. Journal of Pharmacology and Clinical Therapeutics 129:163–171, 1960

Rantakallio P, Laara E, Isohanni M, et al: Maternal smoking during pregnancy and delinquency of the offspring: an association without causation? Int J Epidemiol 21:1106–1113, 1992

Rasanen P, Tiihonen J, Isohanni M, et al: Schizophrenia, alcohol abuse, and violent behavior: a 26-year followup study of an unselected birth cohort. Schizophr Bull 24:437–441, 1998

Rasanen P, Hakko H, Jarvelin M-R, et al: Is a large body size during childhood a risk factor for later aggression? (letter). Arch Gen Psychiatry 56:283–284, 1999

Rasmussen K, Levander S: Symptoms and personality characteristics of patients in a maximum security psychiatric unit. Int J Law Psychiatry 19:27–37, 1996

Ratey JJ, Gutheil CM: The measurement of aggressive behavior: reflections on the use of the Overt Aggression Scale and the Modified Overt Aggression Scale. J Neuropsychiatry Clin Neurosci 3:S57-S60, 1991

Ratey JJ, Morrill R, Oxenkrug G: Use of propranolol for provoked and unprovoked episodes of rage. Am J Psychiatry 140:1356–1357, 1983

Ratey JJ, Mikkelsen EJ, Smith GB, et al: Beta-blockers in the severely and profoundly mentally retarded. J Clin Psychopharmacol 6:103–107, 1986

Ratey JJ, Sovner R, Mikkelsen E, et al: Buspirone therapy for maladaptive behavior and anxiety in developmentally disabled persons. J Clin Psychiatry 50:382–384, 1989

Ratey J, Sovner R, Parks A, et al: Buspirone treatment of aggression and anxiety in mentally retarded patients: a multiple-baseline, placebo lead-in study. J Clin Psychiatry 52:159–162, 1991

Ratey JJ, Sorgi P, O'Driscoll GA, et al: Nadolol to treat aggression and psychiatric symptomatology in chronic psychiatric inpatients: a double-blind, placebo-controlled study. J Clin Psychiatry 53:41–46, 1992

Ratey JJ, Leveroni C, Kilmer D, et al: The effects of clozapine on severely aggressive psychiatric inpatients in a state hospital. J Clin Psychiatry 54:219–223, 1993

Regan D: Human Brain Electrophysiology: Evoked Potentials and Evoked Magnetic Fields in Science and Medicine. New York, Elsevier, 1989

Regier DA, Myers JK, Kramer M, et al: The NIMH Epidemiologic Catchment Area program. Historical context, major objectives, and study population characteristics. Arch Gen Psychiatry 41:934–941, 1984

Regier DA, Boyd JH, Burke JD Jr, et al: One-month prevalence of mental disorders in the United States. Based on five Epidemiologic Catchment Area sites. Arch Gen Psychiatry 45:977–986, 1988

Regier DA, Farmer ME, Rae DS, et al: Comorbidity of mental disorders with alcohol and other drug abuse. Results from the Epidemiologic Catchment Area (ECA) Study. JAMA 264:2511–2518, 1990

Reinisch JM: Prenatal exposure to synthetic progestins increases potential for aggression in humans. Science 211:1171–1173, 1981

Resnick RB, Kestenbaum RS, Schwartz LK: Acute systemic effects of cocaine in man: a controlled study by intranasal and intravenous routes. Science 195:696–698, 1977

Rice ME: Violent offender research and implications for the criminal justice system. Am Psychol 52:414–423, 1997

Rice ME, Harris GT: Psychopathy, schizophrenia, alcohol abuse, and violent recidivism. Int J Law Psychiatry 18:333–342, 1995

Riley EP: The long-term behavioral effects of prenatal alcohol exposure in rats. Alcohol Clin Exp Res 14:670–673, 1990

Riley TL: The electroencephalogram in patients with rage attacks or episodic violent behavior. Mil Med 144:515–517, 1979

Robertson G: Arrest patterns among mentally disordered offenders. Br J Psychiatry 153:313–316, 1988

Robins LN: Deviant Children Grown Up. Melbourne, Robert E. Krieger, 1974

Robins LN: Sturdy childhood predictors of adult antisocial behaviour: replications from longitudinal studies. Psychol Med 8:611–622, 1978

Robins LN, Helzer JE, Croughan J, et al: NIMH Diagnostic Interview Schedule: Version III (unpublished). Rockville, MD, National Institute of Mental Health, Division of Biometry and Epidemiology, 1981

Robins LN, Helzer JE, Weissman MM, et al: Lifetime prevalence of specific psychiatric disorders in three sites. Arch Gen Psychiatry 41:949–958, 1984

Robinson D, Woerner MG, Pollack S, et al: Subject selection biases in clinical trials: data from a multicenter schizophrenia treatment study. J Clin Psychopharmacol 16:170–176, 1996

Rodgers RJ: Differential effects of naloxone and diprenorphine on defensive behavior in rats. Neuropharmacology 21:1291–1294, 1982

Rodin EA: Psychomotor epilepsy and aggressive behavior. Arch Gen Psychiatry 28:210–213, 1973

Rodin EA, Katz M, Lennox K: Differences between patients with temporal lobe seizures and those with other forms of epileptic attacks. Epilepsia 17:313–320, 1976

Rofman ES, Askinazi C, Fant E: The prediction of dangerous behavior in emergency civil commitment. Am J Psychiatry 137:1061–1064, 1980

Rogers R, Seman W: Murder and criminal responsibility: an examination of MMPI profiles. Behav Sci Law 1:90–95, 1983

Rosenbaum A, Hoge SK: Head injury and marital aggression. Am J Psychiatry 146:1048–1051, 1989

Rosenbaum JF, Fava M, Pava JA, et al: Anger attacks in unipolar depression, part 2: Neuroendocrine correlates and changes following fluoxetine treatment. Am J Psychiatry 150:1164–1168, 1993

Rossi AM, Jacobs M, Monteleone M, et al: Violent or fear-inducing behavior associated with hospital admission. Hosp Community Psychiatry 36:643–647, 1985

Rossi AM, Jacobs M, Monteleone M, et al: Characteristics of psychiatric patients who engage in assaultive or other fear-inducing behaviors. J Nerv Ment Dis 174:154–160, 1986

Rosvold HE, Mirsky AF, Pribram KH: Influence of amygdalectomy on social behavior in monkeys. J Comp Physiol Psychol 47:173–178, 1954

Rotondo A, Mazzanti CM, Lunardi A, et al: Evidence for association of the catechol-O-methyltransferase gene with bipolar disorder and aggressive behavior. Paper presented at the World Congress of Psychiatric Genetics, Monterey, CA, October 14–18, 1999

Roy A, Virkkunen M, Linnoila M: Serotonin in suicide, violence and alcoholism, in Serotonin in Major Psychiatric Disorders. Edited by Coccaro EF, Murphy DL. Washington, DC, American Psychiatric Press, 1990, pp 185–208

Royalty J: Effects of prenatal ethanol exposure on juvenile play-fighting and post-pubertal aggression in rats. Psychol Rep 66:551–560, 1990

Ruble DN: Premenstrual symptoms: a reinterpretation. Science 197:291–292, 1977

Ryback R, Ryback L: Gabapentin for behavioral dyscontrol (letter). Am J Psychiatry 152:1399, 1995

Sadoff RL: Political and legal perspectives, in The Premenstrual Syndrome. Edited by Keye WR Jr. Philadelphia, PA, WB Saunders, 1988, pp 15–26

Saito T, Lachman H, Mohr P, et al: Lack of association between violence in schizophrenia and polymorphisms in genes that regulate serotonin transmission (abstract no NR111), in 1999 New Research Program and Abstracts, American Psychiatric Association 152nd Annual Meeting, Washington, DC, May 15–20, 1999. Washington, DC, American Psychiatric Association, 1999, pp 92–93

Salzman C, Kochansky GE, Shader RI, et al: Chlordiazepoxide-induced hostility in a small group setting. Arch Gen Psychiatry 31:401–405, 1974

Salzman C, Kochansky GE, Shader RI, et al: Is oxazepam associated with hostility? Dis Nerv Syst 36:30–32, 1975

Sandor P, Stephens RJ: Risperidone treatment of aggressive behavior in children with Tourette syndrome (letter). J Clin Psychopharmacol 20:710–712, 2000

Sapolsky RM: Hypercortisolism among socially subordinate wild baboons originates at the CNS level. Arch Gen Psychiatry 46:1047–1051, 1989

Sapolsky RM: A.E. Bennett Award paper. Adrenocortical function, social rank, and personality among wild baboons. Biol Psychiatry 28:862–878, 1990

Sapolsky R, Ray J: Styles of dominance and their physiological correlates among wild baboons. Am J Primatol 18:1–13, 1989

Sartorius N, Jablensky A, Korten A, et al: Early manifestations and first-contact incidence of schizophrenia in different cultures. A preliminary report on the initial evaluation phase of the WHO collaborative study on determinants of outcome of severe mental disorders. Psychol Med 16:909–928, 1986

Satterfield JH, Hoppe CM, Schell AM: A prospective study of delinquency in 110 adolescent boys with attention deficit disorder and 88 normal adolescent boys. Am J Psychiatry 139:795–798, 1982

Sayed ZA, Lewis SA, Brittain RP: An electroencephalographic and psychiatric study of thirty-two insane murderers. Br J Psychiatry 115:1115–1124, 1969

Sayegh JF, Kobor G, Lajtha A, et al: Effects of social isolation and the time of day on testosterone levels in plasma of C57BL/6By and BALB/cBy mice. Steroids 55:79–82, 1990

Schaffer CB, Schaffer LC: Gabapentin in the treatment of bipolar disorder (letter). Am J Psychiatry 154:291–292, 1997

Schalling D: Neurochemical correlates of personality, impulsivity, and disinhibitory suicidality, in Mental Disorder and Crime. Edited by Hodgins H. Newbury Park, CA, Sage, 1993, pp 208–226

Schalling D, Edman G, Asberg M, et al: Platelet MAO activity associated with impulsivity and aggressivity. Pers Individ Dif 9:597–605, 1988

Schiavi RC, Theilgaard A, Owen DR, et al: Sex chromosome anomalies, hormones, and aggressivity. Arch Gen Psychiatry 41:93–99, 1984

Schiff HB, Sabin TD, Geller A, et al: Lithium in aggressive behavior. Am J Psychiatry 139:1346–1348, 1982

Schooler NR: Maintenance medication for schizophrenia: strategies for dose reduction. Schizophr Bull 17:311–324, 1991

Schreier HA: Use of propranolol in the treatment of postencephalitic psychosis. Am J Psychiatry 136:840–841, 1979

Schroeder ML, Schroeder KG, Hare RD: Generalizability of a checklist for assessment of psychopathy. J Consult Clin Psychol 51:511–516, 1983

Schuckit MA, Herrman G, Schuckit JJ: The importance of psychiatric illness in newly arrested prisoners. J Nerv Ment Dis 165:118–125, 1977

Schuerman LA, Solomon K: Exposure of community mental health clients to the criminal justice system: client/criminal or patient/prisoner, in Mental Health and Criminal Justice. Edited by Teplin LA. Beverly Hills, CA, Sage, 1984, pp 87–118

Schulte HM, Hall MJ, Boyer M: Domestic violence associated with anabolic steroid abuse (letter). Am J Psychiatry 150:348, 1993

Schulz KP, Newcorn JH, McKay KE, et al: Relationship between central serotonergic function and aggression in prepubertal boys: effect of age and attention-deficit/hyperactivity disorder. Psychiatry Res 101:1–10, 2001

Schuurman T: Hormonal correlates of agonistic behavior in adult male rats, in Adaptive Capabilities of the Nervous System (Progress in Brain Research, Vol 53). Edited by McConnel PS, Boer GJ, Romijn HJ et al. Amsterdam, Elsevier, 1980, pp 415–420

Scott JP, Fredericson E: The causes of fighting in mice and rats. Physiol Zool 24:273–309, 1951

Seidenwurm D, Pounds TR, Globus A, et al: Abnormal temporal lobe metabolism in violent subjects: correlation of imaging and neuropsychiatric findings. AJNR Am J Neuroradiol 18:625–631, 1997

Sellin T, Wolfgang ME: The Measurement of Delinquency. New York, Wiley, 1964

Senault B: Comportement d'aggresivité intraspécifique induit par l'apomorphine chez la rat. Psychopharmacologia 18:271–287, 1970

Sendi IB, Blomgren PG: A comparative study of predictive criteria in the predisposition of homicidal adolescents. Am J Psychiatry 132:423–427, 1975

Sepejak D, Menzies RJ, Webster CD, et al: Clinical predictions of dangerousness: two-year follow-up of 408 pre-trial forensic cases. Bull Am Acad Psychiatry Law 11:171–181, 1983

Serafetinides EA: Aggressiveness in temporal lobe epileptics and its relation to cerebral dysfunction and environmental factors. Epilepsia 6:33–42, 1965

Seroczynski AD, Bergeman CS, Coccaro EF: Etiology of the impulsivity/aggression relationship: genes or environment? Psychiatry Res 81:41–57, 1999

Shader RI, Jackson AH, Harmatz JS, et al: Patterns of violent behavior among schizophrenic inpatients. Dis Nerv Syst 38:13–16, 1977

Shaner A, Khalsa ME, Roberts L, et al: Unrecognized cocaine use among schizophrenic patients. Am J Psychiatry 150:758–762, 1993

Sharif ZA, Raza A, Ratakonda SS: Comparative efficacy of risperidone and clozapine in the treatment of patients with refractory schizophrenia or schizoaffective disorder: a retrospective analysis. J Clin Psychiatry 61:498–504, 2000

Shaywitz SE, Cohen DJ, Shaywitz BA: Behavior and learning difficulties in children of normal intelligence born to alcoholic mothers. J Pediatr 96:978–982, 1980

Sheard MH: Effect of lithium on human aggression. Nature 230:113–114, 1971

Sheard MH: Shock-induced fighting (SIF): psychopharmacological studies. Aggressive Behavior 7:41–49, 1981

Sheard MH, Marini JL, Bridges CI, et al: The effect of lithium on impulsive aggressive behavior in man. Am J Psychiatry 133:1409–1413, 1976

Sheppard GP: High-dose propranolol in schizophrenia. Br J Psychiatry 134:470–476, 1979

Shore D, Filson CR, Rae DS: Violent crime arrest rates of White House Case subjects and matched control subjects. Am J Psychiatry 147:746–750, 1990

Shprintzen RJ, Goldberg RB, Lewin ML, et al: A new syndrome involving cleft palate, cardiac anomalies, typical facies, and learning disabilities: velo-cardio-facial syndrome. Cleft Palate J 15:56–62, 1978

Shprintzen RJ, Goldberg R, Golding-Kushner KJ, et al: Late-onset psychosis in the velo-cardio-facial syndrome (letter). Am J Med Genet 42:141–142, 1992

Shumway RH: Discriminant analysis for time series, in Handbook of Statistics Vol 2. Edited by Krishnaiah PR, Kanal LN. Amsterdam, North-Holland, 1982, pp 1–46

Shupe LM: Alcohol and crime. J Crim Law Criminol Police Sci 44:661–664, 1954

Siever LJ, Buchsbaum MS, New AS, et al: d,l-fenfluramine response in impulsive personality disorder assessed with [18F]fluorodeoxyglucose positron emission tomography. Neuropsychopharmacology 20:413–423, 1999

Silver JM, Yudofsky SC: The overt aggression scale: overview and guiding principles. J Neuropsychiatry Clin Neurosci 3 (suppl):S22–S29, 1991

Silver JM, Yudofsky SC, Kogan M, et al: Elevation of thioridazine plasma levels by propranolol. Am J Psychiatry 143:1290–1292, 1986

Silver JM, Yudofsky SC, Slater JA, et al: Propranolol treatment of chronically hospitalized aggressive patients. J Neuropsychiatry Clin Neurosci 11:328–335, 1999

Simler S, Puglisi-Allegra S, Mandel P: Effects of n-di-propylacetate on aggressive behavior and brain GABA level in isolated mice. Pharmacol Biochem Behav 18:717–720, 1983

Simpson DM, Foster D: Improvement in organically disturbed behavior with trazodone treatment. J Clin Psychiatry 47:191–193, 1986

Singh Y, Jaiswal AK, Singh M, et al: Effect of prenatal diazepam, phenobarbital, haloperidol and fluoxetine exposure on foot shock induced aggression in rats. Indian J Exp Biol 36:1023–1024, 1998

Siris SG: Three cases of akathisia and "acting out." J Clin Psychiatry 46:395–397, 1985

Skirrow MH, Rysan M: Observations on the social behaviour of the Chinese hamster, Cricetulus griseus. Can J Zool 54:361–368, 1976

Small JG: The organic dimension of crime. Arch Gen Psychiatry 15:82–89, 1966

Small JG: Psychiatric disorders and EEG, in Electroencephalography. Basic Principles, Clinical Applications and Related Fields. Edited by Niedermeyer E, Lopes da Silva F. Baltimore, MD, Urban & Schwarzenberg, 1987, pp 528–529

Smith DA, Flynn JP: Afferent projection related to attack sites in the pontine tegmentum. Brain Res 164:103–119, 1979

Smith SE, Pihl RO, Young SN, et al: Elevation and reduction of plasma tryptophan and their effects on aggression and perceptual sensitivity in normal males. Aggress Behav 12:393–407, 1986

Smith SM, Honigsberger L, Smith CA: E.E.G., and personality factors in baby batterers. Br Med J 3:20–22, 1973

Snyder W: Hospital downsizing and increased frequency of assaults on staff. Hosp Community Psychiatry 45:378–380, 1994

Soloff PH, George A, Nathan RS, et al: Paradoxical effects of amitriptyline on borderline patients. Am J Psychiatry 143:1603–1605, 1986

Soloff PH, George A, Nathan RS, et al: Behavioral dyscontrol in borderline patients treated with amitriptyline. Psychopharmacol Bull 23:177–181, 1987

Soloff PH, Lynch KG, Moss HB: Serotonin, impulsivity, and alcohol use disorders in the older adolescent: a psychobiological study. Alcohol Clin Exp Res 24:1609–1619, 2000

Sorgi PJ, Ratey JJ, Polakoff S: Beta-adrenergic blockers for the control of aggressive behaviors in patients with chronic schizophrenia. Am J Psychiatry 143:775–776, 1986

Sorgi P, Ratey JJ, Knoedler DW, et al: Rating aggression in the clinical setting. A retrospective adaptation of the overt aggression scale: preliminary results. J Neuropsychiatry Clin Neurosci 3 (suppl):S52–S56, 1991

Soubrie E, Bizot JC: Monoaminergic control of waiting capacity (impulsivity) in animals, in Violence and Suicidality: Perspectives in Clinical and Biological Research. Edited by Van Praag HM, Plutchik R, Apter A. New York, Brunner/Mazel, 1990, pp 257–272

Spellacy F: Neuropsychological differences between violent and nonviolent adolescents. J Clin Psychol 33:966–969, 1977

Spellacy F: Neuropsychological discrimination between violent and non-violent men. J Clin Psychol 34:49–52, 1978

Spinweber CL, Ursin R, Hilbert RP, et al: L-tryptophan: effects on daytime sleep latency and the waking EEG. Electroencephalogr Clin Neurophysiol 55:652–661, 1983

Spivak B, Roitman S, Vered Y, et al: Diminished suicidal and aggressive behavior, high plasma norepinephrine levels, and serum triglyceride levels in chronic neuroleptic-resistant schizophrenic patients maintained on clozapine. Clin Neuropharmacol 21:245–250, 1998

Spreat S, Behar D, Reneski B, et al: Lithium carbonate for aggression in mentally retarded persons. Compr Psychiatry 30:505–511, 1989

Spunt BJ, Goldstein PJ, Bellucci PA, et al: Drug relationships in violence among methadone maintenance treatment clients. Adv Alcohol Subst Abuse 9:81–99, 1990a

Spunt BJ, Goldstein PJ, Bellucci PA, et al: Race/ethnicity and gender differences in the drugs-violence relationship. J Psychoactive Drugs 22:293–303, 1990b

Stanley B, Molcho A, Stanley M, et al: Association of aggressive behavior with altered serotonergic function in patients who are not suicidal. Am J Psychiatry 157:609–614, 2000

Stanley M, Traskman-Bendz L, Dorovini-Zis K: Correlations between aminergic metabolites simultaneously obtained from human CSF and brain. Life Sci 37:1279–1286, 1985

Stattin H, Magnusson D: The role of early aggressive behavior in the frequency, seriousness, and types of later crime. J Consult Clin Psychol 57:710–718, 1989

Steadman HJ, Cocozza JJ: Careers of the Criminally Insane: Excessive Social Control of Deviance. Lexington, MA, Lexington Books, 1974

Steadman HJ, Felson RB: Self-reports of violence. Ex-mental patients, ex-offenders, and the general population. Criminology 22:321–342, 1984

Steadman HJ, Keveles G: The community adjustment and criminal activity of the Baxstrom patients: 1966–1970. Am J Psychiatry 129:304–310, 1972

Steadman HJ, Morrissey JP: The statistical prediction of violent behavior. Measuring the cost of a public protectionist versus a civil libertarian model. Law Hum Behav 5:263–274, 1981

Steadman HJ, Cocozza JJ, Melick ME: Explaining the increased arrest rate among mental patients: the changing clientele of state hospitals. Am J Psychiatry 135:816–820, 1978a

Steadman HJ, Vanderwyst D, Ribner S: Comparing arrest rates of mental patients and criminal offenders. Am J Psychiatry 135:1218–1220, 1978b

Steadman HJ, Monahan J, Appelbaum PS, et al: Designing a new generation of risk assessment research, in Violence and Mental Disorder: Developments in Risk Assessment. Edited by Monahan J, Steadman H. Chicago, IL, University of Chicago Press, 1994, pp 297–318

Steadman HJ, Mulvey EP, Monahan J, et al: Violence by people discharged from acute psychiatric inpatient facilities and by others in the same neighborhoods. Arch Gen Psychiatry 55:393–401, 1998

Steadman HJ, Gounis K, Dennis D, et al: Assessing the New York City involuntary outpatient commitment pilot program. Psychiatr Serv 52:330–336, 2001

Stein DJ, Hollander E, Liebowitz MR: Neurobiology of impulsivity and the impulse control disorders. J Neuropsychiatry Clin Neurosci 5:9–17, 1993

Steinert T, Wolfle M, Gebhardt R-P: Measurement of violence during in-patient treatment and association with psychopathology. Acta Psychiatr Scand 102:107–112, 2000

Stevens JR, Hermann BP: Temporal lobe epilepsy, psychopathology, and violence: the state of the evidence. Neurology 31:1127–1132, 1981

Stewart JT, Mounts ML, Clark RL Jr: Aggressive behavior in Huntington's disease: treatment with propranolol. J Clin Psychiatry 48:106–108, 1987

Stone AA: Violence and temporal lobe epilepsy (letter). Am J Psychiatry 141:1641–1642, 1984

Stone EM: American Psychiatric Glossary. Washington, DC, American Psychiatric Press, 1988

Streissguth AP, Randels SP, Smith DF: A test-retest study of intelligence in patients with fetal alcohol syndrome: implications for care. J Am Acad Child Adolesc Psychiatry 30:584–587, 1991

Strous RD, Bark N, Parsia SS, et al: Analysis of a functional catechol-O-methyltransferase gene polymorphism in schizophrenia: evidence for association with aggressive and antisocial behavior. Psychiatry Res 69:71–77, 1997a

Strous RD, Bark N, Woerner M, et al: Lack of association of a functional catechol-O-methyltransferase gene polymorphism in schizophrenia (abstract). Biol Psychiatry 41:493–495, 1997b

Stueve A, Link BG: Gender differences in the relationship between mental illness and violence: evidence from a community-based epidemiological study in Israel. Soc Psychiatry Psychiatr Epidemiol 33 (suppl 1):S61–S67, 1998

Surwillo WW: The electroencephalogram and childhood aggression. Aggressive Behavior 6:9–18, 1980

Susman EJ, Inoff-Germain G, Nottelmann ED, et al: Hormones, emotional dispositions, and aggressive attributes in young adolescents. Child Dev 58:1114–1134, 1987

Swanson JW: Mental disorder, substance abuse, and community violence: an epidemiological approach, in Violence and Mental Disorder: Developments in Risk Assessment. Edited by Monahan J, Steadman HJ. Chicago, IL, University of Chicago Press, 1994, pp 101–136

Swanson JW, Holzer CE: Violence and ECA data (letter). Hosp Community Psychiatry 42:954–955, 1991

Swanson JW, Holzer CE, Ganju VK, et al: Violence and psychiatric disorder in the community: evidence from the Epidemiologic Catchment Area surveys. Hosp Community Psychiatry 41:761–770, 1990

Swanson JW, Swartz MS, Borum R, et al: Involuntary out-patient commitment and reduction of violent behaviour in persons with severe mental illness. Br J Psychiatry 176:324–331, 2000

Swartz MS, Swanson JW, Hiday VA, et al: Taking the wrong drugs: the role of substance abuse and medication noncompliance in violence among severely mentally ill individuals. Soc Psychiatry Psychiatr Epidemiol 33 (suppl 1):S75–S80, 1998a

Swartz MS, Swanson JW, Hiday VA, et al: Violence and severe mental illness: the effects of substance abuse and nonadherence to medication. Am J Psychiatry 155:226–231, 1998b

Swartz MS, Swanson JW, Hiday VA, et al: A randomized controlled trial of outpatient commitment in North Carolina. Psychiatr Serv 52:325–329, 2001

Tanke ED, Yesavage JA: Characteristics of assaultive patients who do and do not provide visible cues of potential violence. Am J Psychiatry 142:1409–1413, 1985

Tardiff K: Assault in hospitals and placement in the community. Bull Am Acad Psychiatry Law 9:33–39, 1981

Tardiff K: Characteristics of assaultive patients in private hospitals. Am J Psychiatry 141:1232–1235, 1984

Tardiff K: A survey of assault by chronic patients in a state hospital system, in Assaults Within Psychiatric Facilities. Edited by Lion JR, Reid WH. New York, Grune & Stratton, 1992, pp 3–19

Tardiff K, Deane K: The psychological and physical status of chronic psychiatric inpatients. Compr Psychiatry 21:91–97, 1980

Tardiff K, Koenigsberg HW: Assaultive behavior among psychiatric outpatients. Am J Psychiatry 142:960–963, 1985

Tardiff K, Sweillam A: Assault, suicide, and mental illness. Arch Gen Psychiatry 37:164–169, 1980

Tardiff K, Sweillam A: Assaultive behavior among chronic inpatients. Am J Psychiatry 139:212–215, 1982

Taylor PJ: Motives for offending among violent and psychotic men. Br J Psychiatry 147:491–498, 1985

Taylor PJ: Schizophrenia and crime: distinctive patterns in association, in Mental Disorder and Crime. Edited by Hodgins S. Newbury Park, CA, Sage, 1993, pp 63–85

Taylor PJ, Gunn J: Violence and psychosis. I. Risk of violence among psychotic men. Br Med J (Clin Res Ed) 288:1945–1949, 1984

Taylor PJ, Brown R, Gunn J: Violence psychosis and handedness, in Laterality and Psychopathology. Edited by Flor-Henry P, Gruzelier J. Amsterdam, Elsevier, 1983, pp 181–194

Taylor SP, Vardaris RM, Rawtich AB, et al: The effects of alcohol and delta-9-tetrahydrocannabinol on human physical aggression. Aggressive Behavior 2: 153–161, 1976

Tazi A, Dantzer R, Mormede P, et al: Effects of post-trial administration of naloxone and beta-endorphin on shock-induced fighting in rats. Behav Neural Biol 39:192–202, 1983

Tazi A, Dantzer R, Mormede P, et al: Effects of post-trial injection of beta-endorphin on shock- induced fighting are dependent on baseline of fighting. Behav Neural Biol 43:322–326, 1985

Tec L: Unexpected effects in children treated with imipramin (case report). Am J Psychiatry 120:603, 1963

Teicher MH, Glod C, Cole JO: Emergence of intense suicidal preoccupation during fluoxetine treatment. Am J Psychiatry 147:207–210, 1990

Tengstrom A, Grann M, Langstrom N, et al: Psychopathy (PCL-R) as a predictor of violent recidivism among criminal offenders with schizophrenia. Law Hum Behav 24:45–58, 2000

Teplin LA: Criminalizing mental disorder. The comparative arrest rate of the mentally ill. Am Psychol 39:794–803, 1984

Teplin LA: The criminality of the mentally ill: a dangerous misconception. Am J Psychiatry 142:593–599, 1985

Teplin LA: The prevalence of severe mental disorder among male urban jail detainees: comparison with the Epidemiologic Catchment Area Program. Am J Public Health 80:663–669, 1990

Teplin LA, McClelland GM, Abram KM: The role of mental disorder and substance abuse in predicting violent crime among released offenders, in Mental Disorders and Crime. Edited by Hodgins S. Newbury Park, CA, Sage, 1993, pp 86–103

Thoa NB, Eichelman B, Richardson JS, et al: 6-Hydroxydopa depletion of brain norepinephrine and the function of aggressive behavior. Science 178:75–77, 1972

Thompson JW, Belcher JR, DeForge BR, et al: Changing characteristics of schizophrenic patients admitted to state hospitals. Hosp Community Psychiatry 44: 231–235, 1993

Thompson ML, Miczek KA, Noda K, et al: Analgesia in defeated mice: evidence for mediation via central rather than pituitary or adrenal endogenous opioid peptides. Pharmacol Biochem Behav 29:451–456, 1988

Thompson T, Bloom W: Aggressive behavior and extinction-induced response-rate increase. Psychon Sci 5:335–336, 1966

Thomsen IV: Late outcome of very severe blunt head trauma: a 10–15 year second follow-up. J Neurol Neurosurg Psychiatry 47:260–268, 1984

Thomson GOB, Raab GM, Hepburn WS, et al: Blood-lead levels and children's behaviour—results from the Edinburgh Lead Study. J Child Psychol Psychiatry 30:515–528, 1989

Thornberry TP, Jacoby JE: The Criminally Insane. A Community Follow-up of Mentally Ill Offenders. Chicago, IL, University of Chicago Press, 1979

Tiffany LP, Tiffany M: Nosologic objections to the criminal defense of pathological intoxication: what do the doubters doubt? Int J Law Psychiatry 13:49–75, 1990

Tiihonen J, Eronen M, Hakola P: Criminality associated with mental disorders and intellectual deficiency (letter). Arch Gen Psychiatry 50:917–918, 1993

Tiihonen J, Isohanni M, Rasanen P, et al: Specific major mental disorders and criminality: a 26-year prospective study of the 1966 Northern Finland birth cohort. Am J Psychiatry 154:840–845, 1997

Tiihonen J, Hallikainen T, Lachman H, et al: Association between the functional variant of the catechol-O-methyltransferase (COMT) gene and type 1 alcoholism. Mol Psychiatry 4:286–289, 1999

Tinklenberg JR, Stillman RC: Drug use and violence, in Violence and the Struggle for Existence. Edited by Daniels DN, Gilula MF, Ochberg FM. Boston, MA, Little, Brown, 1970, pp 327–365

Tinklenberg JR, Roth WT, Kopell BS, et al: Cannabis and alcohol effects on assaultiveness in adolescent delinquents. Ann N Y Acad Sci 282:85–94, 1976

Tobin JM, Bird IF, Boyle DE: Preliminary Evaluation of Librium (Ro 5–0690) in the Treatment of Anxiety Reactions. Dis Nerv Syst 21:11–19, 1960

Tolle R: Psychiatrie. Berlin, Springer-Verlag, 1988

Tollefson GD, Rampey AH Jr, Beasley CM Jr, et al: Absence of a relationship between adverse events and suicidality during pharmacotherapy for depression. J Clin Psychopharmacol 14:163–169, 1994

Tompkins EC, Clemento AJ, Taylor DP, et al: Inhibition of aggressive behavior in rhesus monkeys by buspirone. Res Commun Psychol Psychiatr Behav 5:337–352, 1980

Tonkonogy JM: Violence and temporal lobe lesion: head CT and MRI data. J Neuropsychiatry Clin Neurosci 3:189–196, 1991

Torrey EF, Stieber J, Ezekiel J, et al: Criminalizing the Seriously Mentally Ill: The Abuse of Jails as Mental Hospitals. Washington, DC, Public Citizen, 1992

Travin S, Protter B: Mad or bad? some clinical considerations in the misdiagnosis of schizophrenia as antisocial personality disorder. Am J Psychiatry 139: 1335–1338, 1982

Treiman DM: Psychobiology of ictal aggression. Adv Neurol 55:341–356, 1991

Trestman RL, Coccaro EF, Weston S, et al: Biology of impulsivity, suicide and MDD in Axis II (abstract no NR85), in 1992 New Research Program and Abstracts, American Psychiatric Association 145th Annual Meeting, Washington, DC, May 1992. Washington, DC, American Psychiatric Association, 1992, pp 67–68

Tricker R, Casaburi R, Storer TW, et al: The effects of supraphysiological doses of testosterone on angry behavior in healthy eugonadal men—a clinical research center study. J Clin Endocrinol Metab 81:3754–3758, 1996

Troisi A, Vicario E, Nuccetelli F, et al: Effects of fluoxetine on aggressive behavior of adult inpatients with mental retardation and epilepsy. Pharmacopsychiatry 28:73–76, 1995

Tupin JP, Smith DB, Clanon TL, et al: The long-term use of lithium in aggressive prisoners. Compr Psychiatry 14:311–317, 1973

Turner EA: Surgery of the Mind. Birmingham, England, Carmen Press, 1982

Tyrer SP, Walsh A, Edwards DE, et al: Factors associated with a good response to lithium in aggressive mentally handicapped subjects. Prog Neuropsychopharmacol Biol Psychiatry 8:751–755, 1984

U.S. Census Bureau, Administrative and Customer Services Division, Statistical Compendia Branch. Last revised April 25, 2001

Valdiserri EV, Carroll KR, Hartl AJ: A study of offenses committed by psychotic inmates in a county jail. Hosp Community Psychiatry 37:163–166, 1986

Valenstein ES: Review of the literature on postoperative evaluation, in The Psychosurgery Debate: Scientific, Legal, and Ethical Perspectives. Edited by Valenstein ES. San Francisco, CA, WH Freeman, 1980, pp 141–163

Valzelli L: Activity of benzodiazepines on aggressive behavior in rats and mice, in The Benzodiazepines. Edited by Garattini S, Mussini E, Randall LO. New York, Raven, 1973, pp 405–417

Valzelli L: Psychobiology of Aggression and Violence. New York, Raven Press, 1981

Valzelli L, Bernasconi S: Aggressiveness by isolation and brain serotonin turnover changes in different strains of mice. Neuropsychobiology 5:129–135, 1979

Valzelli L, Giacalone E, Garattini S: Pharmacological control of aggressive behavior in mice. Eur J Pharmacol 2:144–146, 1967

Vanezis P: Women, violent crime and the menstrual cycle: a review. Med Sci Law 31:11–14, 1991

Van Woerkom TCAM, Teelken AW, Minderhoud JM: Difference in neurotransmitter metabolism in frontotemporal-lobe contusion and diffuse cerebral contusion. Lancet 1:812–813, 1977

Vartiainen H, Tiihonen J, Putkonen A, et al: Citalopram, a selective serotonin reuptake inhibitor, in the treatment of aggression in schizophrenia. Acta Psychiatr Scand 91:348–351, 1995

Vassout A, Delini-Stula A: Effects of beta-blocking agents (propranolol, oxprenolol) and diazepam on the aggressive behaviour in the rat [in French]. J Pharmacol 8:5–14, 1977

Venables PH: The recovery limb of the skin conductance response in "high-risk" research, in Genetics, Environment and Psychopathology (North-Holland Research Series on Early Detection and Prevention of Behaviour Disorders, Vol 1). Edited by Mednick SA, Schulsinger F, Higgins J, et al. Amsterdam, North-Holland, 1974, pp 117–133

Verebey K, Volavka J, Clouet D: Endorphins in psychiatry: an overview and a hypothesis. Arch Gen Psychiatry 35:877–888, 1978

Virkkunen M: Psychomotor epilepsy and violence. Am J Psychiatry 140:646–647, 1983

Virkkunen M: Insulin secretion during the glucose tolerance test among habitually violent and impulsive offenders. Aggressive Behavior 12:303–310, 1986a

Virkkunen M: Reactive hypoglycemic tendency among habitually violent offenders. Nutr Rev 44 (suppl):94–103, 1986b

Virkkunen M, Huttunen MO: Evidence for abnormal glucose tolerance test among violent offenders. Neuropsychobiology 8:30–34, 1982

Virkkunen M, Linnoila M: Serotonin in early onset, male alcoholics with violent behaviour. Ann Med 22:327–331, 1990

Virkkunen M, Linnoila M: Serotonin in personality disorders with habitual violence and impulsivity, in Mental Disorder and Crime. Edited by Hodgins S. Newbury Park, CA, Sage, 1993, pp 227–243

Virkkunen M, Nuutila A, Goodwin FK, et al: Cerebrospinal fluid monoamine metabolites in male arsonists. Arch Gen Psychiatry 44:241–247, 1987

Virkkunen M, De Jong J, Bartko J, et al: Psychobiological concomitants of history of suicide attempts among violent offenders and impulsive fire setters. Arch Gen Psychiatry 46:604–606, 1989a

Virkkunen M, De Jong J, Bartko J, et al: Relationship of psychobiological variables to recidivism in violent offenders and impulsive fire setters. A follow-up study. Arch Gen Psychiatry 46:600–603, 1989b

Virkkunen M, Rawlings R, Tokola R, et al: CSF biochemistries, glucose metabolism, and diurnal activity rhythms in alcoholic, violent offenders, fire setters, and healthy volunteers. Arch Gen Psychiatry 51:20–27, 1994

Volavka J: Aggression, electroencephalography, and evoked potentials: a critical review. Neuropsychiatry Neuropsychol Behav Neurol 3:249–259, 1990

Volavka J, Citrome L: Atypical antipsychotics in the treatment of the persistently aggressive psychotic patient: methodological concerns. Schizophr Res 35:S23-S33, 1999

Volavka J, Krakowski M: Schizophrenia and violence. Psychol Med 19:559–562, 1989

Volavka J, Dornbush R, Feldstein S, et al: Marijuana, EEG and behavior. Ann N Y Acad Sci 191:206–215, 1971a

Volavka J, Matousek M, Roubicek J, et al: The reliability of visual EEG assessment (abstract). Electroencephalogr Clin Neurophysiol 31:294, 1971b

Volavka J, Matousek M, Feldstein S, et al: The reliability of EEG assessment [in German]. EEG EMG Z Electroenzephalogr Elektromyogr Verwandte Geb 4:123–130, 1973

Volavka J, Levine R, Feldstein S, et al: Short-term effects of heroin in man. Arch Gen Psychiatry 30:677–681, 1974

Volavka J, Mednick SA, Rasmussen L, et al: EEG spectra in XYY and XXY men. Electroencephalogr Clin Neurophysiol 43:798–801, 1977a

Volavka J, Mednick SA, Sergeant J, et al: Electroencephalograms of XYY and XXY men. Br J Psychiatry 130:43–47, 1977b

Volavka J, Mednick SA, Rasmussen L, et al: EEG response to sine wave modulated light in XYY, XXY, and XY men. Acta Psychiatr Scand 59:509–516, 1979

Volavka J, Crowner M, Brizer D, et al: Tryptophan treatment of aggressive psychiatric inpatients. Biol Psychiatry 28:728–732, 1990

Volavka J, Cooper T, Czobor P, et al: Haloperidol blood levels and clinical effects. Arch Gen Psychiatry 49:354–361, 1992a

Volavka J, Martell D, Convit A: Psychobiology of the violent offender. J Forensic Sci 37:237–251, 1992b

Volavka J, Zito JM, Vitrai J, et al: Clozapine effects on hostility and aggression in schizophrenia. J Clin Psychopharmacol 13:287–289, 1993

Volavka J, Mohammad Y, Vitrai J, et al: Characteristics of state hospital patients arrested for offenses committed during hospitalization. Psychiatr Serv 46: 796–800, 1995

Volavka J, Laska E, Baker S, et al: History of violent behaviour and schizophrenia in different cultures. Analyses based on the WHO study on determinants of outcome of severe mental disorders. Br J Psychiatry 171:9–14, 1997

Volkow ND, Tancredi L: Neural substrates of violent behaviour. A preliminary study with positron emission tomography. Br J Psychiatry 151:668–673, 1987

Vom Saal FS: Models of early hormonal effects on intrasex aggression in mice, in Hormones and Aggressive Behavior. Edited by Svare BB. New York, Plenum, 1983, pp 197–222

von Engerth G, Hoff H: Ueber das schicksal der patienten mit schweren characterveranderungen nach encephalitis epidemica. Dtsch Med Wochenschr 55:181–183, 1929

Wakschlag LS, Lahey BB, Loeber R, et al: Maternal smoking during pregnancy and the risk of conduct disorder in boys. Arch Gen Psychiatry 54:670–676, 1997

Walker Z, Seifert R: Violent incidents in a psychiatric intensive care unit. Br J Psychiatry 164:826–828, 1994

Walsh KW: Neuropsychology. A Clinical Approach. Edinburgh, Churchill Livingstone, 1978

Washton AM, Tatarsky A: Adverse effects of cocaine abuse. NIDA Res Monogr 49:247–254, 1984

Wasman M, Flynn JP: Directed attack elicited from hypothalamus. Arch Neurol 6:220–227, 1962

Wassef A, Dott S, Russell J, et al: Divalproex sodium augmentation of neuroleptics in treatment resistant schizophrenia. Paper presented at the 35th Annual Meeting of the American College of Neuropsychopharmacology, San Juan, Puerto Rico, December 9–13, 1996

Wassef AA, Dott SG, Harris A, et al: Critical review of GABA-ergic drugs in the treatment of schizophrenia. J Clin Psychopharmacol 19:222–232, 1999

Wassef AA, Dott SG, Harris A, et al: Randomized, placebo-controlled pilot study of divalproex sodium in the treatment of acute exacerbations of chronic schizophrenia. J Clin Psychopharmacol 20:357–361, 2000

Wassef AA, Hafiz NG, Hampton D, et al: Divalproex sodium augmentation of haloperidol in hospitalized patients with schizophrenia: clinical and economic implications. J Clin Psychopharmacol 21:21–26, 2001

Webster N: Webster's Ninth New Collegiate Dictionary. Springfield, MA, Merriam-Webster, 1991

Wei J, Hemmings GP: Lack of evidence for association between the COMT locus and schizophrenia. Psychiatr Genet 9:183–186, 1999

Weiger WA, Bear DM: An approach to the neurology of aggression. J Psychiatr Res 22:85–98, 1988

Weinberger DR, Bigelow LB, Kleinman JE, et al: Cerebral ventricular enlargement in chronic schizophrenia. An association with poor response to treatment. Arch Gen Psychiatry 37:11–13, 1980

Weinstock M, Weiss C: Antagonism by propranolol of isolation-induced aggression in mice: correlation with 5-hydroxytryptamine receptor blockade. Neuropharmacology 19:653–656, 1980

Weisman AM, Berman ME, Taylor SP: Effects of clorazepate, diazepam, and oxazepam on a laboratory measurement of aggression in men. Int Clin Psychopharmacol 13:183–188, 1998

Weiss G, Hechtman LT: Hyperactive Children Grown Up: Empirical Findings and Theoretical Considerations. New York, Guilford, 1986

Weitzman M, Gortmaker S, Sobol A: Maternal smoking and behavior problems of children. Pediatrics 90:342–349, 1992

Werner E, Simonian K, Bierman JM, et al: Cumulative effect of perinatal complications and deprived environment on physical, intellectual, and social development of preschool children. Pediatrics 39:490–505, 1967

Werner E, Bierman JM, French FE, et al: Reproductive and environmental casualties: a report on the 10-year follow-up of the children of the Kauai Pregnancy Study. Pediatrics 42:112–127, 1968

Werner PD, Yesavage JA, Becker JM, et al: Hostile words and assaultive behavior on an acute inpatient psychiatric unit. J Nerv Ment Dis 171:385–387, 1983

Werner PD, Rose TL, Yesavage JA: Aspects of consensus in clinical predictions of imminent violence. J Clin Psychol 46:534–538, 1990

Wessely S: The Camberwell Study of Crime and Schizophrenia. Soc Psychiatry Psychiatr Epidemiol 33 (suppl 1):S24–S28, 1998

Wessely S, Taylor PJ: Madness and crime: criminology versus psychiatry. Criminal Behaviour and Mental Health 1:193–228, 1991

Wessely S, Buchanan A, Reed A, et al: Acting on delusions. I: prevalence. Br J Psychiatry 163:69–76, 1993

Wettstein RM, Mulvey EP, Rogers R: A prospective comparison of four insanity defense standards. Am J Psychiatry 148:21–27, 1991

White JL, Moffitt TE, Silva PA: A prospective replication of the protective effects of IQ in subjects at high risk for juvenile delinquency. J Consult Clin Psychol 57:719–724, 1989

Whitman JR, Maier GJ, Eichelman B: Beta-adrenergic blockers for aggressive behavior in schizophrenia (letter). Am J Psychiatry 144:538–539, 1987

Whitman S, Coleman TE, Patmon C, et al: Epilepsy in prison: elevated prevalence and no relationship to violence. Neurology 34:775–782, 1984

Widom CS: Child abuse, neglect, and violent criminal behavior. Criminology 27:251–271, 1989a

Widom CS: The cycle of violence. Science 244:160–166, 1989b

Widom CS: A tail on an untold tale: Response to "biological and genetic contributors to violence—Widom's untold tale." Psychol Bull 109:130–132, 1991

Wiener JM, Delano JG, Klass DW: An EEG study of delinquent and nondelinquent adolescents. Arch Gen Psychiatry 15:144–150, 1966

Wigal T, Amsel A: Behavioral and neuroanatomical effects of prenatal, postnatal, or combined exposure to ethanol in weanling rats. Behav Neurosci 104:116–126, 1990

Wilcock GK, Stevens J, Perkins A: Trazodone/tryptophan for aggressive behaviour (letter). Lancet 1:929–930, 1987

Wilcox J: Divalproex sodium in the treatment of aggressive behavior. Ann Clin Psychiatry 6:17–20, 1994

Williams D: Neural factors related to habitual aggression. Consideration of differences between those habitual aggressives and others who have committed crimes of violence. Brain 92:503–520, 1969

Williams DT, Mehl R, Yudofsky S, et al: The effect of propranolol on uncontrolled rage outbursts in children and adolescents with organic brain dysfunction. Am Acad Child Psychiatry 21:129–135, 1982

Wilson EO: Sociobiology: The New Synthesis. Cambridge, MA, Belknap Press, 1976

Wilson JQ: The Moral Sense. New York, Free Press, 1993

Wilson JQ, Herrnstein RJ: Crime and Human Nature. New York, Simon & Schuster, 1986

Wilson WJ: The Truly Disadvantaged. The Inner City, the Underclass, and Public Policy. Chicago, IL, University of Chicago Press, 1987

Wilson WH: Clinical review of clozapine treatment in a state hospital. Hosp Community Psychiatry 43:700–703, 1992

Wilson WH: Addition of lithium to haloperidol in non-affective, antipsychotic non-responsive schizophrenia: a double blind, placebo controlled, parallel design clinical trial. Psychopharmacology 111:359–366, 1993

Wilson WH, Claussen AM: 18-month outcome of clozapine treatment for 100 patients in a state psychiatric hospital. Psychiatr Serv 46:386–389, 1995

Winerip M: Bedlam on the streets. The New York Times, May 23, 1999, Sec 6, pp 42–70

Winslow JT, Miczek KA: Androgen dependency of alcohol effects on aggressive behavior: a seasonal rhythm in high-ranking squirrel monkeys. Psychopharmacology 95:92–98, 1988a

Winslow JT, Miczek KA: Naltrexone blocks amphetamine-induced hyperactivity, but not disruption of social and agonistic behavior in mice and squirrel monkeys. Psychopharmacology 96:493–499, 1988b

Winslow JT, Kozak A, Miczek KA: The effects of naltrexone and amphetamine on squirrel monkey behavior in groups. Neuroscience Abstracts 9:120, 1983

Winslow JT, Ellingboe J, Miczek KA: Effects of alcohol on aggressive behavior in squirrel monkeys: influence of testosterone and social context. Psychopharmacology 95:356–363, 1988

Wistedt B, Rasmussen A, Pedersen L, et al: The development of an observer-scale for measuring social dysfunction and aggression. Pharmacopsychiatry 23:249–252, 1990

Witkin HA, Mednick SA, Schulsinger F, et al: Criminality in XYY and XXY men. Science 193:547–555, 1976

Wolfgang ME: Patterns in Criminal Homicide. Philadelphia, PA, University of Pennsylvania, 1958

Wolfgang ME: Delinquency in two birth cohorts, in Prospective Studies of Crime and Delinquency. Edited by Van Dusen KT, Mednick SA. Boston, MA, Kluwer-Nijhoff, 1983, pp 7–16

Wolfgang ME, Ferracuti F: The Subculture of Violence. London, Tavistock, 1967

Wolfgang ME, Figlio RM, Sellin T: Delinquency in a Birth Cohort. Chicago, IL, University of Chicago Press, 1972

Wolfgang ME, Figlio RM, Tracy P, et al: National Survey of Crime Severity. Washington, DC, National Criminal Justice Reference Service, NCJ-96017, 1985

Wong MTH, Lumsden J, Fenton GW, et al: Electroencephalography, computed tomography and violence ratings of male patients in a maximum-security mental hospital. Acta Psychiatr Scand 90:97–101, 1994

Woods JH, Winger G: Abuse liability of flunitrazepam. J Clin Psychopharmacol 17 (suppl):1S–57S, 1997

Wroblewski BA, Joseph AB, Kupfer J, et al: Effectiveness of valproic acid on destructive and aggressive behaviours in patients with acquired brain injury. Brain Inj 11:37–47, 1997

Yaryura-Tobias JA, Neziroglu FA: Violent behavior, brain dysrhythmia, and glucose dysfunction. A new syndrome. Journal of Orthomolecular Psychiatry 4:182–188, 1975

Yassa R, Dupont D: Carbamazepine in the treatment of aggressive behavior in schizophrenic patients: a case report. Can J Psychiatry 28:566–568, 1983

Yen CY, Stanger RL, Millman N: Ataractic suppression of isolation-induced aggressive behavior. Arch Int Pharmacodyn Ther 123:179–185, 1959

Yesavage JA: Inpatient violence and the schizophrenic patient: an inverse correlation between danger-related events and neuroleptic levels. Biol Psychiatry 17:1331–1337, 1982

Yesavage JA: Bipolar illness: correlates of dangerous inpatient behaviour. Br J Psychiatry 143:554–557, 1983a

Yesavage JA: Inpatient violence and the schizophrenic patient. A study of Brief Psychiatric Rating Scale scores and inpatient behavior. Acta Psychiatr Scand 67:353–357, 1983b

Yesavage JA, Zarcone V: History of drug abuse and dangerous behavior in inpatient schizophrenics. J Clin Psychiatry 44:259–261, 1983

Yesavage JA, Werner PD, Becker JM, et al: Short-term civil commitment and the violent patient. Am J Psychiatry 139:1145–1149, 1982

Yeudall LT: Neuropsychological assessment of forensic disorder. Canada's Mental Health 25:7–15, 1977

Yeudall LT, Fromm-Auch D: Neuropsychological impairments in various psycho-pathological populations, in Hemisphere Asymmetries of Function in Psychopathology. Edited by Gruzelier J, Flor-Henry P. Amsterdam, Elsevier North-Holland, 1979, pp 401–428

Yeudall LT, Fromm-Auch D, Davies P: Neuropsychological impairment of persistent delinquency. J Nerv Ment Dis 170:257–265, 1982

Yorkston NJ, Zaki SA, Pitcher DR, et al: Propranolol as an adjunct to the treatment of schizophrenia. Lancet 2:575–578, 1977

Young SN, Pihl RO, Ervin FR: The effect of altered tryptophan levels on mood and behavior in normal human males. Clin Neuropharmacol 11 (suppl 1):207–215, 1988

Yudofsky S, Williams D, Gorman J: Propranolol in the treatment of rage and violent behavior in patients with chronic brain syndrome. Am J Psychiatry 138:218–220, 1981

Yudofsky SC, Stevens L, Silver JM, et al: Propranolol in the treatment of rage and violent behavior associated with Korsakoff's psychosis. Am J Psychiatry 141:114–115, 1984

Yudofsky SC, Silver JM, Jackson W, et al: The Overt Aggression Scale for the objective rating of verbal and physical aggression. Am J Psychiatry 143:35–39, 1986

Yudofsky SC, Silver JM, Hales RE: Pharmacologic management of aggression in the elderly. J Clin Psychiatry 51 (suppl 10):22–28, 1990

Yuwiler A, Brammer GL, Morley JE, et al: Short-term and repetitive administration of oral tryptophan in normal men. Effects on blood tryptophan, serotonin, and kynurenine concentrations. Arch Gen Psychiatry 38:619–626, 1981

Zander KJ, Fischer B, Zimmer R, et al: Long-term neuroleptic treatment of chronic schizophrenic patients: clinical and biochemical effects of withdrawal. Psychopharmacology 73:43–47, 1981

Zuckerman M: Sensation Seeking: Beyond the Optimal Level of Arousal. Hillsdale, NJ, Erlbaum, 1979

Zuckerman M, Buchsbaum MS, Murphy DL: Sensation seeking and its biological correlates. Psychol Bull 88:187–214, 1980

Index

Page numbers printed in **boldface** type refer to table or figures.